25.00

Ecological Toxicology Research

Effects of Heavy Metal and Organohalogen Compounds

Environmental Science Research

A Continuation Order Plan is available for this series. A continuation order will bring
delivery of each new volume immediately upon publication. Volumes are billed only upon
actual shipment. For further information please contact the publisher.

Ecological Toxicology Research

Effects of Heavy Metal and Organohalogen Compounds

Proceedings of a NATO Science Committee Conference

Edited by

A. D. McIntyre

Department of Agriculture and Fisheries for Scotland
Aberdeen, Scotland

and

C. F. Mills

The Rowett Research Institute
Aberdeen, Scotland

PLENUM PRESS • NEW YORK AND LONDON
Published in cooperation with NATO Scientific Affairs Division

Library of Congress Cataloging in Publication Data

Nato Science Committee Conference on Eco-toxicology, Mont Gabriel, Quebec, 1974.
Ecological toxicology research.

(Environmental science research; v. 7)
"Held under the auspices of the NATO Science Committee."
Includes bibliographical references and index.
1. Heavy metals—Environmental aspects—Congresses. 2. Organohalogen compounds—Environmental aspects—Congresses. 3. Pollution—Toxicology—Congresses. 4. Ecology—Congresses. I. McIntyre, A. D. II. Mills, Colin Frederick, 1926-
III. North Atlantic Treaty Organization. Science Committee. IV. Title.
QH545.M45N37   1974   574.2'4   75-28365
ISBN 0-306-36307-0

Proceedings of the NATO Science Committee Conference on Eco-Toxicology held at Mont Gabriel, Quebec, Canada, May 6-10, 1974

©1975 Plenum Press, New York
A Divison of Plenum Publishing Corporation
227 West 17th Street, New York, N.Y. 10011

United Kingdom edition published by Plenum Press, London
A Division of Plenum Publishing Company, Ltd.
Davis House (4th Floor), 8 Scrubs Lane, Harlesden, London, NW10 6SE, England

Foreword

The Conference on the Ecotoxicity of Heavy Metals and Organohalogen Compounds was held under the auspices of the NATO Science Committee as part of its continuing effort to promote the useful progress of science through international cooperation.

Science Committee Conferences are deliberately designed to focus attention on unsolved problems, with invited participants providing a variety of complementary expertise. Through intensive group discussion they seek to reach a consensus on assessments and recommendations for future research emphases, which it is hoped will be of value to the larger scientific community. The subjects treated in previous Conferences have been as varied as science itself—e.g., computer software, chemical catalysis, oceanography, and materials and energy research.

This volume presents an account of a meeting which evolved from studies within the Science Committee's advisory panel on Eco-Sciences. Environmental monitoring of toxic substances from industrial and agricultural sources is producing a growing volume of data on the quantities of such substances in terrestrial and aquatic milieus. Before this information can be used to assess biological effects, knowledge is required of the chemical form of the pollutants, the mechanisms by which they enter and move through organisms, their concomitant transformations, the nature of the toxic reactions within tissues, and the way in which the physiology and behavior of individuals is affected.

The meeting brought together a number of specialists who critically evaluated their present knowledge and identified those areas of research in which accelerated progress seemed particularly critical.

Some forty-seven papers, either in the form of reprints or specially written reviews, were contributed by the participants for advance circulation. The availability of this material precluded the need for lengthy introductory presentations and permitted rapid initiation of spirited interdisciplinary discussions. All

v

participants gave generously and enthusiastically of their wisdom and knowledge during the week of the meeting, and we extend to them our deep gratitude.

Special thanks go to Dr. A. McIntyre and Dr. C. Mills, for their diligent efforts as Chairman and Co-Chairman of the meeting, to their colleagues on the Organizing Committee, Prof. S. Dalgaard-Mikkelsen, Dr. R. W. Durie, Dr. E. D. Goldberg, Prof. D. H. Remmer, and Prof. R. Truhaut, for their wise counsel, and to the leaders and recorders of the working groups as listed, for their indispensable dedication.

Grateful acknowledgment is also made of the considerable assistance provided to this Conference by Environment Canada. Its concrete and spiritual support contributed significantly to any success which has been achieved.

Eugene G. Kovach

Deputy Assistant Secretary General for Scientific Affairs

Preface

The well-documented increase in pollution from a wide variety of sources presents a potential threat to living organisms, and the term "ecotoxicology" is useful in referring to the study of the distribution and effects of toxic substances in major organic assemblages, from the habitats of mountain ranges to the communities of oceanic abysses. In attempting to assess such effects the ecologist is faced with a bewildering variety of problems. The history of ecological studies is relatively short, and the ecologist has not in the past been particularly concerned with pathology and so has sparse foundations on which to build. Further, the vast assemblage of species with which he has to deal, and their great diversity of reactions, compounds the problem.

By contrast, the medical or veterinary scientist is in an enviable position. He has behind him a long tradition of research providing a detailed understanding of the small number of species on which he is required to concentrate his attention. Consequently he has been able to approach the newer problems of pollution with a substantial background knowledge of a suitable type on which to draw for an assessment of effects on man and domestic animals, and with a significant body of appropriate expertise to guide the design and execution of research.

It is thus reasonable to suggest that the ecologist working in the pollution field would have much to learn from those concerned with these other sciences and with the study of domesticated species. This consideration formed a major part of the rationale behind the NATO Science Committee conference on aspects of ecotoxicology upon which this volume is based. The remit given to participants was as follows:

"The primary task of this interdisciplinary meeting on the ecotoxicology of heavy metals and organohalogen compounds is to identify those areas of this subject in which inadequate knowledge of the processes influencing entry, metabolism, and toxic action of these pollutants is presently hindering assessment of the significance of the hazards they create within ecosystems.

"Specialists from several disciplines have been brought together with the specific objective of facilitating detailed discussion of those physical, biological, and biochemical processes which affect the response to these toxic materials and which thus complicate the interpretation of pollutant survey data.

"It is intended that the report of this meeting shall clearly highlight those areas in which further research activity is particularly desirable to achieve realistic assessment of the hazards presented by individual heavy metals and organohalogen compounds in the environment."

This volume presents an account of the proceedings of the conference. Part I contains the text of eight lectures presented during plenary sessions designed to set the scene for the later activities of specialist Working Groups. Part II contains seven papers selected from among those submitted for circulation to participants before the meeting, these papers illustrating, in differing detail, the wide scope of scientific enquiry that is relevant to the ultimate assessment of the fate and effects of potentially toxic materials present in the environment.

Part III contains the Working Group Reports and their recommendations. Since these were set out in the style of the individual group leaders and rapporteurs, and reflect the separate approaches of each group, no editorial attempt has been made to reduce them to uniformity.

There was general agreement that participation in this multidisciplinary meeting was a stimulating and provocative experience. If this volume reflects the enthusiasm with which the remit of the meeting was handled and concentrates future attention around those topics so clearly felt to be currently hindering assessment of the biological significance of some pollutants, it will have served its purpose. We are confident that it clearly reflects the need for more closely integrated multidisciplinary research effort if satisfactory progress toward control of the adverse effects of pollutants is to be maintained.

C. F. Mills   A. D. McIntyre

Rowett Research Institute   *DAFS Marine Laboratory*
Bucksburn, Aberdeen, Scotland   *Aberdeen, Scotland*

Cochairmen: NATO Science Committee Conference on
Ecotoxicity of Heavy Metals and Organohalogen Compounds

Contents

PART II • INVITED PAPERS

PART III • WORKING GROUP REPORTS

Part I
PLENARY PAPERS

1

Ecotoxicology—A New Branch of Toxicology: A General Survey of its Aims Methods, and Prospects

R. TRUHAUT

Dedicated to my friend, Professor Dr. Hermann Druckrey, who achieved so much in the cause of prevention, on his 70th birthday.

As an introduction it is desirable to define the terms ecology, pollution, toxicology, and ecotoxicology.

Ecology (from the Greek *oikos*, house) is the scientific discipline which studies the relation between living organisms and their milieu. This expression, which means literally "science of the habitat," was coined in 1866 by Haeckel in his work "General Morphology of the Organism."

A more elaborate definition was given by Dajoz in "Precis d'Ecologie," which appeared in 1970: "Ecology is the science which studies the conditions of existence of living creatures, and the interaction of all kinds which exist between these creatures and their environment."

Author's Note: This English version is a translation of the original French text. Interested readers may refer to other articles on the same subject published earlier, notably "Ecotoxicologie et protection de l'environnement," Proceedings of *Colloque Biologie et Devenir de l'Homme*, La Sorbonne, Paris, 18–24 October 1974 (in press).

R. TRUHAUT • Directeur du Centre de Recherches Toxicologiques de la Faculté des Sciences pharmaceutique et biologiques, Université René Descartes, Paris, France.

This young science has made great strides since 1930. It represents a discipline which is more typically multidisciplinary, and is concerned with plant life, animals, and microorganisms, whether terrestrial or aquatic, and, in the latter case, whether fresh-water or marine. Its specialty is concerned with biological problems, not at the level of species or even isolated individuals, such as occurs, for instance, in anatomy and physiology, but at the level of populations of groups of species or ecosystems which constitute the biosphere, taking into consideration the various factors which influence their environment.

Pollution—In a Council of Europe report published in 1967, the following definition of air pollution was put forward: "Pollution of the air occurs when there is present in the air a foreign substance or an important variation in the proportions of its constituents capable of causing a harmful effect or of causing discomfort, bearing in mind the extent of scientific knowledge at the time."

This definition is capable of being extended to the pollution of other parts of the environment: the earth, fresh water, the sea, biota, and food chains. It applies to the harmful effects which can result not only from the introduction of foreign substances, the so-called xenobiotics, but also from the development of imbalance between naturally occurring substances such as, for example, disturbances of the balance between different mineral elements which very often lead to harmful effects. Among such balances can be cited those existing between zinc and cadmium, molybdenum and copper, or selenium and mercury (WHO, 1973). Without entering into details, it seems appropriate to emphasize that, along with the growth of pollution resulting from industrialization and the widespread use of chemical products in different areas of human activity, a characteristic feature of our age, which may truly be called the era of chemistry, the problems faced by specialists in the science of pollution, so called molysmology, have become increasingly manifold and complex.

Toxicology is the scientific discipline which studies toxic or poisonous substances, that is to say, substances which cause alterations or disturbances in the functions of the organism leading to harmful effects of which the most serious is, obviously, the death of the organism in question. For a more elaborate definition, we would refer the reader to a general conference on toxicology given by us on the occasion of the 92nd Congress of the French Association for the Advancement of Science (St. Etienne, July 1973, published in *Science*, 1974, **VL**, No. 2).

Ecotoxicology is the branch of toxicology which studies the toxic effects caused by natural substances or by artificial pollutants on living organisms whether animal or vegetable, terrestrial or aquatic, which constitute the biosphere. It also relates to the interaction of these substances with the physical environment in which these organisms live. In connection with this definition, it must not be forgotten that man is situated at the center of the biosphere. But while human toxicology, that is, the study of directly harmful effects on man of exogenous or xenobiotic agents, has given rise to a great amount of research, coordinated on an international scale (e.g., by WHO), ecotoxicology is still in an embryonic state.

Nevertheless, harmful effects on members of ecosystems other than man usually have an impact on the latter in an indirect way. For example:

1. The decrease in food resources resulting, for example, from the immense slaughter of fish under the influence of the discharge of effluent containing toxic pollutants into rivers or lakes, or the havoc wrought to food crops by air pollution, such as fluoride fumes or the constituents of oxidizing photochemical smog.

2. The indirect effect on agricultural productivity resulting from assaults on organisms which have a beneficial function in the biosphere, such as bees as vehicles for pollen or earthworms and other constituents of the soil fauna which ensure aeration of the soil.

3. The decrease in production of primary source materials, such as textile-producing plants and forest cultures.

4. The toxicity which is bestowed on certain constituents of the food chain, such as the pollution of fish, fresh-water as well as marine, by methylmercury derivatives, and the passage of various residues, notably the residues of organochlorine lipid-soluble pesticides, into the milk of mammals, which constitute, in this connection, spectacular examples. The presence of toxic organic micropollutants in drinking water produced from contaminated river water can pose problems of the same magnitude.

5. The disturbance of biological balance in nature with disastrous consequences on the regenerative possibilities for mankind and, as a result, the quality of life as a whole.

It must be recalled in this connection that in the WHO charter, "health" is defined as not only an absence of infirmity or illness, but also a complete state of physical, mental, and social well-being. Thus, in the context of our forthcoming discussion on the consequences of pollution, we must ultimately consider not only adverse physical responses but also adverse emotional or psychological responses. Although we shall be principally concerned with more direct effects of pollution, it is, for example, worth emphasis that both physical and psychological consequences in man have been claimed to result from prolonged exposure to industrial smog and fumes.

For all these reasons, the term ecotoxicology is applied, sometimes in a more limited way than that given above, to the study of the indirect effects on the health and well-being of man, which can be caused by the harmful effects of chemical pollutants on various living organisms other than man.

Harmful effects on some members of ecosystems may result from beneficial effects upon others, for instance, the injurious effects which can occur in fish due to the stimulation of the growth of aquatic plants by substances such as nitrates and phosphates which cause a decrease in the amount of dissolved oxygen in water.

Man exploits the injurious effects of chemical agents upon certain organisms in his use of pesticides, without which food resources would decline with tragic consequences at a time when increasing population on a world-wide scale poses the problem of a struggle against famine. However, it must not be forgotten that such agents only very exceptionally posses selective toxicity toward such pests, and can thus exercise a harmful effect on other categories of living creatures and in particular on man himself. The choice of compounds to be used and the assessment of methods of application must not, because of this fact, be made without adopting the most rigorous precautions based on adequate scientific information.

All the above comments serve to illustrate that the problems of ecotoxicology must be studied in an *integrated* context.

1.1. Entry, Distribution, and Fate of Pollutants in the Physical Environment

1.1.1. Principal Sources of Pollution

The principal sources of pollution are as follows:

1. Domestic fires and industrial heating devices, generators of, among other materials, carbon dioxide, sulfur dioxide, and unburned matter, whose particles of soot carry polycyclic aromatic hydrocarbons.
2. Industrial effluents, discharged either into the atmosphere or into water, whose nature depends on the activities of the factories producing the effluent. The number of pollutants which can be thus discharged is considerable and increases continually with the rapid progress of the chemical sciences and the manufacture of the products which this progress facilitates.
3. Terrestrial vehicles and aircraft using crude oil or mineral oil and discharging into the atmosphere, in addition to carbon monoxide and dioxide, nitrogen oxides, partially combusted hydrocarbons, and heavy particles of urburned matter, as well as the combustion residues of fuel additives, notably lead particles.
4. The use of a whole series of industrial products such as, to name only a few examples, asbestos, polychlorobiphenyls, and various solvents. Our food itself has not escaped a form of pollution, in that numerous chemical agents, known as food additives, are increasingly and deliberately incorporated in pursuit of various aims (preservation, improvement of organoleptic qualities, and of appearance or coloring).

5. The use of chemical products in agriculture, notably as pesticides, as additives to animal foodstuffs, and as fertilizers, particularly those containing nitrates.
6. The increasing domestic use of solvents, detergents, insecticides, medicines, cosmetics, plastic packaging, and other so-called household products.

We must recognize the urgent need to initiate an accurate objective inventory of these varied types of pollutants. Action of this sort is taking place at the level of the United Nations and international scientific organizations, such as the Scientific Committee on Problems of the Environment (SCOPE) recently created (1970) by the International Council of Scientific Unions (ICSU). Such an international registry is essential to the programing of any action to be undertaken in the struggle against the harmful effects of pollutants.

According to a report presented to an international symposium held in March 1972 at Skolaster in Sweden (Royal Academy of Sciences, 1973), every year 250,000 new chemical compounds, among which about 500 are turned into commercial products, are added to the two million which are already known.

In addition to the pollutants artificially created by man, we must not omit those existing in a natural state, among which, to cite only a few spectacular examples, there are the mycotoxins from certain molds, notably the deadly aflatoxins and the biotoxins which give toxic potential to certain kinds of seafood (mollusks, crustaceans, and fish) and whose origin is increasingly attributed to a pollution of marine plankton.

1.1.2. Entry of Pollutants into the Environment

The principal modes of entry of pollutants into the environment will now be considered briefly.

Discharges into the air are obviously preponderant, not only of gases and fumes, but also of particles. Particularly important are particles small enough to be dispersed in aerosol form, which can be transported for great distances. These particles, apart from their own toxic potential, can play a very important role either as carriers of gases and fumes or as foci for catalytic transformations which eventually create harmful compounds. Atmospheric pollutants can affect both plants and animals adversely. Such particulates are important sources of the fallout which may accumulate in the top layers of soil as well as on the leaf surfaces of growing plants. Examples are many, including pesticides used in agriculture, industrial dusts containing fluoride, and the inorganic lead derivatives formed in the combustion of the organic lead compounds (tetraethyllead and tetramethyllead) used as fuel additives.

Certain compounds of low vapor pressure, such as organochlorine pesticides, have the ability to pass from the surface of the soil to the atmosphere by means of codistillation with the soil water and also with the water of the leaves of plants.

They can then condense as colloidal particles in suspension in the air and form aerosols capable of being carried considerable distances. This is one important process capable of contributing to marine pollution.

In certain cases, pollutants of the atmosphere can dissolve in surface waters. It is in this way that the depletion of the fish population of Swedish lakes has been attributed to the acidulation caused by contamination with sulfur dioxide originating as effluent from industrial complexes as far away as the Ruhr.

Transport by surface waters is an important route of entry of several pollutants into the physical environment. This may arise either as a consequence of deliberate or accidental discharge of effluent from factories or, for example, with herbicides in drainage waters originating from treated land. Harmful effects may arise in aquatic ecosystems, and it must also be appreciated that the chemical and physical procedures used for the purification of water for human consumption may not remove all organic pollutants.

Different investigations have revealed the presence of a considerable number of chemical pollutants in the waters of the great rivers which pass through industrialized areas. Calling upon a combination of biological and physicochemical techniques, Van Esch and his colleagues of the Pharmacology and Toxicology Branch of the National Dutch Institute of Public Health have found evidence of more than a thousand compounds in the waters of the estuary of the Rhine (Van Esch, private communication).

1.1.3. Distribution and Fate in the Physical Environment

After having been released into the physical environment, pollutants are subjected to the influence of many factors which ultimately influence their distribution. Wind, rain, fog, or temperature inversions, play roles that are too widely appreciated to need reiteration. Chemical and physical factors may also induce the transformation of the pollutant into new compounds. A spectacular example is that of the formation of irritant and phytotoxic peracyl nitrate (PAN) in the "oxidizing smog" of the Los Angeles region (for a critical review, see Truhaut, 1962), originating from exhaust gases and subjected to strong solar radiation which induces photochemical reactions between suspended organic matter and nitrogen oxides.

In soil and in water, fungi and bacteria sometimes achieve beneficial biodegradation, but in other situations they may synthesize materials more toxic than the original pollutant. The methylation of mercury by bacteria present in aquatic mud and the subsequent contamination of fish leading ultimately to Minimata disease is a good illustration of just such a possibility. A great deal of research remains to be done on such processes.

Chemical reactions occurring between compounds present at the same location must also be considered. Thus, the purification of water by chlorination may well give rise to unanticipated changes in the nature of organic micropollutants, and the possibility that organochlorine derivatives may form under such circumstances cannot be ruled out. For example, we are already aware that water containing tasteless phenolic compounds develops a particularly unpleasant flavor when chlorinated as a result of the formation of chlorophenols. The organoleptic characteristics of the end products of such interactions may not always give warning of the presence of a toxic material.

1.2. Entry and Fate of Pollutants in the Living Organisms of Ecosystems

1.2.1. Concentrations

Not infrequently, individual members of an ecosystem may achieve a considerable degree of concentration of the pollutant to which the system is exposed. In their study of pollutants of the Rhine, Van Esch et al. used this property of *Daphnia* and certain algae to obtain a biological concentration of pollutants before their nature was examined by physicochemical studies. The concentration of heavy metals and organohalogens by the flora and, especially, the fauna of the sea constitutes another important example. The capacity of plankton for concentrating pollutants is often significant in view of its role in food chains which terminate in man and may result in his food becoming potentially toxic. Such points emphasize the importance of close investigation of the movement of pollutants through food chains.

In some circumstances it is essential to determine the extent to which selective accumulation of a pollutant occurs in certain organs or tissues of an organism, rather than merely measuring total content. For example, significant accumulation of aromatic organohalogens occurs in the gonads of crustaceans and fish, and cadmium and mercury are concentrated in the kidneys of mammals.

Much more information is needed about the biological half-life of relatively persistent pollutants, both within whole organisms and in individual tissues of these organisms.

1.2.2. Metabolic Changes

Once pollutants have penetrated living organisms, they are in contact with enzyme systems which may modify their nature. These changes are of two types:

1. Changes which form products which are less toxic than the molecules from which they are derived, and thus bring about the detoxification of the latter. Such changes may go as far as the complete destruction of xenobiotic compounds, which are then called "biodegradable." Bacteria present in the digestive tract of animals, in plants, in soil, and in water often play an important part in this process of biodegradation. The de-

liberate use of bacteria for this process has been an important recent advance in the fight against pollution, and microbiologists have a considerable part to play in future studies in this direction.

2. Changes which form compounds more toxic than the molecules from which they are derived, and thus play an important role in increasing the severity or modifying the manifestations of the toxic response. Some developments in this subject are to be found in the paper of R. T. Williams (Chapter 4), and many other examples could be cited involving transformation of mercurial pollutants, aromatic amines, nitrosamines, and many carcinogens and mutagens.

Because of the significant consequences of these metabolic modifications, great importance is attached to the study of environmental and chemical factors which may modify such processes by inducing their inhibition or stimulation. It is of paramount importance to gain a better understanding of the significance of enzyme inhibition or stimulation in the response to pollutants and particularly so in situations in which complex patterns of pollutants may be present in the biosphere.

Certain molecules undergo hardly any metabolic changes; if they are relatively insoluble in water and very soluble in lipids they have a tendency to accumulate in living organisms. Such is the case, for instance, with aromatic organochlorine compounds (e.g., insecticides of the DDT type, polychlorobiphenyls), whose concentrations in certain aquatic organisms can reach values 10,000 times higher than those of the water they inhabit, according to a report of the UK Agricultural Research Council (1970).

As examples of such stable and persistent compounds accumulating in the physical as well as the living environment, it is pertinent to mention those compounds which can be present as impurities in association with primary products which are stable. Thus, polychloroparabenzodioxines and particularly tetrachloro-2,3,7,8-parabenzodioxine may be formed in poorly controlled production of trichloro-2,4,5-phenoxyacetic acid (2,4,5T), used widely as a herbicide and a ground-clearing agent in agriculture. This is a highly toxic and teratogenic compound with formidable cumulative toxicity that has enabled us to explain the nature of the chick edema factor and, among other adverse effects, may have given rise to difficulties in poultry breeding.

1.2.3. Reactions of Pollutants or Their Metabolic Products with the Chemical Constituents of Organisms

Many instances of such reactions are known. In certain cases the end result is a true detoxification. For instance, crustaceans accumulate arsenic from sea water to concentrations which would be toxic if the element were not incorporated into compounds which are of relatively low toxicity. This point is well illustrated by the work of Coulson et al. (1935), who showed that rats accumulated considerably less arsenic when it was ingested as the arsenic present in shrimps than when the same quantity of inorganic arsenic was given. It may be concluded that arsenic picked up by shirmps from their marine environment undergoes a metabolic change into less toxic compounds and, during its passage through the rat's digestive tract, releases soluble arsenic derivatives which are rapidly eliminated by renal excretion.

But reactions which generate toxic effects can also be produced. Many carcinogens and mutagens, particularly those belonging to the class of alkylating agents, owe their activity to reactions at the molecular level with certain nucleic macromolecules. The possibility of such reactions which cause biochemical lesions and which create toxic compounds must be considered seriously where constituents in food chains leading to human consumption are concerned. Without going into detail, the following examples may be mentioned:

1. The formation of carcinogenic and mutagenic nitrosamines by the reaction of nitrites at acid pH with secondary amines and even tertiary amines present naturally or incorporated by accident into the edible portions of animals or plants.
2. The formation of dichlorovinylcysteine, with toxic potential for the kidney or the bone marrow, by means of the reaction of trichlorethylene with cysteine residues present in proteins.
3. The formation of toxic chlorhydrines, by the reaction of ethylene oxide with the mineral chlorides that are almost ubiquitous in food chains.
4. The ability of many potentially toxic compounds to combine with proteins can also have a marked influence on the expression of toxicity. Such interactions may directly influence the mechanism of toxic action, are often involved in the tissue accumulation of toxic compounds, or in some cases may result in their sequestration. Species differences in the nature of proteins involved in such interactions may be one of the factors responsible for the manifestation of selective toxicity. Differences in the affinity of the binding sites of proteins for pollutants can lead to competitive interactions and displacement phenomena at such sites when the organism is exposed to more than one pollutant. Such interactions may markedly modify the nature of the response and, in some instances, are involved in the phenomenon of synergistic action to be described later. Some hormones, normally bound to proteins, may also be displaced as a consequence of the interaction between proteins and pollutants, resulting in the manifestation of a pathological disorder (see Truhaut, 1966).

Much remains to be done in the study of such important topics. There is almost total ignorance of their influence upon the pharmacokinetics of pollutants within ecosystems and upon the responses of individuals to pollutants discharged into the environment. Much more information is needed before models valid as predictive aids can be constructed.

1.3. Harmful Effects of Chemical Pollutants on the Constituents of Ecosystems Which Include Man

In order to understand these problems it is essential to present at this point certain general concepts relating to human toxicology which are well established at the present time and whose application to the field of ecotoxicology seems to me to be a useful avenue of approach. These ideas concern:

1. The different forms of toxicity.
2. The influence of various factors on the manifestations of toxicity.
3. The importance attached to the establishment of the relations, qualitative but above all quantitative, between doses and effects, in such a way as to be able to establish thresholds of toxicity and, as a result, allowable limits of exposure.

1.3.1. The Various Forms of Toxicity

1.3.1.1. Acute or Subacute Toxicity

Signs of acute or subacute toxicity arise in animal species immediately or only shortly after sufficiently large amounts of the toxic material are absorbed orally, by inhalation, or through the skin or mucous membranes. They may arise following a single exposure or following several exposures in close succession. They arise, for example, following the ingestion of certain products or the inhalation of many gases or fumes, such as carbon monoxide, chlorine, or hydrogen cyanide. The manifestations of this form of toxicity are spectacular, since they often result in sudden death. Thus it is a widely held view that the term "poison" applies only to those substances which kill in a violent manner!

The experimental assessment of the acute toxicity of a substance is commonly carried out by determination of LD_{50}, the dose needed to kill 50% of the test subjects. In the case of inhalation of toxic materials, the determination of lethal concentrations and especially LC_{50} is greatly influenced by the length of exposure, which should always be indicated. The toxicity of substances in solution (or, occasionally, those in water suspension) to aquatic species and particularly fish is determined by an analogous procedure. Many parameters must be taken into consideration in order to program such experiments. Thus, whereas periods of exposure in these experiments vary generally from 24 to 96 hours, if the product under scrutiny decomposes in the water after several hours, shorter periods of observation are necessary. On the other hand, if the product remains relatively stable in water, it is advisable to carry out the experiments with smaller amounts but for longer periods of exposure, completing them by measuring the residues in the organs or the tissues, so that the dangerous as well as the lethal levels of impregnation may be determined. Interested readers will find, in the third edition of a pamphlet devoted to agricultural pesticides (Council of Europe, 1973), general ideas of some importance, with references relating to methodology concerning the determination of the toxicity of pesticides to wildlife (birds, fish, useful insects, etc.).

Finally, it must be appreciated that the magnitude of lethal doses or concentrations may vary within very wide limits depending on the animal species, and also on variables such as the conditions of exposure.

1.3.1.2. Toxicity Arising over Short or Long Periods by Repeated Absorption of Small Amounts of Toxic Materials

It cannot be overemphasized that toxic effects do not only result from absorption of relatively large amounts over a short period of time; they also frequently arise from the repeated absorption of doses much too small to induce an acute response. Such a situation is more insidious, in that the toxic response often appears without warning signs.

Accumulation of Doses. The cumulative action of poisons upon man and the higher mammals is exhibited following repeated exposure to substances such as methyl alcohol, the heterosides of digitalis, and inorganic derivatives of arsenic, fluorine, and heavy metals (lead, mercury, cadmium, thallium, etc.). These poisons are retained within the organism as a consequence of their physical properties—(e.g., greater solubility in fats (lipids) than in aqueous phases, suitability for adsorption)—or by means of chemical affinities for tissue or cellular components, or even as a result of direct damage to renal excretory mechanisms which thus hinders elimination from the body (e.g., the heavy metals).

Exposure to a cumulative poison to the point that normally tolerable threshold concentrations in tissues are ultimately exceeded may induce a wide range of manifestations of toxicity. These may take the form of effects upon growth rate and behavior, upon the chemical composition of the body fluids, upon histological structure and function of different organs (liver, kidneys, nervous system, bone marrow, endocrine glands), and upon the ability to reproduce or maintain a normal life span.

These forms of poisoning are usually termed "chronic." In my opinion this is not a good description, for, as we shall see, an irreversible (therefore chronic) lesion may result from one acutely toxic phenomenon. That is why it is preferable to use the term "long-term toxicity."

A significant example of long-term toxicity arises from exposure to inorganic fluorine compounds. Doses of sodium fluoride substantially exceeding 1 g are needed before human subjects are adversely affected by a single challenge, but, in contrast, daily doses of only a few centigrams will cause the long-term poisoning called "fluorosis," characterized by damage to teeth and bones and severe cachexia and debilitation. That is why water for human consumption should not have concentrations of fluoride ion that exceed 1.5 mg/liter. Similar differences in the nature of acute and long-term consequences of exposure to organochlorine insecticides such as DDT and hexachlorocyclohexane have been found in work with several species.

Cumulative Effects. Substances endowed with carcinogenic properties appear even more dangerous. According to the findings of Druckrey and Kupfmüller (1949) concerning rats treated with butter yellow, chemically p-dimethyl-aminoazobenzene (an azo dye producing hepatomas, used in the past in some countries to color margarine yellow), we must admit the view, *a priori* paradoxical, that each isolated dose has a cumulative effect throughout the entire life of the animals whatever the extent of elimination and metabolic degradation. In this situation there is both a cumulative effect *and a total summation of irreversible pathological responses.* This theory has been extended to other genotoxic poisons and particularly to compounds having mutagenic effects.

Carcinogenic and mutagenic substances thus occupy a separate place among long-term toxic agents. In their case, threshold doses cannot be determined. Because of the long-lasting effect after the elimination of the product, no dose, however small, would be without danger if it were repeated and if sufficient time were to elapse to allow it to act. However, recent studies have led to the suggestion that the concept of summation of absolutely irreversible damage may have been exaggerated. Observations in the field of molecular biology now indicate the possibility of repair of the damage to nucleic macromolecules which usually conditions the development of malignant growth. These conflicting views are at the present time giving rise to discussion on an international level and to research on dose/effect relations for carcinogenic and/or mutagenic agents, including radiation (WHO, 1974).

Another serious problem is the possibility of cumulative effects occurring over several generations. This possibility is suggested from studies of the toxicity of several compounds. An example of this type of action exists in human subjects, where the administration of diethylstilboestrol during pregnancy has been associated with a high incidence of cancer of the vagina at the onset of puberty in female offspring. Such observations indicate the desirability that studies of long-term toxicity should cover at least two generations, particularly in short-lived species such as the rat and mouse.

Certain members of ecosystems have, in the last few years, shown a sensitivity to long-term effects which were considered until relatively recently to be confined to the higher animal species. This is the case with the hepatomas caused in reared trout by the use of food contaminated by aflatoxins. The cancer of the mantle which occurs frequently in oysters of certain Australian or Californian coasts may well be a manifestation of long-term toxicity. The way these mollusks feed, consisting of the filtering of large amounts of sea water, has perhaps some connection with the appearance of neoplasms. Recently cancers of the skin and of the gills have been noted in a large percentage of fishes living in polluted coastal areas.

1.3.1.3. Effects, More or Less Long-Term, Resulting from the Absorption of a Single Dose

Quite apart from the immediate effects of acute or subacute toxicity and the more or less long-term effects arising from repeated small doses, there are also effects, more or less long-term, which can arise from the absorption of a single dose. In this connection, several materials have been recognized as causing serious effects after a sometimes prolonged latent period, even after they have disappeared from the organism. This is the case with the herbicide Paraquat, a derivative of bipyridinium, which, in man, several weeks after the ingestion of a dose which merely causes minor gastrointestinal disorders, provokes the proliferation of fibroblasts in pulmonary cells and may prove fatal through inhibition of the diffusion of oxygen. This is also the case with certain organophosphorus insecticides endowed with a delayed neurotoxic action, which causes degeneration of the axons of the neurons of the central nervous system and demyelination leading to paralysis. These are, as Bernes has so aptly characterized them, "poisons which hit and run." Research is now under way to try to discover the causative biochemical lesions.

In certain cases the effects of a single dose may be seen after a very long latent period. This is the case with carcinogens such as nitrosamines and related substances (nitrosamides). Thus, the administration of a small dose of methylnitrosourea to a pregnant rat in the middle of gestation, without inducing any signs of poisoning in the dam, will cause brain cancer in the offspring when they reach adulthood—an example of transplacental carcinogenesis.

1.3.1.4. Special Forms of Toxicity: Teratogenic and Mutagenic Effects

The reference just made to assaults within the uterus shows the importance attached to the study of embryotoxic effects. These will be considered later when dealing with the influence of the vital evolutionary stage on toxicity and upon teratogenesis.

Mutagenic effects, that is, the production of mutations which may result in manifestation of genotoxic properties, also require consideration here, if only to emphasize that very active research is now under way in an attempt to establish an adequate experimental methodology for the study of these effects in higher mammals. Other effects to which attention must be drawn are immunosuppressive responses and those on the reproductive system other than the embryotoxic. The complex nature of these effects emphasizes the need for the multiple and multidisciplinary approaches that must be initiated for the toxicological evaluation of the chemical pollutants in the environment.

1.3.1.5. Toxicity Due to Repeated Assaults

Among the more or less long-term effects, mention must finally be made of those which can result from repeated daily exposure at the level of any one particular organ, tissue, or system. Lesions which are of a reversible nature may not have enough time to heal and thus eventually become chronic. This is the case with, for example, the occupational diseases called pneumoconiosis. Chronic bronchitis caused by repeated exposure to the irritating pulmonary action of sulfur dioxide present in the atmosphere of certain industrial cities is another spectacular example. It cannot be discounted that such a form of toxicity could also manifest itself within ecosystems, but, up to now, we know of no such example.

1.3.2. Influence of Various Factors on the Manifestation of Toxicity

Many factors influence the manifestations of toxicity, both qualitative and quantitative. In the interest of brevity I shall examine those considered to be among the more important, namely, species differences, stage of development, genetic characteristics, pathological states, and simultaneous exposure to more than one pollutant.

1.3.2.1. Species Differences in Tolerance and Response

Large species differences exist in the tolerance of living organisms to chemical agents. In human toxicological studies it is thus difficult to extrapolate results obtained with laboratory animals to assess the potential significance of the findings to man. This is why such importance is attached to supporting such studies by epidemiological surveys of effects in groups of human subjects that may have suffered exposure to the potentially toxic agent. Great care is needed in the selection of appropriate criteria to assess the frequency and magnitude of the toxic response in such studies.

Penicillin provides a striking example of species difference in tolerance. In guinea pigs, LD_{50} is approximately 6 mg/kg body weight, whereas in mice it is 1800 mg/kg—i.e., penicillin is about 300 times less toxic to the mouse. Another example is offered by the hamster, which is so tolerant of DDT that it is almost impossible to kill it with this insecticide.

Short-term exposure of human subjects or poultry to a toxic dose of triorthocresyl phosphate causes centripetal degeneration of the axons of neurons and demyelination, but similar doses have no effect upon the rhesus monkey, the rat, or the rabbit. The failure to detect the teratogenic effect of thalidomide in pregnant women was again due to species differences in response; it was not teratogenic in rats used in early "screening" tests, and only later work illustrated its teratogenicity in rabbits and mice.

Cancer of the bladder is a manifestation of long-term toxicity resulting from repeated exposure of dogs and human subjects to β-naphthylamine. It has no such effect upon rats or rabbits. Although aflatoxins do not induce liver cancer in the mouse, hepatomas can readily be induced in this species by repeated exposure to DDT or dieldrin.

Such species differences in response are often explained by suggesting that a metabolite is the primary cause of the lesion and that metabolic pathways differ between species. This is not always the case. Thus, the rat and the hen respond very differently to tricresyl phosphate and yet, as far as is known, this compound is metabolized in the same way in both species.

Such species differences in tolerance and the resulting phenomenon of *selective toxicity* are extremely important in the field of ecotoxicology, as the following examples show. Fish and cats are highly sensitive to aromatic organochlorine compounds; algae and starfish are sensitive to copper; aflatoxins readily induce hepatomas in trout; and conifers and gladioli are extremely intolerant of inorganic fluorides. Conversely, some species are highly tolerant of certain toxins. Thus, slugs and snails readily tolerate the toxic compounds present in *Amanita phalloides*, while quail are not affected by the alkaloid cicutine present in hemlock. Although alkaloids originating from seeds of the *Umbelliferae* are not toxic to the quail, they may accumulate in its flesh and this has in the past given rise to occasional cases of toxicity ("quail poisoning!") in human subjects (Sergent, 1941).

The biochemical mechanisms responsible for these species differences are very poorly understood. In some instances an explanation is available as, for example, from the physicochemical studies indicating that carbon monoxide tolerance in the snail may be associated with the low affinity of its copper-containing respiratory pigment for this gas, compared with the high affinity of hemoglobin in other species. Such plausible explanations are rare and much more research is required on this topic that has important practical consequences in gaining understanding of how chemical pollutants in the environment can disturb the balance within ecosystems.

1.3.2.2. Relationships between Stage of Development and Toxicity

An extensive examination of this important topic would be worthwhile, but in the following paragraphs attention will merely be concentrated upon the hypersensitivity of the embryo and the young.

In human toxicology, it has become a classic notion that the fetus is especially sensitive to certain toxic assaults. In this connection the history of thalidomide is spectacular. When this sedative, possessing slight tranquilizing properties, was launched on the market in 1957, it was considered to be the least toxic of all known sedatives, on the basis of toxicological expertise applied according to classic standards. And yet, when taken by the pregnant woman at the time in pregnancy when the differentiated parts of the embryo were being formed, that is, during the first weeks following conception (23rd to 40th day in human females), it causes anatomical malformation in the fetus, with the consequent birth of malformed babies. The study of these teratogenic effects has therefore been included in the procedure laid down for toxicological evaluation of all medicinal substances. It must be emphasized that teratogenicity is only one example of embryotoxic effects, some of which are long-term or even very long-term. In this connection I have already mentioned the production, at an adult age, of brain cancer in rats born of mothers who had been given only a single very weak dose of nitrosomethylurea during pregnancy.

The importance of prenatal toxicology goes far beyond any particular field of therapy. It must be seriously considered in the context of the field of occupational exposure, industrial or agricultural, where the exclusion of the pregnant woman from certain kinds of work should be recommended. In ecotoxicology, it is no less important to man through his food chain than it is, on a much larger scale, to the various members of the animal world.

It is well known in human toxicology, that infants and very young children are particularly sensitive to many potentially toxic chemical agents. This hyper-sensitivity is due to various factors, among which must be mentioned, first of all, metabolic immaturity and especially deficiency of "detoxifying" enzymes, especially at the level of hepatic microsomes. Other factors, such as the sensi-tivity of the central nervous system and the lack of certain plasma proteins, may also play an important part. In ecotoxicology, the possibility of toxic assaults in the first stages of life, particularly on larval forms, such as fish fry and bird embryos, is obviously of very great importance for the propagation of the species.

1.3.2.3. Influence of Genetic Characteristics

This influence is already illustrated by that of the nature of the living species and strain on its tolerance to toxic agents. The difficulties of extrapolating results obtained from experimental toxicology with other species to man have already been stressed. In human toxicology the difficulties introduced by racial differences in sensitivity have been known for a long time. Thus, for instance, subjects of the yellow or the black race are much less sensitive than those of the white race to toxic effects from the nitrophenols. The existence of individual sensitivity to certain chemical products has also been known for a long time. From this comes the very ancient idea of idiosyncrasy or congenital intolerance, quite distinct from allergy, which represents an acquired intolerance. Over the last thirty years, many advances have been made in the field of toxicogenetics (sometimes known as chemogenetics) which complement those made in pharma-cogenetics. These are the observations that have arisen mainly in the field of therapeutics and have shown the conditioning of certain hitherto inexplicable sensitivities having a genetic origin. For example, a deficiency of erythrocyte glucose 6-phosphate dehydrogenase, an enzyme involved in aerobic catabolism of glucose via pentoses, was the cause of the serious hemolytic disorders observed during the Pacific War in Black Americans following the ingestion in therapeutic doses of an antimalarial compound, primaquin. This deficiency has explained disorders of the same kind in workers exposed to different industrial products, particularly the derivatives of aromatic amines, and toxic reactions following consumption of the common bean in certain groups of population living in the Mediterranean area.

Such genetic influences are certainly of great importance in ecotoxicology, but their study has only just started.

1.3.2.4. Influence of Pathological States

It has been clearly shown, from studies in the field of human toxicology, that pre-existing pathological states can increase sensitivity to toxic effects to a marked degree. This is the case with, for example, hepatic deficiencies which decrease the effectiveness of many detoxication mechanisms; renal deficiencies which limit the possibility of filtration and excretion; certain endocrine glandular deficiencies, particularly of the thyroid and the adrenal cortex (thyroid deficiency makes this organ particularly sensitive to the toxic effect of nitriles); and states of malnutrition. The possible significance of this topic of "pathotoxicology" remains unexplored in an ecological context.

1.3.2.5. Influence of Simultaneous Exposure to Several Pollutants

Conditions in the biosphere are such that members of ecosystems, including man, are not exposed to a single pollutant but to many. From the point of view of the organisms at risk, this can have ameliorating consequences if pollutants interact antagonistically as, for example, in the effect of various organic sulfur derivatives upon acute toxicity caused by ozone or by nitrous fumes in higher mammals. Interaction can, however, potentiate toxic responses. The following examples illustrate the possibility of synergistic reactions: simultaneous exposure to such insecticides as malathion and EPN; exposure to inorganic fluorides and oxides or salts of beryllium; association of carbon monoxide with nitric fumes or hydrogen sulfide; simultaneous exposure to sulfur dioxide or tobacco smoke and to asbestos; exposure of animals to carcinogenic polycyclic aromatic hydrocarbons associated with exposure to solvents such as n-dodecane; association of pesticides with several solvents or agents, known as surfactants, in the liquid formulations used to achieve dispersion.

Many examples of synergists to the action of carcinogenic compounds are known that cannot be described in detail in this paper. However, emphasis must be given to the point that synergistic action may result not only from the interaction of two or more pollutants, but also as a consequence of exposure to compounds normally present in the environment or in food at times when uptake of a toxic pollutant may have modified the activity of enzymes normally involved in their metabolism.

The most outstanding illustration of this possibility is the high incidence of hypertension and cerebral hemorrhage in human subjects eating cheese while receiving the psychotonic drug tranylcypromine. This compound, by its inhibition of the enzyme monoamine oxidase, produces these adverse effects by reducing the rate of destruction of the sympathomimetic substance tyramine present in cheese. (In this context it is relevant that monoamine oxidase activity is greatly influenced by the copper status of animals and thus is probably sensitive to heavy metals that antagonize copper, e.g., cadmium, zinc.) This example illustrates the value of a detailed understanding of the biochemical action of "poisons," or "chemical scalpels," as Claud Bernard has aptly called them.

1.3.3. The Importance of Establishing Dose/Response Relationships

"*Sola dosis fecit venum*" (it is only the dose that makes the poison) wrote Paracelsus many years ago. From this truth comes the golden rule, in pharmacology and toxicology, that the establishment of the relation of dose to effect is the fundamental prerequisite for the ultimate prevention of noxious effects and poisonings. This applies as strongly to ecotoxicology as it does to human toxicology, where the objective of both these fields of endeavor is to reduce the absorbed dose to below the threshold of toxicity. However, in certain cases, exposure to concentrations below the toxic threshold may have a beneficial effect. This is the case with certain oligo-elements such as selenium, whose deficiency in species like cattle, sheep, and poultry causes muscular dystrophy and other pathological changes, or fluoride, which in very small doses proves to be essential to the structural constitution of calciferous tissues (bones and teeth).

Studies on toxic effects must therefore, in ecotoxicology as in human toxicology, be both qualitative and quantitative in order to be able to recommend those limits which are permissible or tolerable.

Although there is still an enormous amount to be done, this quantitative approach has been shown to be particularly fruitful in human toxicology in relation to recommended limits for air pollutants or of foreign substances found in food (Truhaut, 1969). It must be applied to ecotoxicological research, which up to now has concentrated on the qualitative approach. The quantitative approach must employ analytical methods adequate in specificity and accuracy. Adequate definition of dose/response relationships therefore demands careful collaboration between the analytical chemist and the ecotoxicologist if realistic definition of pollutant "doses" is to be achieved.

1.4 Perspectives and Prospects in Ecotoxicology

As in human toxicology, the ultimate objective of research in ecotoxicology must be the establishment of protective measures against the harmful effects of pollutants of the environment upon the various constituents of ecosystems. These harmful effects must first be identified and assessed. In this connection, it cannot be overemphasized that our ecotoxicological information, both qualitative and quantitative, is extraordinarily limited as far as the effects of environmental pollutants on most of the constituents of the biomass are concerned. Data at our disposal concern only a limited number of species and, of these, the greater part are limited to studies of acute or subacute toxicity. In this connection, it is edifying to read a most laborious compilation carried out by the Battelle Laboratories for the US Environmental Protection Agency in 1971. The vast range of problems to be studied makes it essential that there should be a coordination of research on a world-wide scale, involving the cooperation of specialists from a whole series of disciplines (in particular, the various branches of ecology and toxicology), who up to now have continued their work without initiating any exchanges of information concerning methods and results.

It is also essential that specialists in analytical methodology should be actively associated with this work. How, as we have already emphasized, can we establish relations between doses and their effects without having at our disposal methods of analysis which are adequate in their specificity, their sensitivity, and their accuracy to measure the doses of exposure? How can we study the gradual growth of a pollutant in the physical environment, its movements, and those of its possible products of degradation through ecosystems, without having at our disposal subtle techniques for identification and dosage assessment in the complex biological environments which surround living organisms, and where the pollutants and their metabolites usually find themselves considerably diluted? How can we describe the patterns of elimination from tissues and the biological half-life of pollutants? How, in a word, can we establish the pharmacokinetics of the movement of pollutants in the biosphere without having at our disposal adequate analytical tools?

If we wish to avoid a worsening of the already alarming situation where chemical pollutants are flowing into the evironment, it is time for the categories of specialists already mentioned to unite in an effort to program research aimed at combating these pollutants and preventing their effects on the biosphere. First, we must bring into existence an inventory of the pollutants capable of penetrating the environment, by compiling data on the rate of production of the various chemical compounds in different countries, on the nature and modality of their utilization, and on the quantities capable of appearing in different parts of the environment.

An inventory of information on the biological effects, particularly the harmful effects of pollutants on the various living organisms, including man, must then be prepared. The development of data banks at national and international levels should be strongly encouraged. To be profitable, such compilations should provide all the available information needed to facilitate the ecotoxicological evaluation of pollutants, in the form of what we will call ecotoxicological data sheets, and should suggest, at least provisionally, the acceptable limit of exposure.

In the present situation, emphasis should be placed upon those gaps in our knowledge particularly concerning:

- The fate of pollutants in the physical environment and the biosphere, particular attention being paid to their degree of persistence, their eventual chemical transformations, and the eventual extent of their anticipated accumulation.
- Possible manifestations of selective toxicity.
- Relationships between doses and effects without which thresholds of toxicity and permissible limits in various parts of the environment, air, water, food, and living organisms cannot be defined. The possibilities of defining dangerous concentrations in the various animal or plant constituents of ecosystems are much more favorable than in the case of man. For man, except for the limited availability of post-mortem material, it is only possible to define the limits of concentration in those tissues and body fluids which can be sampled, e.g., blood, urine, expelled air, fat reserves, and, possibly, samples of bone tissue (teeth and bone).

The gaps in our knowledge having been clearly defined, we must set up plans for research to fill these gaps. The primary requirements are for:

- the definition of adequate methodological approaches either for routine procedures of testing (studies of acute, subactue, short- or long-term toxicity) or for more specifically directed studies (e.g., functional exploration of organs and systems, biochemical mechanisms of action);
- the development of multidisciplinary studies of toxicity, particularly in so far as this is modified by physiological differences between species, differences in exposure, and mode of penetration of pollutants into organisms;
- the development of predictive models permitting the study of the effects of toxic agents in specific ecosystems.

Among the criteria to be applied in determining priorities for such investigations are:

- the quantities of pollutant discharged into the environment;
- its persistence;
- its tendency to accumulate, either in its original form or as a metabolite, within particular members of ecosystems and food chains;

- appraisal of its toxic potential, particularly its delayed insidious effects (e.g., carcinogenic, teratogenic, or mutagenic potential), and its capacity to influence behavior.

To achieve the progress so urgently needed with this immense task, the following recommendations are made:

- Specialists having a sound knowledge of ecology must receive adequate training in toxicology.
- Adequate financial support must be sought to achieve this, despite present economic problems.
- Machinery must be set up to establish and maintain the essential interdisciplinary approaches to the study of ecotoxicological problems.
- A sufficient number of research centers, well supported by staff and equipment, must be established to investigate the wide range of problems awaiting resolution in this field.

The awareness at various national levels and on an international scale of the serious problems which pollution of the environment poses for the future of man allows us to hope that action will be taken which will give for the benefit of future generations the true realization of the slogan adopted in 1961 by the Conference of the International Union of Pure and Applied Chemistry (IUPAC) and of the International Congress held at New York on the occasion of the celebration of the 75th anniversary of the American Chemical Society: "Chemistry, key to better living."

References

Coulson, E. J., Remington, R. R., and Lynch, K. M. (1935). *J. Nutr.*, **10**, 255–270.

Council of Europe (1973). *Les Pesticides Agricoles*, 3rd ed., Strasbourg.

Drukrey, H., and Kupfmüller, K. (1949). *Dosis und Wirkung*, Cantor, Aulendorf.

Royal Academy of Sciences (1973). "Evaluation of genetic risks of environmental chemicals," Ambio Special Report, Universitetsforlaget, **3**, 327.

Sergent, R. (1941). *Arch. Inst. Pasteur Algérie*, **19**, 161–167.

Truhaut, R. (1962). "Sur les risques pouvant résulter de la pollution de l'air des villes et sur les moyens de lutte à mettre en oeuvre," *Revue de l'APPA*, **4**, 3–19 and 148–186.

Truhaut, R. (1966). "The transportation of toxic compounds by plasma proteins," West European Symposia on Clinical Chemistry (Paris, 1965), Vol. 5, *Transport Function of Plasma Proteins*, pp. 147–171, American Elsevier, New York.

Truhaut, R. (1969). "Dangers of the chemical age," *Pure and Applied Chemistry*, **18**(1–2), 111–128.

UK Agricultural Research Council (1970). *Third Report of the Research Commitee on Toxic Chemicals*. HMSO, London.

WHO (1973). "Trace elements in human nutrition," Technical Reports Series, No. 532.

WHO (1974). "Evaluation de la cancérogénicité et la mutagénicité des produits chimiques," Technical Reports Series, No. 546.

2

Some Effects of Pollutants in Terrestrial Ecosystems

WILLIAM H. STICKEL

2.1. Introduction

As practical biologists, we know that the terrestrial ecosystem is resilient. Minor episodes of pollution are soon corrected or compensated for if nature is given a chance. We know that there is no single, simple balance of nature to be upset. There are many balances, and they shift constantly as summer changes to winter, as drought follows flood, and as erosion follows fire. Among the most powerful factors are our own work: cultivation, exploitation, and construction. Pollution, therefore, is just one factor.

This practical view is true, but it overlooks the fact that pollution can have long-lasting, extremely undesirable effects over whole regions. It also overlooks the fact that troubles caused by pollution are in addition to those caused by all the other factors. Above all, it overlooks the fact that while many conditions are beyond our control, pollution is one factor that we can control.

In this paper, I take up some of the ways in which pollutants affect animals and plants and then comment briefly on the responses of certain groups of organisms. Special attention is paid to organochlorines and their relation to avian reproduction, for this is a field of special concern at our laboratory. Throughout

WILLIAM H. STICKEL ● Patuxent Wildlife Research Center, U.S. Fish and Wildlife Service, Laurel, Maryland 20811.

the paper I try to point out the critical importance of species and group differences in understanding both field and laboratory findings.

Examples are cited freely, but much is necessarily omitted; a paper of this type cannot approach completeness and inevitably reflects the author's interests and limitations. To the many authors whose good work is not mentioned, I can only offer sincere regrets and apologies. Many of the references cited are recent works that lead back into the body of the literature.

2.2. Community Structure and Function

Woodwell (1970) discussed three basic effects of pollutants on ecosystems. (1) As contamination grows, community structure is simplified by the loss of species after species. Simple communities are often less stable—are more subject to wide fluctuations—than are communities that have a wealth of species. (2) Vegetation is lost when pollution reduces the foliage, which is the photosynthetic area, while leaving much of the respiratory area of stems and bark. The larger the plant, the more vulnerable it is to this effect. As Woodwell says, "Thus chronic disturbances of widely different types favor plants that are small in stature, and any disturbance that tends to increase the amount of respiration in proportion to photosynthesis will aggravate the shift." A forest may be changed to a stand of grass or sedge, or even to bare, eroding earth. The animal communities change with it. (3) As the larger plants die, and as animals die or leave the area, the site loses an important part of its nutrients; minerals and decaying organic materials are lost through erosion and leaching. These basic nutrients are not soon replaced. An area may not be able to recover for many years. It may never recover if much erosion has occurred.

These effects can be produced by pollutants as different as herbicides, radiation, or sulfur dioxide from a smelter. They apply primarily to plants, but have many parallels in the animal world. Edwards and Thompson (1973) point out, for example, that radiation and insecticides have similar effects on soil invertebrates.

Numbers of individuals may decline near a pollution source before the number of species drops. Fallout from a kraft paper mill (largely Na_2SO_4) caused 21 species of ground beetles to be scarce near the mill but they were increasingly common out to 1.5 miles. The gradient was shown best by total numbers of individuals. However, a few species were rare or absent at the station that was nearest the mill, although 900 yards from it (Freitag et al., 1973).

2.3. Weedy Species Favored

Among both plants and animals, the species that survive and succeed in the presence of pollution are likely to be hardy, broadly adapted species that have high reproductive potential. The animals are likely to be of diversified food habits. It is fair to call these plants and animals "weedy" species, for they are vigorous exploiters of disturbed sites. We see them as starlings, house sparrows, and herring gulls, as well as domestic rats and mice, which succeed in many outdoor situations. Some of these species may be sensitive to pollutants, as sparrows and starlings are to some common insecticides. But their numbers, their breeding potential, and their adaptability to varied and disturbed habitats easily compensate for this. The more we pollute, and the more we disturb, the more we restrict the biota to weedy species.

2.4. Herbivores Favored over Carnivores

It seems that the birds and mammals that are in trouble because of pollution are almost always of carnivorous groups. True, any kind of animal may be affected near a smelter or on a field treated with a powerful pesticide, but away from known concentrations the problems of mortality, reproduction, and population decline generally strike the flesh-eaters. It is not deer, squirrels, rabbits, quail, grouse, or finches on which pollution problems center. Instead, among birds, it is eagles, ospreys, peregrines, sparrow hawks, Cooper's hawks, sharp-shinned hawks, pelicans, and a number of others (Anderson et al., 1969; Blus et al., 1974a,b; Cade et al., 1971; Gress et al., 1973; Hickey, 1969; Koeman et al., 1972a,b,d; Ratcliffe, 1973; Snyder et al., 1973; L. F. Stickel, 1973). These are bird-eaters or fish-eaters. The worst troubles typically strike animals of these food habits. Indeed, the niche of bird-eating hawks has been nearly emptied in the eastern United States, with the loss of the peregrine and the great reduction of Cooper's and sharp-shinned hawks. Residues of DDE are high in these birds (Cade et al., 1971; Snyder et al., 1973).

Among mammals there is evidence that cats are highly sensitive to pesticides. Mink are sensitive to methylmercury (Aulerich et al., 1974) and are incredibly sensitive to PCBs (Platonow and Karstad, 1973). Raccoons fed 2 ppm dieldrin for long periods fail in reproduction and may die (Morris, 1973). Yet deer fed 25 ppm dieldrin suffer little more than marginal effects (Murphy and Korschgen, 1970). Pheasants are little affected by DDT (or DDE) dosages that may kill kestrels (Azevedo et al., 1965; Porter and Wiemeyer, 1972).

One is tempted to think that the greater sensitivity of carnivores is a general rule, but study of Lehman's compilation of pesticide toxicities (1965) shows that dogs often are no more susceptible than rats.

The reason usually advanced for the herbivore–carnivore difference is that carnivores are more heavily exposed through the food chain. Countless analyses prove that this does happen. Mink, for example, had 10 to 90 times the DDE residues of hares in the same area (Sherburne and Dimond, 1969). It may also be true that herbivores are aided in metabolizing pollutants by their intestinal microflora. It seems likely, however, that there are also more basic, physiological differences. This is shown by the great differences in the rates at which different animals lose a chemical. The shell-thinning suffered by predatory birds, when there is little or none in equally dosed seed-eating birds, suggests sharp physiological differences (Cecil et al., 1973; McLane and Hall, 1972; Wiemeyer and Porter, 1970).

Even among soil invertebrates, predators usually are more readily killed by most pesticides than are herbivores. One reason may be that they move about more and hence come into contact with more chemical (Edwards and Thompson, 1973). The result can be population outbreaks of the herbivores, some of which are pests of crop plants.

Applications of pesticides to crops have often reduced predators and parasites to the point that pest outbreaks occurred. Indeed, observation of this phenomenon provided the most convincing evidence entomologists ever had that parasites and predators are of practical importance in holding down pest populations (Newsom, 1967). Largely because of this, agriculture is now moving toward integrated pest management. In this, parasites and predators are encouraged to the utmost and pesticides are used only in surgical fashion. This means using the smallest amount of the shortest-lived and most specific pesticide that will do the job. Integrated control can also involve the use of scouting to follow pest populations so that pesticides may be employed only when and where they are genuinely needed.

2.5. Substitute Pests

Species and group differences frequently appear in the problem of substitute pests. Harris (1969) gives a good example of this. The black cutworm and the variegated cutworm were well controlled in tobacco by aldrin and heptachlor. A third species, the dark-sided cutworm, was highly tolerant to these chemicals. As the two susceptible species were eliminated, the third species increased to take their places. The outbreak of the dark-sided cutworm soon became extremely serious; years were required to work out new control techniques. An important point here is that cutworms of the same family reacted very differently to the same powerful insecticides.

In one famous example the use of DDT in apple orchards changed spider mites from minor pests to major pests. And, when heptachlor was used to control imported fire ants in the southern United States, it controlled ticks, chiggers, rice water weevils, and some biting flies for a year, but it caused outbreaks of sugar cane borers and rice stink bugs (Newsom, 1967). The fire ants themselves are important predators of caneborers, so much so that after they and certain other predators were reduced by one application of mirex, damage by borers increased by 69%. Use of azinphosmethyl against the borers allows the best predator of the borer, the fire ant, to remain and augment the chemical's action (Negm and Hensley, 1969; Reagan et al., 1972).

2.6. Resistance

Long exposure to lethal pollutants such as insecticides causes selection for resistance, especially in fast-breeding forms of life. Insects may become enormously resistant to chemicals that once controlled them. The carrot rust fly developed 5600-fold resistance to aldrin (Harris, 1969). Resistance to many insecticides has been found in insects, and resistance to any chemical insecticide must be expected to develop in insects. Resistance to one chemical often carries with it cross-resistance to other chemicals.

Chemicals differ sharply in the speed and degree to which they create resistance. Good examples are given for mosquitofish by Culley and Ferguson (1969). As compared to susceptible fish, resistant ones had only 5.1-fold resistance to DDT and 1.7-fold resistance to methoxychlor. But for endrin, their resistance was 523-fold. For strobane, heptachlor, and toxaphene it was 568-, 357-, and 376-fold. Of the 15 organophosphates tested, only one gave as much as 4.8-fold resistance, for these chemicals hydrolyze in water and seldom last long enough to create much selection pressure on fish.

Resistance in frogs and fish living near heavily treated cotton fields has been well established (Ferguson and Gilbert, 1967; Ferguson, 1968, 1969). Resistant cricket frogs and toads had about 100-fold resistance to DDT and also had varying degrees of resistance to toxaphene, aldrin, and dieldrin.

Among mammals, troublesome resistance to the anticoagulant Warfarin has appeared in rats (Drummond and Wilson, 1968). Resistance of pine voles to endrin has made it necessary to seek new control methods (Webb et al., 1973). Apparently, resistance to pesticides has not yet been found in mammals other than rodents.

No birds are known to have developed resistance in the wild, but approximately twofold resistance to DDT was created experimentally in *Coturnix* (Poonacha et al., 1973). It has been suggested that we should seek to develop resistance in wild birds. There are several difficulties in this. One is that there is a large number of chemicals to which resistance would be needed. Secondly, the amount of mortality that would be necessary for selective pressure would be unacceptable to large sections of the public. The most crucial objection is that it is almost certain that numerous scarce species that are high on the food chain would be eliminated in the process of causing selection in other species.

Geneticists report that resistance is not wholly to an animal's advantage: a genetic price must be paid for it. This may involve smaller size or poorer physiological adaptation to some environmental condition. As an example of this, endrin-resistant pine voles were more susceptible to the organophosphate Gophacide than were nonresistant voles (Webb et al., 1973).

Resistance may depend upon metabolizing and/or excreting the chemical or upon becoming able to tolerate it. "The physiological mechanism seems to differ depending upon the type of pesticide involved. For DDT and parathion, only low levels of resistance have been recorded in fishes, and there is evidence that the toxicants are degraded in the tissues. With most compounds, such as endrin and toxaphene, the mechanism seems to be one of physiological toleration which permits the fish to survive massive body burdens of the toxicant" (Ferguson, 1969).

Resistant, pesticide-laden animals—whether fish, insects, or other animals— offer a serious threat to susceptible individuals. At the minimum, they add enormously to the residues in the food web. At the worst, they can kill outright. Black bass and green sunfish have been killed by prolonged feeding on wild-caught resistant mosquitofish. It is believed that bass have been eliminated from some waters because of this (Ferguson, 1968; Finley· et al., 1970). An endrin-tolerant mosquitofish was able to carry as much as 1042 ppm of endrin, if experimentally exposed. When the experimental residues of endrin averaged 180 ppm, as in the study of Finley et al. (1970), a single fish would kill a nonresistant green sunfish that ate it. Residues are far lower than these at most places, of course, but it is clear what can happen where persistent toxic chemicals are commonly present.

Some groups of animals are naturally resistant to many chemicals and can accumulate them to dangerous levels. The trait seems common among the Mollusca and Annelida, and slugs, snails, and earthworms are well known examples. Slugs near treated orchards have been found carrying as much as 134 ppm of endrin (dry weight) and at the same time carrying high levels of dieldrin and DDT (Gish, 1970). The threat to predators is obvious. Earthworms have insecticide residues that average about nine times those of the soil. Barker (1958) found that pools of earthworms of various species from an area treated heavily with DDT contained from 33 ppm to 164 ppm DDT and 14 ppm to 59 ppm DDE (wet weight). He was the first to point out that this was the route by which many birds were being killed. In proving this, he was also the first to use brain residues of a pesticide diagnostically.

2.7. Delayed Mortality

When birds drop dead—even fall from the sky—and prove to have lethal brain residues of an organochlorine although there was no known treatment in the vicinity, one must always suspect that lethal mobilization occurred. The organochlorines are stored in fat and may be carried in large amounts after heavy, but sublethal, exposure. Small amounts of the chemical can be found in the blood, but no effects appear as long as fat is maintained or increased. But when fat is drawn upon suddenly, as in starvation, illness, or migration, the chemical content of the blood increases more rapidly than the body can cope with it and residues in the brain rise. Indeed, residues in the brain tend to vary as the mirror image of the fat content of the body, even in seemingly healthy birds (W. H. Stickel et al., 1973). If stored residues are great enough, mobilization may cause death with typical signs of poisoning and with residues in the brain that are typical of death.

This has occurred at various places in the wild with individual birds. In early April of 1974, numbers of blue and snow geese died in Missouri with lethal levels of dieldrin in their brains. No other cause of death could be determined and no local source of dieldrin was known. The source suspected was aldrin used on rice seed on the Gulf Coast of Texas, 600 miles to the south, where similar mortality had occurred in late March.

A classic example of lethal mobilization was reported by Koeman (1971) for eider ducks on the Dutch coast. Eiders go without food for long periods during incubation and thus live on their fat. Many of them died on their nests in the early 1960s. They proved to have high levels of telodrin, dieldrin, and endrin. These were traced to effluent from a distant pesticide plant. The effluent was corrected and the mortality dropped gradually over a period of years.

Experimental proof of mobilization was given by Dale et al. (1962) for DDT in rats. Van Velzen et al. (1972) demonstrated it conclusively in birds and proved that lethal mobilization of DDT could occur at least four months after dosage ceased. L. F. Stickel (1973) summarized much evidence on this subject.

As mobilization can be severe enough to cause death, it must be severe enough to affect reproduction and behavior far more often. Weight losses sufficient to raise residues in blood appear to be frequent in nature and certainly are in our experimental birds. Birds commonly have a large weight loss in the spring at about the time of the breeding season.

Moriarty (1969) reviewed the evidence for delayed mortality and other sublethal phenomena in insects, where it is termed "latent toxicity." Apparently it is not uncommon for insects to die from mobilized pesticide at the time of metamorphosis, when they are calling upon energy stores. Moriarty points out that insects of incomplete metamorphosis seldom show this effect, and that the effect appears to be unknown with organophosphate and carbamate insecticides. Storage of these chemicals is far less than that of the organochlorines.

2.8. Mutagenesis

It is well established that selenium can be carcinogenic in large amounts, although it is also a necessary trace element. There is much evidence that methylmercury is mutagenic at levels that can occur in polluted areas. It is less well known that some of the common pesticides have appeared mutagenic in certain test systems. The significance of this is not clear, for what happens in a cell culture at heavy dosages may not happen in a living animal exposed only to environmental levels. As Epstein and Legator (1971) said in their monograph on this subject, "Although we can point to no pesticide now in wide use that has been demonstrated to be mutagenic, the overwhelming majority have not been adequately tested, although appropriate methodologies are now available."

Proper testing of this type is one of the most critical needs in the pollution field. Methods of testing, and of interpreting results, should be agreed upon by responsible groups to avoid damning useful chemicals unfairly and needlessly. A harmful effect of some sort can be shown for any substance, necessary as it may be for our nutrition, if it is tested at extreme concentrations in a sensitive test system.

We have little idea how many mutagenic compounds are being released in industrial exhausts and effluents, but we can be sure that no strongly mutagenic compound would be released into the environment as a pesticide. The danger is known and tests are made to prevent it. What we cannot be sure of is the possibility of weak mutagens among our pesticides. Most mutations are harmful, and the mild ones, which are easily overlooked and may be transmitted through the generations, are at least 10 times as common as the more severe and more easily detected ones (Epstein and Legator, 1971). The US Environmental Protection Agency ruled in 1974 that dieldrin is a carcinogen, and carcinogens are often mutagens. Dahlgren and Linder (1974) claim that behavioral effects of dieldrin in pheasants persisted through three generations when either the male or female of the first generation was dosed. It is difficult to construe this as anything but a genetic effect. One is reminded of Lederberg's words (in Epstein and Legator, 1971): "If the malformation induced by thalidomide were a mental retardation of 10 percent of the I.Q. . . . we would be unaware of it to this day."

We must also remember the work of Peakall et al. (1972), which demonstrated chromosomal aberrations and severe hatching failure in the third generation of ring doves fed only 10 ppm of a PCB, Aroclor 1254.

DDT is now known to cause chromosomal damage in living mice, when given in high but sublethal dosages, and is suspected of causing point mutations as well (Johnson and Jalal, 1973).

Is it not possible that certain long-lived animals such as bald eagles, which do not breed until five years old, and are often loaded with pollutants, might have enough accumulated genetic defects to interfere with reproduction? There are areas in Maine and around the Great Lakes where no eagle eggs can hatch.

Fortunately, we need not worry about the effects of weak mutagens on most forms of life, for an occasional genetic or carcinogenic event would be lost without trace in the enormous population turnover that occurs in most wildlife. Few animals live for long, and natural selection is still vigorous in the wild.

2.9. Behavior

The reality and importance of behavioral changes in birds was demonstrated by Peakall and Peakall (1973). They fed ring doves (*Streptopelia*) 10 ppm of a PCB, Aroclor 1254, and studied incubation behavior by recording egg temperatures automatically. Eggs of treated parents varied wildly in temperature, reflecting erratic incubation behavior. Hatching success was greatly reduced. Eggs of the same group did well when incubated artificially. The average egg residue was only 16 ppm (wet weight), an amount of PCB that has often been exceeded in eggs of wild birds.

In the most highly contaminated British bird, the gray heron (*Ardea*), Prestt (1970) found that eggs contained up to 80 ppm PCB, 6.3 ppm dieldrin, and 26 ppm DDE. Means for the colony that he chiefly studied were 5.75, 2.2, and 5.45 ppm, respectively, Eggshells were thin and, according to Prestt, over a third of the pairs broke their own eggs. The evidence suggested that the breaking was behavioral rather than accidental. The herons were maintaining their numbers only by virtue of determined renesting.

Egg eating by contaminated parents has been witnessed or suspected in wild peregrine falcons, ospreys, and other falconiform birds. This could be triggered by accidental perforation or cracking of thinned shells, but there is unpublished evidence that a pesticide-induced behavioral factor can be important.

When mallards and their young were fed methylmercury at approximately 0.1 ppm or 0.6 ppm, wet weight (0.5 and 3.0 ppm, dry weight), the ducklings were hyperresponsive to a frightening stimulus. They also differed from controls in their reaction to the mother's call (Heinz, 1975).

In mammals, low levels of DDT have reduced the normal aggressiveness of laboratory mice, an effect that would be of no help in the wild (Peterle and Peterle, 1971; Scudder and Richardson, 1970). Young mice were slow to acquire a conditioned avoidance response if their mothers had received 2.5 mg/kg of DDT during mid- or late pregnancy (Al-Hachim and Fink, 1968). DDT-treated rats that seemed otherwise normal had reduced ability to swim in cold water (Durham, 1967). One-month-old mice that appeared normal, but whose mothers had been exposed to methylmercury during pregnancy, behaved abnormally when placed in water (Spyker, et al., 1972).

Insects also display behavioral effects. Ground beetles (*Harpalus rufipes*), which are relatively resistant to DDT, had their feeding rate markedly reduced when exposed to DDT at well below the lethal level. They recovered rapidly when exposure ceased. This beetle is an important predator of certain crop pests, and the investigator (Dempster, 1968) believed that "the persistence of DDT may be a considerable disadvantage in that it may prevent *Harpalus* from controlling the numbers of *Pieris* after spraying . . . the survival of *Pieris* caterpillars is greatly improved after spraying with DDT and this is primarily due to the reduction in the effect of arthropod predators." Other examples of behavioral effects on insects are summarized by Moriarty (1969).

Behavioral changes in fishes are found both in the field and with very low experimental exposures. The subject is beyond the scope of the present paper, but good examples have been reported by Anderson (1971), Davy et al. (1972), Hatfield and Johansen (1972), McKim et al. (1973), Rongsriyam et al. (1968), Saunders (1969), and Warner et al. (1966).

In general, behavioral changes in birds and mammals are exceedingly difficult to prove in the field, for multiple factors are present, individual variability is high, and alternative explanations seldom can be ruled out. Laboratory work often reveals little unless high dosages (or high tissue residues) are used. Even then, the findings usually can be interpreted as stemming from an increase or decrease in activity or irritability. Whether there is an increase or a decrease may depend more upon dosage level than upon chemical. A decrease often appears as dullness, or slowness to learn or relearn. Faster learning is sometimes observed as one aspect of increased irritability.

Too much behavioral work is done with lethal or nearly lethal dosages; the reader often feels that he is simply learning how sick animals act. We need much more work with dosage levels that are both environmentally realistic and well below the long-term lethal level. Such work usually requires statistically valid tests with large numbers of individuals.

Another crucial need is to relate both dosages and results to residues in the body. Knowledge of residues in tissues often permits extrapolation of experimental findings to the field, where residues may be the only solid clues in a complex picture of poor reproduction and declining populations. And as aquatic animals can acquire large and effective residues very quickly when exposed to minute concentrations in the water, it is far more significant to know the amount in the body than the amount in the water.

2.10. Reproduction

Reproduction is often affected at levels of pollution well below those that kill adults. The reproductive success of mallard ducks was reduced by half when parents received methylmercury in their diet at 3 ppm, dry weight, which is approximately 0.6 ppm wet weight, a level that can be found in food organisms of mercury-contaminated areas. The decrease in reproductive success resulted from a sequence of reduced egg production, poorer hatching success, and increased mortality of young (Heinz, 1974). Stepwise effects such as this appear to be common (Heath et al., 1969). They are difficult to prove in the field, but can be critical to maintenance of a population.

The vast literature on mammalian reproduction in relation to pollutants points in different directions. Considerable resistance was shown in studies of DDT in rats (Ottoboni, 1972), dieldrin in deer (Murphy and Korschgen, 1970), and dieldrin in wild rabbits (Malecki et al., 1974). Yet in laboratory mice, a DDT dosage that created residues of only 1.2 ppm in liver caused small but significant changes in reproduction: a prolongation of the estrus cycle and a decrease in the percentage of implanted ova (Lundberg, 1973). The mouse is surprisingly sensitive to mirex, a chemical of high persistence but low toxicity: 5 ppm in the diet reduced the number of young (Ware and Good, 1967).

The danger to mammals seems to be greatest in carnivores. For instance, 2 ppm dieldrin in the diet of raccoons upset reproduction in both males and females (Morris, 1973) to a greater extent than 25 ppm dieldrin did in deer (Murphy and Korschgen, 1970).

A demonstration of effects on another carnivore was given by Deichmann et al. (1971), who dosed dogs with low levels of aldrin and/or DDT for 14 months. The dogs seemed normal, except for increases in residues and alkaline phosphatase activity. They were not bred until dosage ceased and residues fell to levels found in exposed people. "Attempts were made to breed all experimental female dogs with experimental males during the 19-month post-feeding period. Because of suppression of libido, only eight of the 11 experimental male dogs could be used for reproduction. In six of the 15 females, estrus was delayed (7-12 months). Mammary development and production of milk associated with the first litters were severely depressed in all dogs, regardless of the pesticide administered. . . . Also, regardless of the compound fed, stillbirths (usually one pup) occurred with half of the deliveries. Two females, in spite of two and three copulations, respectively, did not become pregnant. Two other females and their fetuses died during delivery. . . . Compared with a normal weaning survival rate of 84% of pups born to 16 control . . . dogs, the survival rate of the first litters of eight experimental females was 32% . . . the absorbed pesticides in all dogs had induced rather long-lasting metabolic changes that influenced reproduction adversely." Here again we see that the total effect stemmed from a cumulative series of adverse changes of systemic origin.

Insects that survive applications of insecticides may have reduced egg production, reduced fertility of eggs, and even complete sterility of adults. At some dosages, however, reproduction may be stimulated (Moriarty, 1969).

Early life stages are often sensitive to pollutants. Herbicides usually work best on the youngest vegetation. Many insecticides and miticides are most effective on eggs or larvae. Unfortunately, the young of valuable, nontarget organisms are also vulnerable. Whole runs of young salmon or trout in both eastern and western Canada were virtually eliminated by DDT applied to forests (Crouter and Vernon, 1959; Elson, 1967). Lake trout eggs tended to die at the sac-fry stage if they contained as much as 2.9 ppm of DDT + DDD; all of the sac-fry died if eggs contained 5 ppm (Burdick et al., 1964). Eggs of the winter flounder (*Pseudopleuronectes*) had many abnormalities and almost complete hatching failure if they contained about 2-4 ppm DDT. Eggs of this species also failed if they contained 1-2 ppm dieldrin (Smith and Cole, 1973).

Most striking of all, however, is the report of Cuerrier et al. (1967) that a mortality of 30-90% occurred among trout fry when DDT compounds were 0.4 to 1.4 ppm in eggs and averaged 0.18 ppm in feed. This represents an extreme, for eggs of various other kinds of fishes will succeed despite containing several ppm of DDT compounds. It is clear that species differences are important and it is likely that species of cold clean water, particularly salmonids, are the most sensitive.

2.11. Biostimulatory Effects of Small Doses

Many people fear that any toxic chemical may be dangerous in trace amounts, especially if exposure is prolonged and if effects are measured sensitively. In truth, one of the oldest precepts of medicine is that the dose makes the poison. Any investigator who has examined toxicological data extensively has seen studies in which metals, herbicides, or insecticides were beneficial to life and to reproductive success when fed at less than toxic levels. The principle has been discovered many times, especially by microbiologists, and given many names, but is still too little known. Horne et al. (1972) and Smyth (1967) discuss the concept and provide references. Dr. Wayland J. Hayes devotes to it a section of his book on pesticides (1975).

The gist of it is that any chemical can be toxic at some level and that most chemicals become biostimulatory at a subtoxic level. This holds as true for poisons as for nutrients and drugs. It holds true for animals as well as plants. Furthermore, the difference between a beneficial (or necessary) amount and a toxic amount may be small. Vitamin A can be toxic and pesticides can improve reproduction. Toxic heavy metals that are necessary for life include vanadium, iron, manganese, cobalt, nickel, copper, and zinc (Horne et al., 1972).

Below the stimulatory level, chemicals tend to be neutral. We must, therefore, be cautious about viewing with alarm the usual, low, environmental residues that occur away from pollutant sources. No doubt these low, ambient residues are often far down in the neutral zone, well below even the stimulatory level.

This comforting outlook can be in error, however, for there are at least three problems that we must keep in mind. (1) Minute residues of such chemicals as organochlorines in water can be multiplied thousands of times in aquatic life within hours, chiefly through adsorption and lipid partitioning. Some chemicals can then be multiplied further through food chains. (2) Certain forms of life are surprisingly sensitive to small residues. Calanoid crustaceans may die with as little as 5 parts per trillion of DDT in sea water, which is far less than the amount in rain (Goldberg et al., 1971). And a fraction of a part per billion of DDE in water can be concentrated in fish to levels that affect reproduction of fish-eating birds, some of which are amazingly sensitive to this effect of DDE. (3) Many experts maintain that there can be no safe level for a carcinogen. The same claim can be made for mutagens, for in theory one molecule striking a chromosome can start trouble. Other experts believe that in practice there are safe (but very low) levels even for carcinogens. Both groups agree, however, that there are dose–effect relationships with carcinogens and mutagens, for heavy dosages produce effects more frequently than light dosages and very light dosages often fail to produce measurable effects.

2.12. Food Chain Concentrations

Accumulation in food chains is one of the most dangerous traits of persistent pollutants. It is easy to misunderstand this factor, however, for the great concentration of fat-soluble pollutants that occurs in aquatic life is not primarily a food chain effect. Chemicals such as organohalogens are barely soluble in water and consequently adsorb quickly to particles of sediments, filaments of algae, or gills of animals. As much may adsorb to a dead filament as to a living one. The amount entering an animal is largely a function of the amount of water passing over the gills. The amount stored is likely to depend on the lipid content of the animal, and this often increases with age and size. Concentration factors of a thousand, or a hundred thousand, from water to animal are often found. These are not food chain results, but they do provide a great set-up of residues for the beginning of food chains.

The problem of residue accumulation has been confused by many workers who used noncomparable bases, as by comparing residues in total food to residues in fat. When one uses comparable bases, as dry weight in feed compared to dry weight of whole body, the reality of food chain build-up is readily seen. In American kestrels fed 10 ppm DDE (dry weight), carcasses contained approximately 12–24 times this much. Eggs contained about 12 times as much as food (S. N. Wiemeyer, personal communication).

Hanko et al. (1970) found several times as much methylmercury in tissues of ferrets killed by this chemical as in the flesh fed to them. Borg et al. (1970) found a four- or fivefold concentration of methylmercury from chicken to goshawk. Secondary poisoning occurred in both studies.

Gary Heinz (personal communication) has shown that the concentration factor for methylmercury in mallards, from food to eggs, both dry weight, is approximately six to nine times.

Haney and Lipsey (1973) used a model ecosystem to study the concentration of methylmercury up a food chain in which tomato plants grew in treated solution, aphids fed upon the plants, and lace-winged fly larvae fed upon the aphids. When the concentration in the solution was 0.06 ppm, there was a 16-fold concentration in the plant. The concentration from plant to aphid was 3.5 times; the concentration from aphid to lacewing larva was 4.6 times. Overall, from solution to lacewing, the concentration was 262 times. Some test groups in the study gave more extreme results that ranged up to 4178 times from solution to lacewing.

Food chain build-ups occur when the chemical is persistent and the organisms in the chain are not efficient at getting rid of it. Certainly, decreases in food chains must be far commoner than build-ups, for few chemicals, even most organohalogen insecticides, are very persistent and many organisms are adept at metabolizing or excreting them. With really persistent chemicals such as DDE, mirex, methylmercury, and the higher PCBs, however, food chain build-ups must be expected.

Lead accumulates in vegetation and the concentration increases in animal food chains. This has been noted along highways (Giles et al., 1973; Price et al., 1974). It also is stored by marine mussels (Schulz-Baldes, 1974). Waterfowl commonly obtain lead both from their food organisms and from ingestion of shot. Bones from waterfowl wings supplied by hunters are analyzed in the United States to determine the frequency and severity of lead contamination in different states.

It is not generally understood that short-lived chemicals can kill through very short food chains. Fenthion, for example, disappears in a day or two after it is applied lightly for mosquito control. It lasts long enough, however, for struggling insects and small fishes to be consumed by various birds, often shore birds, some of which die of secondary poisoning. When highly toxic phosphates that have a moderate length of life, such as fensulfothion and parathion, are used for control of grubs in pastures, hundreds of birds may be killed by eating the struggling grubs (Mills, 1973). This sort of thing may happen with any chemical that has high toxicity and moderate persistence. If a chemical is highly persistent, it need not even be very toxic. This was shown by the deaths of thousands of birds of many species that ate earthworms and insects heavily contaminated by DDT used for control of the beetle vector of Dutch elm disease (Bernard, 1963; Wallace et al., 1961). Toxic and persistent chemicals can be used safely, but it is easy to use them unsafely.

2.13. Bases of Terrestrial Food Chains

The food chain began at a high level when DDT at ¾ lb per acre was applied to a California forest in 1964. Insects collected on the day of application contained 206 ppm (wet weight) of DDT + DDE. One and two days later they contained 84 ppm (Keith and Flickinger, 1965). Such highly contaminated organisms commonly shower down after insecticidal applications. Struggling, intoxicated insects attract the attention of birds, frogs, and other animals, which are likely to gorge on the sudden food supply. Even birds that are mainly seedeaters take advantage of the opportunity. The result is death if the chemical is highly toxic, or prolonged high residues if the chemical is persistent.

This is one of the major bases of terrestrial contamination, one that investigators too often ignore. They put birds in wire cages in fields that are to be treated for insect control. There are, of course, few insects in a small cage containing several birds, so there is hardly any highly contaminated food in the cage as a result of the application. As only the severest treatments can kill by other routes, birds usually survive and the treatments are thereby whitewashed. The error is a critical one in this era of toxic but short-lived phosphates and carbamates.

Flying insects that survive applications of persistent pesticides may carry the chemicals far and wide. Some have been known to contain as much as 90 ppm DDE. Long after an application, sometimes months, grubs and other insects become intoxicated through mobilization at the time of metamorphosis and writhe about on the surface, attracting predators.

Rodents affected by thallium rodenticide move slowly and are extremely attractive to all sorts of predators, great numbers of which may die (Mendelssohn, 1972).

Facts such as these have been observed or deduced in many field studies. Experienced workers are convinced that contaminated foods, especially animal foods in which chemicals are concentrated, are the chief source of trouble, even in directly treated areas in which other routes of exposure also occur. And in untreated areas, where residues are relatively low, the oral route probably is the only route. This means that the oral route is the main route at the great majority of times and places.

Litter feeders are one of the most important bases of the terrestrial food chain. Contaminated foliage falls to the ground and is consumed by many kinds of creatures. Slugs, snails, and earthworms consume litter and build up amazing concentrations of persistent chemicals. These animals are eaten by many predators, including birds, mammals, amphibians, and reptiles. The consequences range up to lethality in heavily treated areas, as with the mass mortality of American robins in neighborhoods where elms were soaked with DDT.

Plant-eating birds and mammals generally have low residues, for they have little exposure unless feeding in or near a treated field or near a source of industrial contamination. Also, it is possible that herbivores are better able to rid themselves of various chemicals than carnivores. These considerations should not lead us to underrate vegetation as the beginning of food chains. Plants pick up lead, certain pesticides, and other chemicals from the soil and thus make them available to herbivores. Vegetation receives pesticides by direct application and catches fallout of many pollutants. Because of these routes, undesirable residues often appear in milk and meat. Lead along highways is picked up by plants and concentrated in animal food chains. Poisoning by fallout of chemicals such as cadmium and fluorine affects livestock and wildlife in wide zones around smelters.

Although residues usually are low in herbivores, these animals can be killed or heavily contaminated by eating foliage recently treated with insecticide. Carbofuran on alfalfa killed 2450 widgeon ducks that ate the alfalfa at one locality in California in 1974. After a forest spraying of 1 lb per acre DDT, the rumen contents of deer collected one month after spraying averaged 119 ppm DDT (dry weight basis) (Pillmore et al., 1965).

Veld sprayed with one or two ounces per acre of dieldrin for control of harvester termites has killed antelope (Wiese et al., 1973). The dieldrin went largely to the more toxic photodieldrin, and both persisted on grass for months. The antelope killed were far more sensitive than domestic stock because of their low stores of body lipid, a factor that is of primary importance in governing effects of lipophilic toxicants.

Some of the most serious food chain contamination of air-breathing animals arises from the aquatic environment. Waters become contaminated with pesticides, PCBs, mercury, and other chemicals from urban industrial sources. Pesticides may wash from agricultural lands, mainly adsorbed to particulates. Physical and biological factors often cause an enormous increase of concentration in fish and other aquatic animals. Fish pick up pesticides efficiently and hold them strongly for long periods. Bald eagles, ospreys, herons, mink, seals, and many other animals eat the fish. Reproductive failure and death have followed in the more polluted areas. More will be said of this later.

Although the oral route is the major one, it is not the only one, even for wild animals. Birds, with their vast air exchange, are singularly exposed to air pollutants. Pigeons in cities have been found to have elevated lead levels. Animals that are in fields at the time of pesticide applications undergo respiratory and dermal exposure, but the effects rarely can be separated from those of oral intake. At times, however, the dermal route seems dominant. Rudd and Genelly (1956) mention several observations of toxaphene seeming to kill more readily by contact than by intake. Toxaphene is well absorbed through the skin, but so are many insecticides. The foot-licking and the grooming of fur or feathers that animals commonly practice confuse matters by adding the oral route to the dermal route.

Fowle (1972) has shown that birds can be killed by perching on phosphamidon-treated twigs and believes that this occurs in the wild. Birds can absorb chemicals through their feet; fenthion and endrin have been applied to roosts to control nuisance birds. This involves heavy treatment of perches with chemicals that are highly toxic to birds. In the field, where there is rarely any comparable exposure, it is likely that respiratory and dermal exposure generally are of secondary importance.

2.14. Soil Organisms and Insects

What are pesticides doing to microbes that are essential to the health of soil, especially nitrifying and nitrogen-fixing bacteria? There is an extensive literature on this subject (Corke and Thompson, 1970; Fletcher, 1961; Martin, 1963). Agricultural scientists know that the action of pesticides and their metabolites on the soil microflora must be tested systematically, but they agree that normal uses of herbicides and insecticides have little effect on it. The microbes vary widely, from species to species, in sensitivity to given chemicals. Environmental conditions play a large role in altering toxicity. Certain herbicides or their metabolites can reduce populations or inhibit their action, especially if applied in large amounts, but the results are not lasting. Insecticides seldom have much effect. Fungicides and fumigants have the most severe effects on many forms of life, but these chemicals are seldom applied heavily to large outdoor areas, and even their effects are not likely to persist for years. In all, the available evidence gives no reason to worry about lasting or widespread damage to nitrogen bacteria or other soil microflora.

Soil invertebrates are also important to soil fertility and texture. An excellent review of the effects of pesticides on them has recently been prepared by Edwards and Thompson (1973). Results of treatments vary sharply depending upon the animal group and upon the specific chemical. Persistent pesticides can have serious effects because they last for years in the soil, especially if mixed in rather than applied to the surface, so that a large proportion of the individual invertebrates will come into contact with them. Shorter-lived chemicals usually have less effect. On the other hand, certain short-lived chemicals, particularly the soil fumigant D-D, can have drastic and long-lasting effects. The authors conclude that the overall effect of any pesticide is a product of its toxicity to soil animals and its persistence in soils. Their general conclusion, however, is that there is little evidence that microorganisms, soil animals, plants, or soil fertility have been adversely affected to a significant extent. Cultivation itself has such severe effects on soil invertebrates that most pesticide applications have little additional effect. Edwards believes that the greatest problem is in natural ecosystems, where pesticide applications may interfere with processes of decay and soil formation.

Most of the older pesticides had little effect on earthworm populations, but as Harris (1969) points out, some of the substitute chemicals are more lethal to earthworms. He particularly mentions chlordane, phorate, and carbaryl. Carbamates in general, particularly carbofuran, are toxic to earthworms, and so are some of the organophosphates, notably fensulfothion (Thompson, 1971). Both fensulfothion and carbofuran are also fairly long lived in the soil, remaining highly active for at least four weeks (Harris, 1969). Such chemicals can be used to reduce populations of earthworms, but they have strong potential for causing secondary poisoning. This has been shown by Mills (1973) for fensulfothion in grubs. Earthworms are vulnerable to copper-based fungicides and may be virtually eliminated from orchards in which these are used (van Rhee, 1969). Perhaps copper compounds should be used rather than insecticides where it is desirable to reduce earthworm populations, as on golf greens and along airport runways.

Turning to invertebrates above ground, we find the infinite literature of economic entomology. A key finding is that resistance to almost any chemical may appear. Another key finding is that the complex of natural control factors—predators, parasites, and diseases—often gives partial control and sometimes gives an acceptable degree of control. The present trend, therefore, is toward integrated control, or pest management, in which natural factors are encouraged to do as much as they can and relatively short-lived pesticides are used only when needed. Short-lived insecticides are less able to cause resistance than persistent ones because they are present for less of the time. Furthermore, they tend to be less hard on parasites and predators of economic pests.

"Phytophagous mite populations may be altered to almost prescribed levels with pesticides when the predator populations are known. This allows selective chemicals to be used to complement the predator effect and maintain red mites below the threshold of damage" (Sanford and Herbert, 1970). This example comes from the apple areas of Nova Scotia, where much fine research has been done.

Another interesting finding of this research is that, "Fungicides have more effect on parasites and predators than might be expected. Sulfur sprays are known to have insecticidal action on some pests but most other fungicides have been considered harmless to insects. However, these studies have shown that not only sulfur but also other fungicides heretofore considered innocuous are very injurious to certain beneficial species and have interfered with the natural control of some important pest species. Therefore, it is considered necessary to determine the effects of a chemical on each pest and on beneficial species before it is safe to conclude that in a spray schedule its useful effects sufficiently offset its harmful ones" (MacPhee and Sanford, 1954).

With pest management requiring so much knowledge and professionalism, and so many changes in practice, it is not surprising that new systems are coming slowly. Instead, it is gratifying how much solid progress has been made with many pests. A brief but impressive review of this progress in citrus orchards in the United States is given by Jeppson (1974).

It should be remembered as a baseline fact that pest management systems will require the use of chemicals as far into the future as we can see. Biological controls alone cannot always give acceptable control of native (nonintroduced) pests. Indeed, even persistent pesticides are needed—and will continue to be needed—in places such as plant nurseries and airports, from which pests may spread. In view of resistance and the other multiple problems of insect control, it seems likely that we should not discard any of our chemical weapons. Each may find an appropriate place on prescription lists of the future.

Honeybees are a worrisome part of the pesticide problem. Regrettably, they are more sensitive to some of the shorter-lived materials such as malathion and carbaryl than to some of the more presistent compounds, including DDT. Apiculturists often lose heavily. Enough notice should be given so that hives can be protected in advance of a treatment.

Surprisingly little is known about the fate and status of other nontarget invertebrate populations after applications. What, for example, happens to the natural pollinators other than honeybees when large blocks of land are treated? Is it true, as alleged, that butterfly populations are down? If so, why? This is an enormous field that has received little attention.

2.15. Amphibians and Reptiles

Amphibians and reptiles are less sensitive to insecticides than are fish, but those in heavily treated areas may be killed (Ferguson, 1963; Herald, 1949; Smith and Glasgow, 1965). Wilson (1972) lists many lizards and snakes killed by dieldrin used for tsetse fly control in Africa. In view of the high oral and dermal toxicity of dieldrin, such mortality was to be expected.

Fashingbauer (1957) studied wood frogs in pools before and after an aerial application of 1 lb per acre of DDT to the forest. The frog population appeared to be wiped out; many dead frogs were found. The frogs fed heavily on treated caterpillars and may also have been exposed through an oily film that appeared on the pools.

Mulla (1962) found that a large percentage of organophosphate and some organochlorine insecticides were relatively harmless to tadpoles at dosages that were high relative to mosquito-control applications. Tadpoles were killed, however, by relatively low applications of some of the more toxic pesticides such as endrin, endosulfan, dieldrin, and trithion. Young toads were all killed by endosulfan at 1 lb per acre or by a mixture of toxaphene and DDT at 1 and 2 lb per acre.

A number of papers report tests of various pesticides against amphibians; they confirm Mulla's impression that amphibians are not hypersensitive. These studies are difficult to relate to the field, or to one another, for they were not done in comparable ways and employed immersion or contact rather than oral intake.

The most intensive work with amphibians was done in Britain by Cooke (1970, 1971, 1972, 1973a, b), who investigated the belief that pesticides may well be one reason why amphibian populations have declined in areas where either breeding waters or feeding grounds for adults have been treated. Working with tadpoles, Cooke found that 2,4-D had no effect, and dieldrin had less effect than DDT. Working further with DDT, he found that tadpoles could acquire high levels from the environment, but could lose them quickly, given a chance. A sudden sublethal exposure caused hyperactivity, which made the tadpoles more vulnerable to predation by newts. Delayed mortality occurred when tadpoles drew upon their fat stores at the time of metamorphosis. Small tadpoles were more vulnerable to these effects than larger ones. Mortality, and the frequency of abnormalities, increased in treated groups. In the field, high acute treatment levels tended to delay metamorphosis, whereas low residues, acquired slowly, tended to increase the speed of metamorphosis. In all, Cooke's studies proved that DDT applications can be extremely dangerous to frog tadpoles, but that the usual low ambient levels of DDT seem relatively harmless to them.

Species differences again appeared strongly: Cooke and other workers found that toads are far more resistant than frogs. Indeed, Cooke found some toads living with residues of DDT in excess of 300 ppm.

Healthy amphibians and reptiles have extensive fat bodies. Because of this, and because they are not outstandingly sensitive to insecticides, they often accumulate surprisingly large residues. The highest residue that Meeks (1968) found in any animal of a marsh treated with 0.2 lb per acre DDT was 41.6 ppm (dry weight) in a tadpole. As much as 172 ppm (dry weight) of heptachlor epoxide was found in a turtle, *Pseudemys* (Rosene et al., 1961). Korschgen (1970) found 14 ppm (wet weight) of dieldrin in a garter snake from an aldrin-treated field. Hundreds of parts per million of DDE, up to 1009 ppm, were found in fat melted from fat bodies of various snakes from an agricultural area in Texas (Fleet et al., 1972). It is certain that such levels represent food chain dangers, but it is not known what effect residues in female reptiles and amphibians have upon their reproduction.

2.16. Birds and Mammals

Work with the usual laboratory and domestic animals can lead to a relaxed view of pollutant problems in wild birds and mammals. One sees that these animals are relatively resistant as compared to crustaceans and fishes. They easily tolerate the low ambient levels of pollution found at most places. They may benefit at times from the biostimulatory effect. We know that all chemicals are gradually lost from the body, many of them rapidly, and that a low intake can result only in a relatively low equilibrium level in the body. It is reasonable, therefore, to assume that the common, low environmental levels are not likely to be harmful even after prolonged intake.

Why, then, the heated controversy? There are three major reasons. (1) Heavy kills still occur in and near pesticide-treated areas, probably a great many more than are reported. Corresponding to pesticide-treated areas are areas where PCBs, lead, mercury, and other chemicals are concentrated. These, if they do not kill, cause dangerous residues, often for long periods. (2) Food chain accumulations cause far higher residues in carnivorous species than would be expected from ambient levels. (3) Many animals, especially carnivorous ones, are exceedingly sensitive to lethal and/or reproductive effects. Local and regional populations have been lost and some continental populations are in danger. Let us look at a few examples of kills and then examine the reproductive problem.

Species after species of hawk, kite, and eagle that were "common" or "very common" in Israel before 1950 are now rated "no recent observations" or "very rare" (Mendelssohn, 1972). The greatest source of trouble was thallium sulfate, which was used for rodent control over large areas until 1965, when its use was stopped. Dead and half-paralyzed rodents attracted birds of prey of many kinds. Secondary poisoning of a scale and intensity rarely seen wiped out national populations of a number of species, reduced others to a fringe existence away from cultivation, and cut deeply into populations migrating from Europe.

Seed-eating birds of several kinds, including skylarks, were attacked widely by use of endrin-treated seeds. Endrin reduced populations of the target birds to some extent, but it added to the thallium problem by causing much secondary poisoning among several kinds of birds of prey and in various mammals (Mendelssohn, 1972). This may be questioned in view of the short half-time of endrin in the rat, which is 2–4 days (Klein et al., 1968), but our own unpublished experiments support Mendelssohn's report. Apparently endrin is still used against seed-eating birds in Israel.

Thallium was replaced by fluoracetamide, which is very toxic, but has only a small danger of secondary poisoning. It killed nontarget animals in large numbers, but with thallium gone, a few of the hawks began to do a little better. Populations of certain insectivorous birds were still down in 1972.

Insectivorous bats were nearly exterminated by fumigation of caves to kill fruit bats. As might be expected where pesticides are used so intensively, Israeli animals, like Israeli people, have exceptionally high residues of chlorinated hydrocarbon insecticides. However, Mendelssohn found the consequences difficult to work out in the presence of so many other adverse factors.

While the falconiform birds of Israel were perishing wholesale, many other birds did well and some flourished under heavy exposure to pesticides. One can understand about the bulbul, for it is a fruit-eater, but certain insectivorous species, including hoopoe, white-breasted kingfisher, and cattle egret, also flourished in treated areas. One must suspect physiological resistance as well as high reproductive potential.

Another program that has caused heavy outright mortality of birds, mammals, and reptiles is the eradication of tsetse flies by spraying habitat with dieldrin (Koeman et al., 1971; Wilson, 1972). Not only were many kinds of animals killed, but certain local populations appeared to be exterminated.

Mortality caused by pollutants in the wild is probably overlooked most of the time, for it usually affects only part of the fauna, is scattered in space and time, and generally occurs where there is no biologist to record it. It is remarkable, therefore, that we have as many records of kills as we do. Some of the American examples were mentioned earlier in this paper. Prestt and Ratcliffe (1972), in their excellent review of effects of insecticides on European birds, cite many examples of kills, especially from aldrin, dieldrin, and heptachlor used as seed dressings. Numerous seed-eaters were killed and secondary poisoning seriously reduced populations of raptorial birds, partly through death, partly through reduced reproduction.

In Sweden, methylmercury used as a seed dressing caused wholesale mortality of seed-eating birds and drastic secondary poisoning of predators, both birds and mammals (Borg et al., 1969). This led to the discovery of the great importance of mercury in industrial effluent. In America, seed dressing with methylmercury led to undesirably high residues in game birds, but is not known to have had drastic ecological effects; the real trouble has been mercury from effluent in water.

Today, methylmercury is not used on seed in Sweden or the United States; the use of dieldrin and heptachlor on seeds is reduced and regulated in Britain; and the use of persistent organochlorine pesticides has been, or is being, controlled in many countries. Mortality from these chemicals is less often reported today, but the chemicals are still used freely in numerous nations. They still enter the world ecosystem, and migratory birds still pick them up, often in substantial amounts. The significance of these residues in avian reproduction is a major problem that has been solved only in part.

The importance of the reproductive problem lies in the fact that a healthily breeding population can rebound quickly from heavy mortality. The common game animals are famous for this. But if the reproductive base of a population is eroded, the population is likely to decline and may vanish.

The erosion of reproduction was seldom noted in birds until after World War II. Indeed, immediately after the war, peregrines made a good return in southern Britain, where they had been eliminated for military reasons. Soon, however, ornithologists noted that peregrines and sparrow hawks (*Accipiter nisus*) were in trouble in Britain and Europe (Koeman et al., 1972d; Newton, 1974; Prestt and Ratcliffe, 1972; Ratcliffe, 1973). In America, the peregrine proved to be gone from the eastern United States and adjacent Canada (Hickey, 1969). Two bird-eating accipiters, sharp-shinned and Cooper's hawks, had suddenly become rare in the eastern United States. Ospreys and bald eagles in parts of the northeastern United States were unable to hatch their eggs and their populations declined. Ornithologists and falconers blamed DDT. Others, including the writer, disagreed because DDT residues in the hawks were trivial by comparison with those that meant trouble in experimental birds, such as pheasants, and because the effects were different. Much of this background was detailed by specialists in Hickey's peregrine volume (1969).

The breakthrough came in 1967, when Ratcliffe announced the discovery of eggshell thinning in British peregrines, sparrow hawks, and golden eagles. Hickey and Anderson (1968) soon demonstrated shell thinning in several American birds, especially bald eagle, osprey, and peregrine. In both studies, the trouble began in 1947, soon after DDT came into common use.

In the flood of studies that followed Ratcliffe's discovery, it became clear that shell thinning occurred in many kinds of birds and was severe in fish-eating and bird-eating species, particularly those of the hawk and pelican orders (Anderson and Hickey, 1972). Herons too were affected (Faber et al., 1972; Prestt, 1970). The full extent of the problem still is far from known and new examples are reported frequently. We do know that shell thinning has been demonstrated in at least 54 species of 10 orders. Thinning reached 10% or more in 27 of these species. It reached 20% in 9 species, at some time and place. Reproductive trouble tends to increase as shells become thinner, and thinning of 20% or more is likely to result in reproductive failure and population decline.

It was soon found that many birds were not sensitive to shell thinning. Eggshells of seed-eaters such as chickens, quail, grouse, finches, doves, and others did not thin in the field and would thin but little under environmentally realistic dosages of toxicants. Indeed, it was the earlier work with these birds that misled us as to what might be expected with raptors. Unfortunately, much of the experimentation with shell thinning has been done—and is being done—with these birds, for reasons of availability, despite the risk of obtaining results that do not apply to birds that are senstitive to shell thinning. In this connection we should keep in mind Jefferies' statement (1969), "It is known that thyroxine has opposite effects on the concentration of calcium in the plasma of laying ducks and hens." Ducks are sensitive to thinning, hens are not.

Once shell thinning was discovered, the next step was to correlate the degree of thinning with the kinds and amounts of residue in eggs. This has been done successfully for several wild species, including falcons and pelicans (Anderson et al., 1969; Blus et al., 1974a; Cade et al., 1971; Enderson and Wrege, 1973; Fyfe et al., 1969; Gress et al., 1973; Koeman et al., 1972a; Snyder et al., 1973).

The only known residues that are commonly present are DDE, dieldrin, and PCBs. It is DDE that correlates by far the best with shell thinning in nearly every study. At times the correlation is so clear that individual eggs of a single good series will show it (Cade et al., 1971).

More often it is necessary to have series from different areas in which the ratios of DDE, dieldrin, and PCBs differ, for these compounds are correlated in nature: in any one area, as one goes up, the others tend to go up. But with samples from different areas, and with the use of stepwise regression analysis, the importance of DDE usually appears. One study pointed to different pollutants in different groups of aquatic birds, but sample sizes were small and the results require confirmation (Faber and Hickey, 1973). Otherwise, neither field correlations nor valid experiments have supported the idea of dieldrin, PCBs, mercury, lead, cadmium, or other recognized pollutants being the primary explanation of thinning (Haegele et al., 1974; Haegele and Tucker, 1974). Dieldrin does not correlate well with shell thinning in the wild and is known to be a weak shell thinner in ducks (Lehner and Egbert, 1969). We may yet, however, be surprised by species differences, as the Faber and Hickey paper suggests.

The idea of DDE causing shell thinning has been criticized on the grounds that too little DDT had been used by 1947, when thinning appeared. This claim does not hold up, for Peakall (1974) has shown that California peregrine eggs contained enough DDE to account for thinning at least as early as 1948.

Field correlations are strongly indicative, but they are not proof in science or law. Our Center has, therefore, devoted great effort to experimental tests of DDE and other chemicals in the reproduction of birds. We now have definite proof that serious shell thinning can be produced with 3 ppm (wet weight) of DDE in the diet of mallards, black ducks, American kestrels, and screech owls (Heath et al., 1969, Longcore et al., 1971a, b; McLane and Hall, 1972; Wiemeyer and Porter, 1970). The mallard findings were recently confirmed by Davison and Sell (1974). With black ducks, which were allowed to incubate their own eggs, the thinned shells commonly broke under the parents; reproductive success declined to one-fifth that of controls (Longcore and Samson, 1973). In the mallard study, the number of ducklings per treated hen was only 24% of the number in the controls.

No other chemical tested has had equivalent effects. Only DDE has caused serious thinning and great drops in reproduction at low, realistic dosages. Other chemicals may sicken a bird and cause it to lay thin-shelled eggs for a few days, but the DDE effect persists (Haegele and Tucker, 1974). DDE has a half-time of 8.3 months in the pigeon (Bailey et al., 1969), and we found it nearly as persistent in grackles. It accumulates and mobilizes so readily that some kestrels died with high residues in their brains after long dosage of only 2.8 ppm (wet weight) (Porter and Wiemeyer, 1972). Regardless of when and where a bird acquires

DDE or DDT in its travels, it will have a substantial proportion of DDE left at the next breeding season.

A striking example is that of the peregrines nesting along the Colville, the northernmost large river of Alaska, far from any DDT application. In 1967–69, the eggs of these falcons averaged higher in DDE than did eggs of kestrels, birds of the same genus, that had been on a dosage of 2.8 ppm DDE (wet weight) for over a year (50.4 ppm *vs.* 32.4 ppm, wet weight) (Cade et al., 1971; Wiemeyer and Porter, 1970). How could this happen? The answer is that these peregrines migrate southward to lands where residues are high and perhaps to lands where DDT is still freely applied. When they return to Alaska, they feed partly upon migratory birds, such as ducks and shore birds, which contain enough DDE to help maintain the residues of the falcons (Lincer et al., 1970). The consequence is that "The tundra and taiga peregrines now lay eggs with shells as thin as those associated with the decimated populations of Great Britain, California, and the eastern United States." In 1970, 72% of the Colville nests failed: ". . . pairs have begun to disappear from their historic nesting crags on the Colville and Yukon rivers, just as they did 20 years ago along the Hudson and Susquehanna" (Cade et al., 1971).

Species differences appear strongly in the degree to which shells will thin. Eggshells of chickens, pheasants, and quail will thin little or not at all under DDE or DDT dosage. *Coturnix* eggshells can scarcely be made to thin more than 8%. Gulls and terns will undergo shell thinning to a limited extent, but only when egg residues are very high. Mallard eggshells thin enough to make mallards good test animals, but they will thin only so far—usually not over 22%. Hawks are more sensitive, but the brown pelican may be the most sensitive of all, for with 5 ppm DDE in the egg there is an average of 15% shell thinning. Only when DDE in the egg declines to about 0.5 ppm does thinning disappear, to judge from the regression line (Blus et al., 1974a). And when pelican eggs were excessively loaded with DDE, as they were from industrial effluent at Anacapa Island, California, they became virtually shell-less and spilled over the rocks and sticks (Keith et al., 1970; Risebrough et al., 1971). This gradation of sensitivity between species has been discussed by Keith and Gruchy (1972) with different examples and a graph.

"Shell thinning" has become a short-hand expression for a complex of events including lowered egg production, cracking, changes in shell structure, changes in incubation behavior, embryonic death, destruction of eggs by parents, and disappearance of eggs. These factors are often linked, but not always. Egg production is often normal, for example, and eggs with thin shells have been known to hatch in the wild (Prestt, 1970).

Thinned shells of three species had a smaller number of pores per unit area and also displayed more globular inclusions than did normal shells. Surprisingly, eggs with thinned shells had a lower rate of water loss than control eggs (Peakall et al., 1973). The mineral content of thinned shells was altered in ducks (Longcore et al., 1971a). The weakened shells tend to crack or perforate from contact with parental beaks and feet, and this may cause eggs to be eaten or discarded. Often, however, the egg simply fails to hatch.

It is uncertain whether thinning, embryonic mortality, and other features of the thin eggshell syndrome are all phases of one process caused by one chemical or whether specific chemicals have separate effects. If eggs with thinned shells can hatch well, it is just possible that DDE causes thinning and dieldrin or PCB causes embryonic mortality. We must remember that Peakall has shown both changes in incubation behavior and chromosomal damage from a PCB, Aroclor 1254, a chemical that does not appear to account for most (if any) shell thinning in the wild.

Blus et al. (1974b) suggest that brown pelican embryos die if the egg contains more than about 2.5 ppm DDE or 0.54 ppm dieldrin. This recalls the Scottish golden eagles, whose eggs were said to fail if their dieldrin content was over 0.5 ppm (Lockie et al., 1969). Yet eggs of various herbivorous birds such as gallinules and pheasants have been shown to hatch well, or to have no shell thinning, when they contain several ppm of dieldrin (Dahlgren and Linder, 1970; Fowler et al., 1971; Graves et al., 1969; Mick et al., 1973; Peakall, 1970; Walker et al., 1969; Wiese et al., 1969). It appears that many of these problems cannot be settled without tests of species that are likely to be sensitive to the syndrome.

A possibility that requires more study in connection with shell thinning is additivity. We know that DDE, dieldrin, and PCBs are generally present in thinned eggs, that other pollutants are present occasionally, that DDE usually accounts for most of the thinning. But dieldrin is at least a weak shell thinner in ducks and PCBs will cause some shell thinning in chickens. In a paper that should be better known, Sprague (1970) assembled much information to show that when fish are subjected to more than one toxicant the general rule is that additivity will prevail, with each chemical contributing to death in proportion to its toxicity and its amount. This holds even when the chemicals are totally unlike, as with copper and phenol. Synergism and antagonism occur far less often than additivity. Other references that support this view are cited by Kreitzer and Spann (1973). In studies of shell thinning, most workers have studied the chemicals separately or have simply lumped all organochlorines. The latter seems self-defeating, for there is no likelihood that the chemicals are at all similar in shell thinning power. What is needed are careful, quantitative tests with species that are truly susceptible to shell thinning.

A high degree of synergism between a PCB (Aroclor 1254) and the carbamate insecticide carbaryl in houseflies was reported by Plapp (1972). Lichtenstein et al. (1969) found that Aroclors from 1221 to 1254 increased the toxicity of dieldrin or DDT to two kinds of flies. Aroclor 1248 significantly increased the toxicity of oxygen analogs of five organophosphorus insecticides to houseflies

(Fuhremann and Lichtenstein, 1972). We cannot assume that these results apply to vertebrates. Ringer et al. (1972) found that DDT and dieldrin did not increase the effect of PCB on mink. Heath et al. (1972) tested the subacute toxicity of combinations of Aroclor 1254 and DDE in *Cortunix;* nothing more than additivity was found. The same workers compared reproduction in bobwhite quail fed 50 ppm of Aroclor 1254 or 30 ppm of DDE, or 25 ppm of 1254 + 15 ppm of DDE. None of these treatments had a significant effect in the 80-day test. Risebrough and Anderson (1971) found no additive effect of Aroclor 1254 in thinning of mallard eggshells caused by DDE dosage.

Another interaction, and one that must affect survival and reproduction in the wild, is the tendency of one chemical to alter the amount of another chemical that is stored in the body. Ludke (1974) reported that a small amount of dieldrin doubled the storage of DDE in *Coturnix*. This certainly could be important in the field. References by J. C. Street and others (cited by Ludke) show that these interactions vary sharply and unpredictably, even between animals of similar food habits.

The mechanism of shell thinning arouses much curiosity. The process is not well understood, but it seems clear that both thyroids and parathyroids are involved and that a final action is interference with carbonic anhydrase in forming calcium carbonate in the shell gland. Most of the papers on this subject are listed by Jefferies in his 1973 review, or by Haseltine et al. (1974).*

The press and the public tend to think that some one factor is the real cause of an animal's troubles. Eagles are a good example of how oversimplified this view is. We have seen how the eagles of Israel were virtually eliminated by secondary poisoning by both thallium sulfate and endrin (Mendelssohn, 1972). The white-tailed sea eagles of the Baltic were killed outright and suffered reproductively because of methylmercury (Borg et al., 1969; Henriksson et al., 1966). Decline of this species in northern Germany was attributed to reproductive effects of DDE; also, PCB residues were very high in these birds (Koeman et al., 1972b). Studying bald eagles in the United States, our laboratory found that half of the dead were shot, some were killed by dieldrin, two were killed by mercury, one was killed by DDT, and one by DDE (Belisle et al., 1972; Mulhern et al., 1970). In addition, their eggs are thin shelled, contain pesticides and PCBs, and fail to hatch in some parts of the United States (Wiemeyer et al., 1972). All of this came in addition to loss of habitat and severe contraction of range. By contrast, the golden eagle of the western United States has been shot and poisoned frequently in the past to protect lambs, but, thanks to much remaining habitat and little contamination in its diet, the bird still breeds well and maintains its numbers.

A significant sidelight is the discovery of Cooke and Pollard (1973) that birds are not alone in having DDT–calcium problems. Snails (*Helix pomatia*) had

---

*See note on page 74.

lighter shells and opercula when exposed to relatively low levels of DDT. And reminiscent of the egg-eating reported for affected birds, affected snails tended to eat their opercula.

Mammals are often killed by heavy applications of the more toxic pesticides. This is best known for dieldrin, but also occurs with endrin, toxaphene, and heptachlor. The first three, especially endrin, have been used for agricultural rodent control, a purpose for which safer techniques will generally serve. The more toxic organophosphates, such as azodrin, are also known to kill wild mammals, but most of the reports are unpublished. From the paucity of published reports, one gathers that the more toxic phosphates and carbamates seldom persist long enough in the field, and in the body, to kill many mammals. However, mammals are secretive, which makes mortality easy to miss, and discovery of an occasional dead shrew or mouse would seldom be reported. These facts suggest that effects on wild mammals are poorly known. But there is more to it than that: carnivores, which would be relatively vulnerable, are scarce, secretive, and range widely. Thus they would have little exposure to a single small, treated area. Any that were affected would seldom be found. Some of the commonest mammals, in contrast, are the least likely to be affected, as we shall see later.

One of the best-described kills occurred when dieldrin was used at 3 lb per acre in Illinois (Scott et al., 1959). Some 90% of farm cats perished. "Ground squirrels, muskrats, and rabbits were virtually eliminated, and short-tailed shrews, fox squirrels, woodchucks, and meadow mice appeared to have taken heavy losses. White-footed mice . . . seemed to exhibit a relatively high resistance to dieldrin poisoning. Wildlife populations appeared to have recovered or to have been well on the way toward recovery by the following year." Sheep were killed by drift of dieldrin from across a road. It is not surprising, therefore, that large numbers of hares were killed by dieldrin applications in the Netherlands (van Klingeren et al., 1966).

Secondary poisoning occurs with dieldrin. Numerous British foxes were killed by eating wood pigeons and other animals that died from eating dieldrin-dressed seed wheat (Blackmore, 1963). Even today, when dieldrin may not be used on spring-sown wheat in Britian, mice (*Apodemus*) eat treated seed in fall and winter to the point that some may be killed and others carry burdens of dieldrin (and some mercury) that endanger carnivorous birds and mammals that eat them (Jefferies et al., 1973).

Heptachlor, applied at 2 lb per acre for control of fire ants in the southern United States, killed many mammals: raccoons, foxes, skunks, armadillos, opossums, nutria, many rabbits, cotton rats, rice rats, and some mice (principally from Allen et al., 1959). Oral reports from the fire ant country indicate that the faster breeding of these species had a strong resurgence in the year after treatment.

This is in line with the finding of Malecki et al. (1974) that although granular dieldrin at 2 lb per acre killed some cottontail rabbits in large enclosures, the survivors bred normally. In contrast, dogs bred poorly even after low dosage ceased, as described in the quotation from Deichmann et al. (1971) in the "Reproduction" section of this paper. And raccoons fed 2 ppm dieldrin over long periods suffered reproductive failure and even some mortality (Morris, 1973). A study of deer reproduction revealed far less damage from 25 ppm dieldrin in the diet (Murphy and Korschgen, 1970).

Clearly, animals such as deer and rabbits could tolerate, or quickly recover from, severe applications of cyclodiene pesticides. We must remember, however, that antelope of two lipid-poor species were killed by small amounts of dieldrin and photodieldrin on the veld (Wiese et al., 1973).

Small rodents are surprisingly resistant, at least American cricetids, and particularly the most ubiquitous and most numerous of American rodents, the white-footed mouse, *Peromyscus*. We have seen that few were killed in the heavy dieldrin application in Illinois. In Kansas, there was little effect on rodent populations when a crop field was treated with diazinon, endrin, heptachlor, parathion, methyl parathion, and aldrin (Robel et al., 1972). The rodents were chiefly *Peromyscus*. Most mice had no residues and the residues that did exist were low. Marked individual *Peromyscus* survived nearly as well in the treated field as in the untreated field. Our laboratory has an unpublished study that supports this work in showing that a relatively heavy application of a cyclodiene insecticide had little effect upon marked populations of cricetid rodents.

The explanation of this remarkable tolerance probably has been given in large part by Cordes (1971). Starting with the knowledge that *Peromyscus* could withstand thousands of ppm of DDT in the diet, whereas house mice can be controlled with DDT tracking powder, he studied the loss rates of DDT in *Peromyscus*, wild *Mus*, and laboratory *Mus*. Loss rates were amazingly rapid. In males, the mean half-times were 3.7 days for *P. leucopus*, 3.0 days for *P. maniculatus*, 3.8 days for laboratory mice, and 5.5 days for wild *Mus*. Females lost residues a little more slowly: 5.3 days for *P. leucopus* and 7.8 days for *P. maniculatus*. *P. leucopus* tolerated 10 times as much DDT in the diet as did laboratory *Mus*. *P. leucopus* stored far less and lost more with feces. To judge from field data, *Peromyscus* and its relatives are able to cope with many chemicals besides DDT.

For this reason, small rodents may be the poorest forms that could be selected as indicators of pesticide effects. And because they lose residues so rapidly, and so often lack residues after exposure (according to Robel et al., 1972), they are also very poor for the purpose of monitoring residues in the environment. Unfortunately, their abundance and trappability have led numerous people to try to use them in both ways.

Sublethal and indirect effects must be far commoner than actual kills, but it is extremely difficult to obtain reliable proof of them in the field. An indication of such an effect was noted by Barrett (1968), who applied 2 lb per acre of carbaryl to an enclosure in which millet was grown and in which cotton rats (*Sigmodon*), wild house mice, and white-footed mice (*Peromyscus*) were stocked. He observed a four-week delay in reproduction of cotton rats and a consequent lag in population growth. The other species were not so affected. A laboratory test with *Sigmodon* suggested that the effect was real. The point is challenging and worth further study.

Bats are at the center of a current controversy. Students of bats in both Europe and America are convinced that bat populations have declined sharply in recent years and that pesticides are responsible. The situation is not clear, but part of the pattern is appearing, thanks to Jefferies (1972) and Luckens (1973). Luckens' first tests led him to consider the big brown bat (*Eptesicus*) the most sensitive of all mammals to DDT. Yet this bat was no more sensitive to dieldrin and endrin than the rat. Later tests with dietary DDT revealed not sensitivity but a great tolerance. The difference was in time of year. The first tests were made in May, with single doses given to thin bats. The dieldrin–endrin tests were made in late summer. The later DDT-feeding tests were made in the fall, when bats were putting on fat.

Jefferies found that the fall fattening had a serious consequence: his bats, collected from an agricultural area of England, accumulated DDT with the fat; by spring the fat was low and the residue concentration was high, far higher than at any other time of year. Indeed, it was high enough to suggest that some individuals might be killed. Certainly bats were in poor condition to withstand DDT from crop applications in early spring, for when they left hibernation they were low in lipids and had peak residues. Jefferies' bats, pipistrelles, were exceedingly sensitive to single doses of DDT. They tended to hold it as DDT, converting less to DDE than would a small bird. However, they stored no gamma BHC despite heavy use of it in the area, presumably because it breaks down rapidly in the body.

Clark et al. (1975) studied a colony of Mexican free-tailed bats (*Tadarida*) in Texas and concluded that the residues of DDT, DDE, and dieldrin that were present were too low to account for the observed decline of an Arizona population in which these residues were even lower.

Braaksma (1973) described the decline of bat populations and pointed out another hazard—preservatives used on timbers of buildings in which bats roost. Chemicals used in various preservatives include lindane, dieldrin, DDT, pentachlorophenol, and chlorinated naphthalenes. Hundreds of bats are known to have been killed, as many as 100 at a single place. Analyses of a few bats revealed chiefly lindane, with whole-body residues up to 267 ppm and 463 ppm. As so many buildings must be treated, this could be a serious factor in Europe. The extent of the problem in America, if there is one, is unknown. However, DDT has been used in the United States to free lofts of bats. This can now be done only with special permission from the Environmental Protection Agency, as is true of other DDT uses in the United States.

Further experimentation on the bat problem requires determination of pre-experimental residues, thorough consideration of lipid levels, a statement of dates when the work was done, and discrimination between DDT and DDE residues. As Jefferies suggests, whole-body residues in micrograms should be determined for comparison with amounts reaching target organs.

Marine mammals are high on the food chain and have a layer of blubber in which to carry residues. Residues are present even in Antarctica, but they are often surprisingly small. Off the shores of industrial nations, however, residues of pesticides, PCBs, and mercury can reach worrisome levels, as they do in the Baltic, North Sea, Irish Sea, and in some areas off North America. Koeman et al. (1972c) provide a good recent guide to this subject, and L. F. Stickel (1973) tabulates much of the data published by 1970.

Such figures as 150 ppm or 310 ppm of DDT in Swedish seals are less frightening when one realizes that they represent blubber lipids, not wet weight of blubber, and that they are chiefly DDE. Still, they mean that there are many thousands of micrograms in the body and that much of this is always in the blood and entering the milk, possibly representing a danger when the animal has to draw upon its fat. But one could argue as well that blubber is a perpetual safety factor, a safe sponge for lipophilic pollutants. In all, the biological significance of most records is uncertain.

Koeman et al (1972c), however, found dead seals (*Phoca vitulina*), from the Dutch coast, in which PCBs ranged from 385 to 2530 ppm (wet weight) in blubber and from 13 to 89 ppm in brain. These levels in brain would be far from lethal if judged by several bird studies, but, as the authors point out, they may be serious in aquatic mammals in view of the extreme sensitivity of mink to PCBs, as discussed later. The authors also suggest that PCB contamination should be considered in connection with the reproductive troubles and high juvenile mortality recently noted in Dutch seals.

Mercury also ran high in dead Dutch seals: 257 ppm to 326 ppm (wet weight) in livers (Koeman et al., 1972c). As it was probably methylmercury in large part, these residues are high in the lethal range. Residues of 9.6 ppm to 30 ppm in brains also support the idea that these seals may have been killed by mercury. Even living and supposedly healthy seals had from 40 to 218 ppm of mercury in livers. Residues in several dolphins and porpoises from European waters also fell in this range, while others were as low as 2.2 ppm. It is evident that the mercury levels are perilously high, but it is also evident that surprisingly high concentrations can be found in living seals.

High mercury residues are found in adults of the endangered landlocked subspecies of seal, *Pusa hispida saimensis*, of the Saimaa Lake system in Finland.

Perhaps 250 individuals exist. One found sick and ataxic proved to have 197 ppm of mercury in muscle and 210 ppm in liver, ample to account for its condition. Yet mercury levels were low in local fish. Tests with *Pusa hispida* revealed that this seal had a rate of loss of mercury slower than that known for any other mammal and similar to that of fish (Tillander et al., 1970). With this slow loss, even a low concentration of mercury in food could cause high concentration in seals. There is no reason to think that *P. hispida* is unique. Other fatty, highly aquatic animals may prove to have equally low rates of loss.

Sea lions off Southern California produced a small percentage of premature young, most of which died (DeLong et al., 1973). Analyses revealed that affected females had several times as much DDT (chiefly DDE) and PCBs in blubber and liver as did normal females and that the brains of the premature pups had more DDE and PCBs than those of normal pups. Still, DDT compounds in livers of affected females ranged only from 22 to 30 ppm (wet weight) and PCBs ranged only from 3.4 to 9.7 ppm. Mercury in livers of three affected females varied from 38 to 64 ppm. This study has attracted much attention, but it should be regarded not as proof, but as a lead to further study. Possibly the key to the situation is less in the residues than in the percentages of fat reported for livers of affected and normal females (1.7 *vs.* 4.4) and for the brains of their pups (3.3 *vs.* 4.8). Depletion of unknown origin seems to have occurred.

Residues in big game mammals are of much interest to the public and to regulatory authorities. Many sets of analyses were tabulated by L. F. Stickel (1973). It is surprising how low residues usually are, even in fat, the tissue that is most often analyzed because legal limits for livestock are based on residues in fat, at least in the United States. Residues rise sharply in treated areas, of course, but rarely to levels at which population effects might be suspected in ungulates.

One of the most surprising of all pollution stories began in the 1960s when mink ranchers around the Great Lakes found litter size slipping from around 4 to less than 0.5. This happened when coho salmon, a fish new to the Great Lakes, began to be used in mink rations. Tests by Aulerich et al. (1971) demonstrated that reproduction failed if whole raw coho made up 30% of the diet. An equal percentage of coho by-products was worse; it killed breeders within three months. Other fish from Lake Michigan had similar effects, but coho from the Pacific Coast caused no trouble. Analyses proved that neither rancidity nor mercury was to blame. Feeding trials proved that neither DDT nor dieldrin could create the effects, even at levels far higher than those in the fish.

The authors next studied PCBs alone and with pesticides (Ringer et al., 1972). The first test revealed that a mixture of PCBs at 30 ppm in the diet killed all breeders.

Dietary dosages of 5 and 10 ppm of Aroclor 1254 were then tried. No reproduction occurred on either diet; five of the six breeders died on 10 ppm.

In the next and largest trial, the inclusion of either raw or cooked coho in the diet eliminated reproduction. A dosage as low as 1 ppm of PCB in the diet reduced reproductive success from 5 living kits per living female to 3.5. At 5 ppm of PCB, reproduction was nearly eliminated: there was only 0.25 living kit per living female. At 15 ppm of PCB, there was no reproduction and some breeders died. Addition of DDT and dieldrin to the 5 ppm PCB diet did not make the results worse; there was no sign of additive or synergistic action.

More drastic results were observed by Platonow and Karstad (1973). They dosed cows with Aroclor 1254 and used the meat as part of the mink ration. The concentration of PCB in the two diets was 3.57 ppm and 0.64 ppm. When the 3.57 ppm diet was fed to mink, there was no reproduction and all breeders (12 females and 4 males) died within 105 days. With the 0.64 ppm diet 2 of the 12 females died. Of the rest, only one produced a litter and those kits died at once. Among the many controls, reproduction fell from the expected 4 per litter to 1.81. Analysis of the control diet revealed 0.3 ppm PCB, and this the authors considered responsible. The authors, veterinary research men, sought signs of disease but found none.

In both sets of mink studies, material from cohos or cows was more toxic than might have been expected from the amount of PCB detected in it, to judge from the results of feeding PCB itself in the Aulerich and Ringer work. It could be argued that some unknown pollutant in coho was acting on mink, but this would not apply to the other work, in which cows were used. We will return to this point later.

If 3-10 ppm of PCBs in the diet are lethal to mink, how much is found in wild fish? Near urban industrial sources of PCBs, as at Milwaukee, Wisconsin, fish may carry 405 ppm; in Lake Michigan, residues run 18.6-22.4 ppm (Veith and Lee, 1971). Ringer and Aulerich suggest that their coho had about 15 ppm. Fish from many areas carry 2-10 ppm, but fish from lightly polluted areas usually have less than 1 ppm (Henderson et al., 1971).

Clearly, mink would be endangered in numerous areas in the wild. It is not likely that mink are unique in their reaction to PCBs, but no one knows what other animals are similar. Does the susceptibility extend to all mustelids, to all aquatic mammals, or to scattered members of many groups? We may never know, but the urgency of keeping PCBs out of the environment is evident.

At least two distinct modes of death from PCBs are apparent. When we killed various small birds with heavy dietary dosages of Aroclor 1254, they displayed signs of neurotoxicity—tremors and traces of convulsive behavior. Residues in brains were highly diagnostic: from 349 ppm to 763 ppm (wet weight) in the dead and not above 301 ppm in survivors (unpublished). Other workers have reported high PCB residues in brains of dead birds (Dahlgren et al., 1972; Koeman, 1971; Koeman et al., 1972a; Prestt et al., 1970; Vos and Koeman, 1970).

Mink, however, died with about 11 ppm of PCBs in the brain in the Ringer-Aulerich study, with about 5 ppm in the Platonow-Karstad animals fed 3.57 ppm, and about 0.52 ppm in those fed 0.64 ppm. Residues in brain were roughly proportional to dosage and did not appear to correlate with, or account for, death. Furthermore, neurotoxic signs were not mentioned. Platonow and Karstad carefully sought cause of death, but findings were nonspecific. Most mink had hemorrhages of a seepage type (diapedesis) and several had nephrosis. In our birds killed by heavy dosage and neurotoxicity, the liver often had hemorrhagic spots or streaks and the gastrointestinal tract often contained blackish fluid (presumably from blood) in all or part of its length. We may have been seeing the beginning of the condition described by Platonow and Karstad. The implication is that sudden heavy intake may cause death from neurotoxicity with high and diagnostic brain residues and that long, low intake may kill by causing diapedesis and related phenomena, with the signs varying between individuals and between species. Authors describe many types of pathology, but emphasize liver, kidney, and vascular changes.

Long, low intake would be usual in the field. If this causes death with low residues, as in mink, effects probably are overlooked or misinterpreted in nearly all cases. No good diagnostic technique can be suggested at present, for the signs are nonspecific and the significant residue levels seem to vary enormously between groups of animals and between dosage levels. We have here a major field problem to which we know no good approach.

What PCB levels in food are safe for animals as sensitive as mink? Ringer et al. (1972) found reduced reproductive success, but no mortality, at 1 ppm. Platonow and Karstad (1973) had a little mortality and no successful reproduction at 0.64 ppm. They suspected that reproduction was halved by 0.3 ppm. Perhaps a safe level would be around 0.1 ppm. By this standard, nearly all fish samples from the United States would be deemed highly unsafe (Henderson et al., 1971). Before this idea is accepted, however, confirmation of the Platonow and Karstad findings is essential.

The Interdepartmental Task Force on PCBs (1972) points out that PCBs can concentrate from water to aquatic animals by at least 75,000 times. To keep fish residues below the United States interim action level of 5 ppm, residues in water "should be less than 0.07 part per billion, or to allow some safety factor, 0.01 ppb." If the 0.01 ppb is multiplied by 75,000, the result is 750 ppb, or 0.75 ppm. As this amount in fish is several times too great to be safe for animals such as mink, it seems that the level considered safe in water should be 0.001 ppb rather than 0.01 ppb.

Chickens are sensitive to PCBs, as serious accidents and numerous good studies have revealed. These studies demand attention here, for some wild birds surely must resemble chickens in their reactions to PCBs, and PCB residues in the wild are often high enough to suggest trouble.

The chief reproductive effects in chickens are reduced hatchability and lowered egg production. Deformities in chicks are common. Growth of young may be depressed. But these effects are not caused by all PCBs. Lillie et al. (1974) tested several Aroclors at 2 ppm and 20 ppm in the diet. A dosage of 2 ppm had no effect, but 20 ppm yielded excellent comparisons. Aroclors 1221 and 1268 did not affect egg production or hatchability. The worst effects were from 1248, which caused some mortality of adults and nearly eliminated hatchability. Effects of 1242 were nearly as bad. Aroclor 1232 was less active and 1254 was the least effective of the active forms. This is vital to remember, for most experiments have been done with 1254 because residues from the field often resemble it. The Aroclor most used commercially is 1242, and there can be no doubt that what looks like 1254 in field samples stems largely from lower PCBs from which the more easily metabolized portions are gone.

As Lillie et al. (1974) point out, the trouble comes from Aroclors in the middle of the range—from 1232 through 1254. Hence it certainly is not merely the degree of chlorination that counts. In a related paper (Cecil et al., 1974), the authors point out that the exceedingly toxic dioxins and dibenzofurans are not known from Aroclors, although dibenzofurans occur in PCBs of other manufacturers. It is possible, however, that minute amounts of highly toxic impurities occur in certain Aroclors. Unless this is true, one must conclude that certain PCB compounds contained in the mid-range Aroclors are especially embryotoxic, or have metabolites that are (Bush et al., 1974).

The finding that 2 ppm of dietary PCB had no effect on chicken reproduction was supported by the 39-week feeding test with Aroclor 1254 conducted by Platonow and Reinhart (1973). With a dosage of 5 ppm, 1254 did no more than reduce egg production erratically over the 39-week period. With 50 ppm, however, mortality began and dosage was stopped at 14 weeks. Egg production fell sharply. Hatchability dropped nearly to zero; residues in eggs were then about 25–50 ppm. As residues in eggs dropped after 6 weeks of clean food, hatchability rose. Residues over 15 ppm in eggs meant heavy embryotoxicity, but those below 5 ppm had no effect. At the start of the 50 ppm dosage, deaths of embryos came late in development, but deaths came progressively earlier as residues built up. The same progression was observed by Tumasonis et al. (1973). These authors also noted that many deformities appeared when residues of 1254 in yolks were 10–15 ppm or more.

Bush et al. (1974) gave 50 ppm of Aroclor 1254 in water for 6 weeks and then studied the chickens during 20 weeks of clean food. Hatchability dropped to zero within 3 weeks after dosage began and stayed nearly at zero through 8 weeks of clean food, then rose to approximately normal levels after 16 weeks of clean food. Deformities appeared and one of them, a toe condition, was inherited by some birds, supporting the claim of Peakall et al. (1972) of chromosomal changes. As in all the other studies of PCBs and chickens mentioned here, there was no drop in fertility.

The most interesting finding of Bush et al. was that the amount of embryonic mortality associated with a given amount of PCB residue in the egg became far higher as the study went on. In other words, PCB that had time to age in the hen seemed much more embryotoxic than did fresh PCB. Thus, 50% mortality of embryos correlated with 50 ppm in the yolk at 1.6 weeks of dosage, but with 10 ppm at 18.7 weeks, a five-fold difference. The greatest toxicity per unit of PCB came after 11 weeks of clean food. Late in the study, 6-8 ppm in yolks correlated with 14-36% mortality of embryos. As yolk is about 36% by weight of egg content in chickens, 10 ppm in yolk would be about 3.6 ppm in egg. Levels greater than this are common in the wild.

Bush et al. concluded that the increase of toxicity with time was caused by the accumulation of some persistent isomer or homolog of 1254, or by a metabolite.

The statement by Bush et al. that a given amount of PCB is more dangerous after being altered in the hen is consistent with (a) the comment by Ringer et al. (1972) that coho salmon was more toxic to mink than the amount of PCB in it would account for, and (b) the extreme toxicity found by Platonow and Karstad (1973), who put the PCB into cattle before feeding it to mink. The implications for future experimentation are evident. Furthermore, we should guard against judging the importance of PCB residues in field samples from short-term studies in which PCBs were fed directly.

PCB residues in wild birds are often at levels that would mean trouble in a chicken flock. To cite only a few examples, 11 eggs of bald eagles from the United States had from 2.2 ppm to 27.7 ppm of PCB with a median of 9.7 ppm (Wiemeyer et al., 1972). In the same period, 1969-70, bodies of numerous bald eagles had from a trace to 400 ppm; medians were 10 ppm in 1969 and 20 ppm in 1970 (Belisle et al., 1972). For eggs of German white-tailed eagles, Koeman et al. (1972b) reported from 6.1 ppm to 97 ppm, wet weight. Blus et al. (1974b) found from 1.9 ppm to 36.5 ppm, wet weight, of PCB in brown pelican eggs from the eastern United States, with many readings over 5 ppm.

What do these field residues mean? Apparently they mean less than the chicken work would predict, at least in some of the species studied. Species differences seem to be great. Blus et al. (1974b) found no significant correlation between PCB residues and embryotoxicity; instead, DDE and dieldrin residues (which were themselves correlated) best explained hatching failure in brown pelicans. Heath et al. (1972) found no effect on mallard reproduction in long dosage with 25 ppm of Aroclor 1254. DDE fed at 10 ppm had far more effect. In contrast, Hays and Risebrough (1972) suspected that PCBs or related chemicals were the cause of deformities in a small number of young in a tern colony in which PCB residues were high. Koeman et al. (1972a) concluded that PCBs killed cormorants in the Netherlands and that other aquatic birds had dangerously high residues.

At present, the significance of PCB residues in the wild is very uncertain. PCBs must do to some wild species what they do to mink and chickens, but this is far from being understood, much less proved. Instead, most reproductive troubles that have been studied in wild birds can be attributed best to DDE and/or dieldrin. Still, much of this work has focused on shell thinning and far too little is known about embryotoxicity and genetic damage as phenomena distinct from shell thinning.

This paper has touched only selected facets of the vast PCB literature. Production, use, and biological effects have been reviewed at length by the Interdepartmental Task Force on PCBs (1972) and also by the Panel on Hazardous Trace Substances (Nelson et al., 1972). Peakall (1972) reviewed biological effects. Fishbein (1974) reviewed the toxicology of PCBs. In addition, there are at least two symposium volumes on PCBs, edited by Namovicz (1972) and Lundström (1973).

2.17. Persistence

Persistence is an admirable trait where it is needed, as it is in pesticides that are sprayed in buildings to stop malaria or in pesticides that are used to prevent the spread of pests from plant nurseries. It is also needed in countless industrial products, including the PCBs used in capacitors and transformers. Yet the more one studies pollutants in the ecosystem, the more one sees that persistence itself is a major cause of trouble.

A nonpersistent pollutant may cause serious damage at its point of release, but its danger drops sharply with both distance and time. A persistent pollutant remains in the soil for years. It persists in living animals for months or years. Its residues are likely to occur in the foods of man and in the bodies of man. It can accumulate in food chains and cause serious damage at places that are hundreds or even thousands of miles away from the point of origin, as in Alaskan peregrines. Its residues are almost certain to occur in the eggs of birds and fishes, with severe consequences for those that are sensitive to it. If resistance to the pollutant appears, resistant individuals may carry such high residues as to become living poisoned bait.

When persistent chemicals become widespread and enter species that are sensitive to their reproductive effects, they can destroy the reproductive core of whole populations. If recovery is possible, it comes slowly, for the chemical is lost so slowly from the animals and their foods. And, as Goodman (1974) has pointed out, as persistent chemicals move through the ecosystem, even in minute amounts, they are almost certain to encounter certain forms of life that are sensitive to them. These may well be some of the thousands of species that no one is watching. We cannot forget that the development of the calanoid copepod is completely blocked when egg-bearing females are maintained in sea water containing 10 parts per trillion of DDT, and that significant mortality occurs at 5 parts per trillion (Goldberg et al., 1971). These concentrations are 8 and 16 times lower than those expected in rain water falling into the sea. Species differences being as enormous as they are, we must expect that some groups will be affected seriously by residues that would be judged harmless by nearly all standards.

The only safe course is to eliminate persistent pollutants to the greatest extent possible. It seems foolhardy to apply them deliberately to large open areas or to allow them to be discharged into our waters.

In judging a chemical's environmental dangers, we need to know its toxicity and its persistence. Toxicity data are always available for several species at an early date, and there are standardized protocols for determining toxicity. Yet ecologically, persistence may be more important. Neither DDE nor PCBs are especially toxic; they would have caused little trouble if nonpersistent. Even chemicals like dieldrin would cause less concern if they did not keep appearing in man and animals.

Despite the importance of persistence, there is no standard expression for it and one often finds it incredibly difficult to find out how persistent a given chemical is. Try, for example, to look up the half-times of any given set of herbicides in living animals. It is true, of course, that persistence varies widely with conditions: an organophosphate that remains active on foliage for 100 days may be lost rapidly enough from a living bird to be tolerated in large amounts. The greatest need, therefore, is to know the chemical's half-time in some one species, age, and sex of animal. This would give a standard base for comparisons, and, for many of the shorter-lived chemicals, it would be enough for practical purposes. Problems of metabolites and chemical methodology would be less than one might think, for regulatory authorities require that these be worked out for each pesticide and they are among the first topics studied for other pollutants. Furthermore, much can be done at relatively low cost by use of isotopes with suitable chemical cross-checks.

As nearly all chemicals are tested extensively in rats, even in the most preliminary toxicological studies, it would seem both simple and highly desirable to have a standard expression of half-time based on rats of a given age and sex. The data could be obtained as part of the early toxicological work on a chemical and released as commonly as LD_{50} and LC_{50} data now are.

2.18. Summary

Pollutants tend to simplify plant and animal communities by causing a progressive loss of species. At the extreme, this leads to erosion and loss of soil fertility. Weedy, broadly adapted species increase. Among animals, carnivorous species and groups are often the first to suffer. This is partly because of their exposure at the top of the food chain, and partly, it appears, because of physiological differences.

Species differences in susceptibility are abundant and are often critical. One result is that when one pest is controlled another is likely to flare up. Resistance appears commonly in insects and is known in other fast-breeding forms, including fishes, frogs, and rodents. Resistant individuals can carry toxicant loads that make them dangerous food for other animals. Some groups, including mollusks and annelids, are naturally resistant to many organohalogens and tend to accumulate them.

Animals such as birds may carry lipophilic pollutants in large amounts with apparent safety until forced to draw upon their fat. They may then suffer delayed mortality, and no doubt suffer reproductive or behavioral effects at sublethal levels. Lipophilic pollutants in the brain rise when body lipids decrease and fall when body lipids increase.

Mutagenesis can be caused by some common pollutants and the mutagenic properties of most chemicals are far too little known. Fortunately, common pesticides are not likely to be strong mutagens. Mutagenicity may be affecting certain long-lived and slow-breeding species in the wild, but most species have enough population turnover to swamp an occasional mutagenic event.

Behavioral changes can be caused by relatively low levels of contaminants, but it is often hard to demonstrate them without using high dosages. Reproduction may or may not be affected adversely by low exposures. At certain exposures that are below the toxic levels of a chemical, a biostimulatory effect is to be expected.

Food chain accumulations definitely do occur when persistent chemicals enter organisms that eliminate them poorly. However, loss of chemicals in the food chain must be more common than accumulation. The great concentration from water to aquatic organism is chiefly a physical phenomenon, not a food chain effect, but it affords high starting levels for these chains. Terrestrial food chains often start at a high level with heavily contaminated, struggling prey. Litter feeders are another important base. Vegetation may be contaminated enough to be dangerous to animals that eat it. Dermal and respiratory routes of intoxication occur in the wild, but the oral route is far more important at most times and places.

The organisms that govern soil fertility and texture are affected more by cultivation than by pesticides. Above ground, growing knowledge of resistance, species differences, and biological controls is leading to integrated control, in which use of chemicals is limited and specific. We do not know what is happening to most nontarget invertebrates.

Amphibians and reptiles may be killed by applications of insecticides, but are not highly sensitive and can carry large residues. Effects of these residues on reproduction are little known.

Heavy kills of birds by pesticides still occur in the field. Fish-eating and bird-eating birds also undergo shell thinning and related reproductive troubles in many areas, sometimes to the point of population decline and local or regional extermination. DDE most often correlates with shell thinning in the wild and in experiments. No other known chemical approaches DDE in causing severe and lasting shell thinning. Herbivorous birds seem to be largely immune to this effect. It is uncertain how much dieldrin and PCBs contribute to embryotoxicity in carnivorous birds.

Mammals may be killed by the more toxic pesticides, but some of the commonest small rodents are so resistant, and lose their residues so rapidly, that they are of little value in monitoring effects or residues. Bat populations are declining and pesticides have been blamed. One study in the United States does not support this idea. Bats are sensitive to DDT when thin, but resistant when fat. Bats have not seemed unusually sensitive to BHC, endrin, or dieldrin. Marine mammals of polluted coasts carry large DDE residues in blubber, but the significance of this is unknown. They may also carry levels of PCBs and methylmercury that kill or endanger them.

Mink are exceedingly sensitive to PCBs, so much so that numerous areas are unsafe for mink and any animals of equal sensitivity. It is clear that PCBs kill in at least two distinct ways: neurotoxicity, with high residues in brain; and through liver, kidney, and circulatory system, with low residues in brain.

Certain PCBs of medium chlorination cause chickens to lay fewer eggs, many or all of which fail to hatch, and to have deformed young. Some of the deformities are heritable, which supports other evidence of genetic damage. A given amount of PCB in the egg correlates with a much greater effect on hatchability after being in the hen for some weeks than when dosage begins. This suggests accumulation of some toxic component or metabolite of PCB. Evidence from mink work supports this view. We do not know what wild birds are affected by low levels of PCBs. Study of residues in pelican eggs and experimentation with mallards suggest that reproduction of these species is not very sensitive to PCBs.

Persistence in living animals is one of the chief traits that make chemicals troublesome away from their points of release. Yet we have no standard way to measure and express this trait. It is suggested that half-times of chemicals be determined in rats of a given size and sex, preferably when the early toxicological testing of a chemical is done.

Acknowledgments

The author is indebted to Dr. Lucille F. Stickel for providing references and for reviewing the manuscript. Miss Marian N. Kulp typed all drafts of the manuscript and also assisted with portions of the bibliographic work.

References

Al-Hachim, G. M., and Fink, G. B. (1968). "Effect of DDT or parathion on condition avoidance response of offspring from DDT or parathion treated mothers," *Psychopharmacologia*, 12, 424–427.

Allen, R. H., and others (1959). Papers on the fire ant program and how it affects wildlife, *Proc. 12th Annual Conf. Southeast. Assoc. Game Fish Comm.*, 227–260.

Anderson, D. W., and Hickey, J. J. (1972). "Eggshell changes in certain North American birds," *Proc. XVth Int. Ornithol. Congr.*, 514–540.

Anderson, D. W., Hickey, J. J., Risebrough, R. W., Hughes, D. F., and Christensen, R. E. (1969). "Significance of chlorinated hydrocarbon residues to breeding pelicans and cormorants," *Can. Field Nat.*, 83(2), 91–112.

Anderson, J. M. (1971). "Assessment of the effects of pollutants on physiology and behavior," *Proc. Roy. Soc. Lond.*, B177, 307–320.

Aulerich, R. J., Ringer, R. K., Seagran, H. L., and Youatt, W. G. (1971). "Effects of feeding coho salmon and other Great Lakes fish on mink reproduction," *Can. J. Zool.*, 49(5), 611–616.

Aulerich, R. J., Ringer, R. K., and Iwamoto, S. (1974). "Effects of dietary mercury on mink," *Arch. Environ. Contam. Toxicol.*, 2(1), 43–51.

Azevedo, J. A., Jr., Hunt, E. G., and Woods, L. A., Jr. (1965). "Physiological effects of DDT on pheasants," *Calif. Fish Game*, 51(4), 276–293.

Bailey, S., Bunyan, P. J., Rennison, B. D., and Taylor, A. (1969). "The metabolism of 1,1-di(p-chlorophenyl)-2,2-dichloroethylene and 1,1-di(p-chlorophenyl)-2-chloroethylene in the pigeon," *Toxicol. Appl. Pharmacol.*, 14, 23–32.

Barker, R. J. (1958). "Notes on some ecological effects of DDT sprayed on elms," *J. Wildl. Manage.*, 22(3), 269–274.

Barrett, G. W. (1968). "The effects of an acute insecticide stress on a semi-enclosed grassland ecosystem," *Ecology*, 49(6), 1019–1035.

Belisle, A. A., Reichel, W. L., Locke, L. N., Lamont, T. G., Mulhern, B. M., Prouty, R. M., DeWolf, R. B., and Cromartie, E. (1972), "Residues of organochlorine pesticides, polychlorinated biphenyls, and mercury and autopsy data for bald eagles, 1969 and 1970," *Pestic. Monit. J.*, 6(3), 133–138.

Bernard, R. F. (1963). "Studies on the effects of DDT on birds," *Mich. State Univ., Publ. of Mus., Biol. Ser.*, 2(3), 155–192.

Blackmore, D. K. (1963). "The toxicity of some chlorinated hydrocarbon insecticides to British wild foxes (*Vulpes vulpes*)," *J. Comp. Pathol. Ther.*, 73, 391–409.

Blus, L. J., Belisle, A. A., and Prouty, R. M. (1974a). "Relations of the brown pelican to certain environmental pollutants," *Pestic. Monit. J.*, 7(3/4), 181–194.

Blus, L. J., Neely, B. S., Jr., Belisle, A. A., and Prouty, R. M. (1974b). "Organochlorine residues in brown pelican eggs: relation to reproductive success," *Environ. Pollut.*, 7(2), 81–91.

Borg, K., Wanntorp, H., Erne, K., and Hanko, E. (1969). "Alkyl mercury poisoning in terrestrial Swedish wildlife," *Viltrevy*, 6(4), 301–379.

Borg, K., Erne, K., Hanko, E., and Wanntorp, H. (1970). "Experimental secondary methyl mercury poisoning in the goshawk (*Accipiter g. gentilis* L.)," *Environ. Pollut.*, 1, 91–104.

Braaksma, S. (1973). "Some details about the occurrence of bats in summer and winter resorts in the Netherlands and about the risks caused by wood preservation activities in buildings," *Period. Biol.*, 75, 125–128.

Burdick, G. E., Harris, E. J., Dean, H. J., Walker, T. M., Skea, J., and Colby, D. (1964). "The accumulation of DDT in lake trout and the effect on reproduction," *Trans. Am. Fish. Soc.*, 93(2), 127–136.

Bush, B., Tumasonis, C. F., and Baker, F. D. (1974). "Toxicity and persistence of PCB homologs and isomers in the avian system," *Arch. Environ. Contam. Toxicol.*, 2(3), 195–212.

Cade, T. J., Lincer, J. L., White, C. M., Roseneau, D. G., and Swartz, L. G. (1971). "DDE residues and eggshell changes in Alaskan falcons and hawks," *Science*, 172, 955–957.

Cecil, H. C., Bitman, J., Fries, G. F., Harris, S. J., and Lillie, R. J. (1973). "Changes in egg shell quality and pesticide content of laying hens or pullets fed DDT in high or low calcium diets," *Poult. Sci.*, 52(2), 648–653.

Cecil, H. C., Bitman, J., Lillie, R. J., Fries, G. F., and Verrett, J. (1974). "Embryotoxic and teratogenic effects in unhatched fertile eggs from hens fed polychlorinated biphenyls (PCBs)," *Bull. Environ. Contam. Toxicol.*, 11(6), 489–495.

Clark, D. R., Jr., Martin, C. O., and Swineford, D. M. (1975). "Organochlorine insecticide residues in the free-tailed bat (*Tadarida brasiliensis*) at Bracken Cave, Texas," *J. Mammal.* 56(2), 429–443.

Cooke, A. S. (1970). "The effect of *pp'*-DDT on tadpoles of the common frog (*Rana temporaria*)," *Environ. Pollut.*, 1, 57–71.

Cooke, A. S. (1971). "Selective predation by newts on frog tadpoles treated with DDT," *Nature (Lond.)*, 229, 275–276.

Cooke, A. S. (1972). "The effects of DDT, dieldrin and 2,4-D on amphibian spawn and tadpoles," *Environ. Pollut.*, 3, 41–68.

Cooke, A. S. (1973a). "The effects of DDT, when used as a mosquito larvicide, on tadpoles of the frog *Rana temporaria*," *Environ. Pollut.*, 5, 259–273.

Cooke, A. S. (1973b). "Response of *Rana temporaria* tadpoles to chronic doses of *pp'*-DDT," *Copeia*, 1973(4), 647–652.

Cooke, A. S., and Pollard, E. (1973). "Shell and operculum formation by immature Roman snails *Helix pomatia* L. when treated with *pp'*-DDT," *Pestic. Biochem. Physiol.*, 3(3), 230–236.

Cordes, C. L. (1971). "Comparative study of the uptake, storage, and loss of DDT in small mammals," Ph.D. Thesis, North Carolina State University.

Corke, C. T., and Thompson, F. R. (1970). "Effects of some phenylamide herbicides and their degradation products on soil nitrification," *Can. J. Microbiol.*, 16(7), 567–571.

Crouter, R. A., and Vernon, E. H. (1959). "Effects of black-headed budworm control on salmon and trout in British Columbia, *Can. Fish Culturist*, 24, 23–40.

Cuerrier, J.-P., Keith, J. A., and Stone, E. (1967). "Problems with DDT in fish culture operations," *Nat. Can. (Que.)*, 94, 315–320.

Culley, D. D., Jr., and Ferguson, D. E. (1969). "Patterns of insecticide resistance in the mosquito fish, *Gambusia affinis*," *J. Fish. Res. Board Can.*, 26(9), 2395–2401.

Dahlgren, R. B., and Linder, R. L. (1970). "Eggshell thickness in pheasants given dieldrin," *J. Wildl. Manage.*, 34(1), 226–228.

Dahlgren, R. B., and Linder, R. L. (1974). "Effects of dieldrin in penned pheasants through the third generation," *J. Wildl. Manage.*, 38(2), 320–330.

Dahlgren, R. B., Bury, R. J., Linder, R. L., and Reidinger, R. F., Jr. (1972). "Residue levels and histopathology in pheasants given polychlorinated biphenyls," *J. Wildl. Manage.*, 36(2), 524–533.

Dale, W. E., Gaines, T. B., and Hayes, W. J., Jr. (1962). "Storage and excretion of DDT in starved rats," *Toxicol. Appl. Pharmacol.*, 4, 89–106.

Davison, K. L., and Sell, J. L. (1974). "DDT thins shells of eggs from mallard ducks maintained on *ad libitum* or controlled-feeding regimens," *Arch. Environ. Contam. Toxicol.*, 2(3), 222–232.

Davy, F. B., Kleerekoper, H., and Gensler, P. (1972). "Effects of exposure to sublethal DDT on the locomotor behavior of the goldfish (*Carassius auratus*)," *J. Fish. Res. Board Can.*, 29(9), 1333–1336.

Deichmann, W. B., MacDonald, W. E., Beasley, A. G., and Cubit, D. (1971). "Subnormal reproduction in beagle dogs induced by DDT and aldrin," *Ind. Med. Surg.*, 40(2), 10–20.

DeLong, R. L., Gilmartin, W. G., and Simpson, J. G. (1973). "Premature births in California sea lions: association with high organochlorine pollutant residue levels," *Science*, 181, 1168–1169.

Dempster, J. P. (1968). "The sublethal effect of DDT on the rate of feeding by the ground-beetle *Harpalus rufipes*," *Entomol. Exp. Appl.*, 11, 51–54.

Drummond, D. C., and Wilson, E. J. (1968). "Laboratory investigations of resistance to warfarin of *Rattus norvegicus* Berk. in Montgomeryshire and Shropshire," *Ann. Appl. Biol.*, 61, 303–312.

Durham, W. F. (1967). "The interaction of pesticides with other factors," *Residue Rev.*, 18, 21–103.

Edwards, C. A., and Thompson, A. R. (1973). "Pesticides and the soil fauna," *Residue Rev.*, 45, 1–79.

Elson, P. F. (1967). "Effects on wild young salmon of spraying DDT over New Brunswick forests," *J. Fish. Res. Board Can.*, 24(4), 731–767.

Enderson, J. H., and Wrege, P. H. (1973). "DDE residues and eggshell thickness in prairie falcons," *J. Wildl. Manage.*, 37(4), 476–478.

Epstein, S. S., and Legator, M. S. (1971). *The Mutagenicity of Pesticides*, MIT Press, Cambridge, Mass.

Faber, R. A., and Hickey, J. J. (1973). "Eggshell thinning, chlorinated hydrocarbons and mercury in inland aquatic bird eggs, 1969 and 1970," *Pestic. Monit. J.*, 7(1), 27–36.

Faber, R. A., Risebrough, R. W., and Pratt, H. M., (1972). "Organochlorines and mercury in common egrets and great blue herons," *Environ. Pollut.*, 3, 111–122.

Fashingbauer, B. A. (1957). "The effects of aerial spraying with DDT on wood frogs," *Flicker*, 29(4), 160.

Ferguson, D. E. (1963). "Notes concerning the effects of heptachlor on certain poikilotherms," *Copeia*, 1963(2), 441–443.

Ferguson, D. E. (1967). "The ecological consequences of pesticide resistance in fishes," *Trans. 32nd N. Am. Wildl. Nat. Resour. Conf.*, 103–107.

Ferguson, D. E. (1968). "Characteristics and significance of resistance to insecticides in fishes," *Reservoir Fish. Resour. Symp., Athens, Ga. 1967*, 531–536.

Ferguson, D. E. (1969). "The compatible existence of non-target species to pesticides," *Bull. Entomol. Soc. Am.*, 15(4), 363–366.

Ferguson, D. E., and Gilbert, C. C. (1967). "Tolerances of three species of anuran amphibians to five chlorinated hydrocarbon insecticides," *Miss. Acad. Sci. J.*, 13, 135–138.

Finley, M. T., Ferguson, D. E., and Ludke, J. L. (1970). "Possible selective mechanisms in the development of insecticide-resistant fish," *Pestic. Monit. J.*, 3(4), 212–218.

Fishbein, L. (1974). "Toxicity of chlorinated biphenyls," *Annual Rev. Pharmacol.*, 14, 139–156.

Fleet, R. R., Clark, D. R., Jr., and Plapp, F. W., Jr. (1972). "Residues of DDT and dieldrin in snakes from two Texas agro-systems," *BioScience*, 22(11), 664–665.

Fletcher, W. W. (1961). "Effect of organic herbicides in soil microorganisms," *Pest Technol.* (now *Int. Pest Control*), 3, 272–275.

Fowle, C. D. (1972). "Effects of phosphamidon on forest birds in New Brunswick," *Can. Wildl. Serv. Rep. Ser. No. 16*, 1–25.

Fowler, J. F., Newsom, L. D., Graves, J. B., Bonner, F. L., and Schilling, P. E. (1971). "Effect of dieldrin on egg hatchability, chick survival and eggshell thickness in purple and common gallinules," *Bull. Environ. Contam. Toxicol.*, 6(6), 495–501.

Freitag, R., Hastings, L., Mercer, W. R., and Smith, A. (1973). "Ground beetle populations near a kraft mill," *Can. Entomol.*, 105, 299–310.

Fuhremann, T. W., and Lichtenstein, E. P. (1972). "Increase in the toxicity of organophosphorus insecticides to house flies due to polychlorinated biphenyl compounds," *Toxicol. Appl. Pharmacol.*, 22, 628–640.

Fyfe, R. W., Campbell, J., Hayson, B., and Hodson, K. (1969). "Regional population declines and organochlorine insecticides in Canadian prairie falcons," *Can. Field Nat.*, 83(3), 191–200.

Giles, F. E., Middleton, S. G., and Grau, J. G. (1973). "Evidence for the accumulation of atmospheric lead by insects in areas of high traffic density," *Environ. Entomol.*, 2(2), 299–300.

Gish, C. D. (1970). "Organochlorine insecticide residues in soils and soil invertebrates from agricultural lands," *Pestic. Monit. J.*, 3(4), 241–252.

Goldberg, E. D., chairman (1971). *Chlorinated Hydrocarbons in the Marine Environment.* National Academy of Sciences, Washington, D.C.

Goodman, G. T. (1974). "How do chemical substances affect the environment?," *Proc. Roy. Soc. Lond.*, B185, 127–148.

Graves, J. B., Bonner, F. L., McKnight, W. F., Watts, A. B., and Epps, E. A. (1969). "Residues in eggs, preening glands, liver, and muscle from feeding dieldrin-contaminated rice bran to hens and its effect on egg production, egg hatch, and chick survival," *Bull. Environ. Contam. Toxicol.*, 4(6), 375–383.

Gress, F., Risebrough, R. W., Anderson, D. W., Kiff, L. F., and Jehl, J. R., Jr. (1973). "Reproductive failures of double-crested cormorants in Southern California and Baja California," *Wilson Bull.*, 85(2), 197–208.

Haegele, M. A., and Tucker, R. K. (1974). "Effects of 15 common environmental pollutants on eggshell thickness in mallards and Coturnix," *Bull. Environ. Contam. Toxicol.*, 11(1), 98–102.

Haegele, M. A., Tucker, R. K., and Hudson, R. H. (1974). "Effects of dietary mercury and lead on eggshell thickness in mallards," *Bull. Environ. Contam. Toxicol.*, 11(1), 5–11.

Haney, A., and Lipsey, R. L. (1973). "Accumulation and effects of methyl mercury hydroxide in a terrestrial food chain under laboratory conditions," *Environ. Pollut.*, 5, 305–316.

Hanko, E., Erne, E., Wanntorp, H., and Borg, K. (1970). "Poisoning in ferrets by tissues of alkyl mercury fed chickens," *Acta. Vet. Scand.*, 11, 268–282.

Harris, C. R. (1969). "Insecticide pollution and soil organisms," *Proc. Entomol. Soc. Ont.*, 100, 14–29.

Haseltine, S., Uebelhart, K., Peterle, T., and Lustick, S. (1974). "DDE, PTH and eggshell thinning in mallard, pheasant and ring dove," *Bull. Environ. Contam. Toxicol.*, 11(2), 139–145.

Hatfield, C. T., and Johansen, P. H. (1972). "Effects of four insecticides on the ability of Atlantic salmon parr (*Salmo salar*) to learn and retain a simple conditioned response," *J. Fish. Res. Board Can.*, 29(3), 315–321.

Hayes, W. J. (1975). *Toxicology of Pesticides*, Williams & Wilkins, Baltimore.

Hays, H., and Risebrough, R. W. (1972). "Pollutant concentrations in abnormal young terns from Long Island Sound," *Auk*, 89, 19–35.

Heath, R. G., Spann, J. W., and Kreitzer, J. F. (1969). "Marked DDE impairment of mallard reproduction in controlled studies," *Nature (Lond.)*, 224, 47–48.

Heath, R. G., Spann, J. W., Kreitzer, J. F., and Vance, C. (1972). "Effects of polychlorinated biphenyls on birds," *Proc. 15th Int. Ornithol. Congr.*, 475–485.

Heinz, G. (1974). "Effects of low dietary levels of methyl mercury on mallard reproduction," *Bull. Environ. Contam. Toxicol.*, 11(4), 386–392.

Heinz, G. (1975). "Effects of methylmercury on approach and avoidance behavior of mallard ducklings," *Bull. Environ. Contam. Toxicol.*, 13(5), 554–564.

Henderson, C., Inglis, A., and Johnson, W. L. (1971). "Organochlorine insecticide residues in fish–Fall 1969," *Pestic. Monit. J.*, 5(1), 1–11.

Henriksson, K., Karppanen, E., and Helminen, M. (1966). "High residue of mercury in Finnish white tailed eagles," *Ornis Fenn.*, 43, 38–45.

Herald, E. S. (1949). "Effects of DDT-oil solutions upon amphibians and reptiles," *Herpetologica*, 5, 117–120.

Hickey, J. J., ed. (1969). *Peregrine Falcon Populations, Their Biology and Decline*, University of Wisconsin Press.

Hickey, J. J., and Anderson, D. W. (1968). "Chlorinated hydrocarbons and eggshell changes in raptorial and fish-eating birds," *Science*, 162, 271–273.

Horne, R. A., Lockeretz, W., Appleby, A. P., and Dinman, B. D. (1972). "Biological effects of chemical agents," *Science*, 177, 1152–1154.

Interdepartmental Task Force on PCBs (1972). *Polychlorinated Biphenyls and the Environment*, National Technical Information Service, Springfield, Va. (Accession No. COM-72-10419).

Jefferies, D. J. (1969). "Induction of apparent hyperthyroidism in birds fed DDT," *Nature (Lond.)*, 222, 578–579.

Jefferies, D. J. (1972). "Organochlorine insecticide residues in British bats and their significance," *J. Zool.*, 166, 245–263.

Jefferies, D. J. (1973). "The effects of organochlorine insecticides and their metabolites on breeding birds," *J. Reprod. Fert. Suppl.*, 19, 337–352.

Jefferies, D. J., Stainsby, B., and French, M. C. (1973). "The ecology of small mammals in arable fields drilled with winter wheat and the increase in their dieldrin and mercury residues," *J. Zool.*, 171, 513–539.

Jeppson, L. R. (1974). "Pest management in citrus orchards," *Bull. Entomol. Soc. Am.*, 20(3), 221–222.

Johnson, G. A., and Jalal, S. M. (1973). "DDT-induced chromosomal damage in mice," *J. Hered.*, 64(1), 7–8.

Keith, J. A., and Gruchy, I. M. (1972). "Residue levels of chemical pollutants in North American birdlife," *Proc. XVth. Int. Ornithol. Congr.*, 437–454.

Keith, J. O., and Flickinger, E. L. (1965). "Fate and persistence of DDT in a forest environment," *U.S. Fish Wildl. Serv. Circ.*, 226, 44–46.

Keith, J. O., Woods, L. A., Jr., and Hunt, E. G. (1970). "Reproductive failure in brown pelicans on the Pacific Coast," *Trans. 35th N. Am. Wildl. Nat. Resour. Conf.*, 56–64.

Klein, W., Müller, W., and Korte, F. (1968). "Ausscheidung, Verteilung und Stoffwechsel von Endrin-[14C] in Ratten," *Liebigs Ann. Chem.*, 713, 180–185.

Koeman, J. H. (1971). "The occurrence and toxicological implications of some chlorinated hydrocarbons in the Dutch coastal area in the period from 1965 to 1970" (in Dutch, English summary), Ph.D. Thesis, University of Utrecht.

Koeman, J. H., Rijksen, H. D., Smies, M., Na'Isa, B. K., and MacLennan, K. J. R. (1971). "Faunal changes in a swamp habitat in Nigeria sprayed with insecticide to exterminate Glossina," *Neth. J. Zool.*, 21(4), 443–463.

Koeman, J. H., Bothof, T., de Vries, R., van Velzen-Blad, H., and Vos, J. G. (1972a). "The impact of persistent pollutants on piscivorous and molluscivorous birds," *TNO-Nieuws*, 27, 561–569.

Koeman, J. H., Hadderingh, R. H., and Bijleveld, M. F. I. J. (1972b). "Persistent pollutants in the white-tailed eagle (*Haliaetus albicilla*) in the Federal Republic of Germany," *Biol. Conserv.*, **4**(5), 373–377.

Koeman, J. H., Peeters, W. H. M., Smit, C. J., Tjioe, P. S., and de Goeij, J. J. M. (1972c). "Persistent chemicals in marine mammals," *TNO-Nieuws*, **27**, 570–578.

Koeman, J. H., van Beusekom, C. F., and de Goeij, J. J. M. (1972d). "Eggshell and population changes in the sparrow hawk (*Accipiter nisus*)," *TNO-Nieuws*, **27**, 542–550.

Korschgen, L. J. (1970). "Soil–food-chain–pesticide wildlife relationships in aldrin-treated fields," *J. Wildl. Manage.*, **34**(1), 186–199.

Kreitzer, J. F., and Spann, J. W. (1973). "Tests of pesticidal synergism with young pheasants and Japanese quail," *Bull. Environ. Contam. Toxicol.*, **9**(4), 250–256.

Lehman, A. J. (1965). *Summaries of Pesticide Toxicity*, Association of Food and Drug Officials of the United States.

Lehner, P. N., and Egbert, A. (1969). "Dieldrin and eggshell thickness in ducks," *Nature (Lond.)*, **224**, 1218–1219.

Lichtenstein, E. P., Schulz, K. R., Fuhremann, T. W., and Liang, T. T. (1969). "Biological interaction between plasticizers and insecticides," *J. Econ. Entomol.*, **62**(4), 761–765.

Lillie, R. J., Cecil, H. C., Bitman, J., and Fries, G. F. (1974). "Differences in response of caged white leghorn layers to various polychlorinated biphenyls (PCBs) in the diet," *Poult. Sci.*, **53**, 726–732.

Lincer, J. L., Cade, T. J., Devine, J. M. (1970). "Organochlorine residues in Alaskan peregrine falcons (*Falco peregrinus* Tunstall), rough-legged hawks (*Buteo lagopus* Pontoppidan) and their prey," *Can. Field Nat.*, **84**(3), 255–263.

Lockie, J. D., Ratcliffe, D. A., and Balharry, R. (1969). "Breeding success and organochlorine residues in golden eagles in West Scotland," *J. Appl. Ecol.*, **6**(3), 381–389.

Longcore, J. R., and Samson, F. B. (1973). "Eggshell breakage by incubating black ducks fed DDE," *J. Wildl. Manage.*, **37**(3), 390–394.

Longcore, J. R., Samson, F. B., Kreitzer, J. F., and Spann, J. W. (1971a). "Changes in mineral composition of eggshells from black ducks and mallards fed DDE in the diet," *Bull. Environ. Contam. Toxicol.*, **6**(4), 345–350.

Longcore, J. R., Samson, F. B., Whittendale, T. W., Jr. (1971b). "DDE thins eggshells and lowers reproductive success of captive black ducks," *Bull. Environ. Contam. Toxicol.*, **6**(6), 485–490.

Luckens, M. M. (1973). "Seasonal changes in the sensitivity of bats to DDT," in *Pesticides and the Environment: A Continuing Controversy* (ed. Deichmann, W. B.), pp. 63–75, Intercontinental Medical Book Corp., New York.

Ludke, J. L. (1974). "Interaction of dieldrin and DDE residues in Japanese quail *(Coturnix coturnix japonica)*, *Bull. Environ. Contam. Toxicol.*, **11**(4), 297–302.

Lundberg, C. (1973). "Effects of long-term exposure to DDT on the oestrus cycle and the frequency of implanted ova in the mouse," *Environ. Physiol. Biochem.*, **3**, 127–131.

Lundström, S., ed. (1973). *PCB Conference II*. Natl. Swed. Environ. Prot. Board Publ. 1973: 4E.

MacPhee, A. W., and Sanford, K. H. (1954). "The influence of spray programs on the fauna of apple orchards in Nova Scotia. VII. Effects on some beneficial arthropods," *Can. Entomol.*, **86**, 128–135.

Malecki, R. A., Allen, S. H., Elliston, J. O., Sadler, K. C., Goforth, W. R., and Baskett, T. S. (1974). "Cottontail reproduction related to dieldrin exposure," *U.S. Bur. Sport Fish Wildl., Spec. Sci. Rep. Wildl.*, **177**, 1–61.

Martin, J. P. (1963). "Influence of pesticide residues on soil microbiological and chemical properties," *Residue Rev.*, **4**, 96–129.

McKim, J. M., Cristensen, G. M., Tucker, J. H., Benoit, D. A., and Lewis, M. J. (1973). "Effects of pollution on freshwater fish," *J. Water Pollut. Control Fed.*, **45**(6), 1370–1407.

McLane, M. A. R., and Hall, L. C. (1972). "DDE thins screech owl eggshells," *Bull. Environ. Contam. Toxicol.*, 8(2), 65–68.

Meeks, R. L. (1968). "The accumulation of ^{36}Cl ring-labeled DDT in a fresh-water marsh," *J. Wildl. Manage.*, **32**(2), 376–398.

Mendelssohn, H. (1972). "The impact of pesticides on bird life in Israel," *Int. Counc. Bird Preserv. XI Bull.*, 75–104.

Mick, D. L., Long, K. R., and Aldinger, S. M. (1973). "The effects of dietary dieldrin on residues in eggs and tissues of laying hens and the effects of phenobarbital and charcoal on these residues," *Bull. Environ. Contam. Toxicol.*, 9(4), 197–203.

Mills, J. A. (1973). "Some observations on the effects of field applications of fensulfothion and parathion on bird and mammal populations," *Proc. N. Z. Ecol. Soc.*, **20**, 65–71.

Moriarty, F. (1969). "The sublethal effects of synthetic insecticides on insects," *Biol. Rev.*, **44**, 321–357.

Morris, J. E. (1973). "Effects of dieldrin on reproduction in raccoons," Ph.D. Thesis, University of Missouri.

Mulhern, B. M., Reichel, W. L., Locke, L. N., Lamont, T. G., Belisle, A., Cromartie, E., Bagley, G. F., and Prouty, R. M. (1970). "Organochlorine residues and autopsy data from bald eagles 1966–68," *Pestic. Monit. J.*, 4(3), 141–144.

Mulla, M. S. (1962). "Frog and toad control with insecticides!," *Pest Control*, **30**(10), 20 and 60.

Murphy, D. A., and Korschgen, L. J. (1970). "Reproduction, growth, and tissue residues of deer fed dieldrin," *J. Wildl. Manage.*, **34**(4), 887–903.

Namovicz, R. M., ed. (1972). PCB Symposium issue, *Environ. Health Perspect.* No. 1.

Negm, A. A., and Hensley, S. D. (1969). "Effect of insecticides on ant and spider populations in Louisiana sugarcane fields," *J. Econ. Entomol.*, **62**(4), 948–949.

Nelson, N., Chairman, Panel on Hazardous Trace Substances. (1972). "Polychlorinated biphenyls—environmental impact," *Environ. Res.*, 5(3), 249–362.

Newsom, L. D. (1967). "Consequences of insecticide use on nontarget organisms," *Annual Rev. Entomol.*, **12**, 257–286.

Newton, I. (1974). "Changes attributed to pesticides in the nesting success of the sparrow-hawk in Britain," *J. Appl. Ecol.*, **11**(1), 95–102.

Ottoboni, Alice (1972). "Effect of DDT on the reproductive life-span in the female rat," *Toxicol. Appl. Pharmacol.*, **22**, 497–502.

Peakall, D. B. (1970). "*p,p'*-DDT: effect on calcium metabolism and concentration of estradiol in the blood," *Science*, **168**, 592–594.

Peakall, D. B. (1972). "Polychlorinated biphenyls: occurrence and biological effects," *Residue Rev.*, **44**, 1–19.

Peakall, D. B. (1974). "DDE: its presence in peregrine eggs in 1948," *Science*, **183**, 673–674.

Peakall, D. B., and Peakall, M. L. (1973). "Effect of polychlorinated biphenyl on the reproduction of artificially and naturally incubated dove eggs," *J. Appl. Ecol.*, **10**, 863–868.

Peakall, D. B., Lincer, J. L., and Bloom, S. E. (1972). "Embryonic mortality and chromosomal alterations caused by Aroclor 1254 in ring doves," *Environ. Health Perspect.*, **1**, 103–104.

Peakall, D. B., Lincer, J. L., Risebrough, R. W., Pritchard, J. B., and Kinter, W. B. (1973). "DDE-induced eggshell thinning: structural and physiological effects in three species," *Comp. Gen. Pharmacol.*, **4**, 305–313.

Peterle, A. F., and Peterle, T. J. (1971). "The effect of DDT on aggression in laboratory mice," *Bull. Environ. Contam. Toxicol.*, 6(5), 401–405.

Pillmore, R. E., Robison, W. H., and Wilson, R. A. (1965). "Persistence of DDT on forage species," *U.S. Fish Wildl. Serv. Circ.*, 226, 40–43.

Plapp, F. W., Jr. (1972). "Polychlorinated biphenyl: an environmental contaminant acts as an insecticide synergist," *Environ. Entomol.*, 1(5), 580–582.

Platonow, N. S., and Karstad, L. H. (1973). "Dietary effects of polychlorinated biphenyls on mink," *Can. J. Comp. Med.*, 37(4), 391–400.

Platonow, N. S., and Reinhart, B. S. (1973). "The effects of polychlorinated biphenyls (Aroclor 1254) on chicken egg production, fertility and hatchability," *Can. J. Comp. Med.*, 37(4), 341–346.

Poonacha, K. B., Wentworth, B. C., and Chapman, A. B. (1973). "Genetic resistance to DDT in the Japanese quail *Coturnix coturnix japonica*," *Poult. Sci.*, 52, 841–846.

Porter, R. D., and Wiemeyer, S. N. (1972). "DDE at low dietary levels kills captive American kestrels," *Bull. Environ. Contam. Toxicol.*, 8(4), 193–199.

Prestt, I. (1970). "Organochlorine pollution of rivers and the heron (*Ardea cinerea* L.)," *Pap. Proc., IUCN 11th Tech. Meet.*, 1, 95–102.

Prestt, I., and Ratcliffe, D. A. (1972). "Effects of organochlorine insecticides on European birdlife," *Proc. 15th Int. Ornithol Congr.*, 486–513.

Prestt, I., Jefferies, D. J., and Moore, N. W. (1970). "Polychlorinated biphenyls in wild birds in Britain and their avian toxicity," *Environ. Pollut.*, 1, 3–26.

Price, P. W., Rathcke, B. J., and Gentry, D. A. (1974). "Lead in terrestrial arthropods: evidence for biological concentration," *Environ. Entomol.*, 3(3), 370–372.

Ratcliffe, D. A. (1967). "Decrease in eggshell weight in certain birds of prey," *Nature (Lond.)*, 215, 208–210.

Ratcliffe, D. A. (1973). "Studies of the recent breeding success of the peregrine, *Falco peregrinus*," *J. Reprod. Fert. Suppl.*, 19, 377–389.

Reagan, T. E., Coburn, G., and Hensley, S. D. (1972). "Effects of mirex on the arthropod fauna of a Louisiana sugarcane field," *Environ. Entomol.*, 1(5), 588–591.

Ringer, R. K., Aulerich, R. J., and Zabik, M. (1972). "Effect of dietary polychlorinated biphenyls on growth and reproduction of mink," *Preprints of Papers Presented, 164th Natl. Meet. Am. Chem. Soc.*, 12(2), 149–154.

Risebrough, R. W., and Anderson, D. W. (1971). Aroclor 1254 did not increase effect of DDE in thinning mallard eggshells, *PCB Newsletter*, 3, 17.

Risebrough, R. W., Sibley, F. C., and Kirven, M. N. (1971). "Reproductive failure of the brown pelican on Anacapa Island in 1969," *Am. Birds*, 25(1), 8–9.

Robel, R. J., Stalling, C. D., Westfahl, M. E., and Kadoum, A. M. (1972). "Effects of insecticides on populations of rodents in Kansas—1965-69," *Pestic. Monit. J.*, 6(2), 115–121.

Rongsriyam, Y., Prownebon, S., and Hirakoso, S. (1968). "Effects of insecticides on the feeding activity of the guppy, a mosquito-eating fish, in Thailand," *Bull. WHO*, 39(6), 977–980.

Rosene, W., Jr., Stewart, P., and Adomaitis, V. (1961). "Residues of heptachlor epoxide in wild animals," *Proc. 15th Annual Conf. Southeast Assoc. Game and Fish Comm.*, 107–113.

Rudd, R. L., and Genelly, R. E. (1956). "Pesticides: their use and toxicity in relation to wildlife," *Calif. Dept. Fish Game, Game Bull.*, 7, 1–209.

Sanford, K. H., and Herbert, H. J. (1970). "The influence of spray programs on the fauna of apple orchards in Nova Scotia. XX. Trends after altering levels of phytophagous mites or predators," *Can. Entomol.*, 102(5), 592–601.

Saunders, J. W. (1969). "Mass mortalities and behaviour of brook trout and juvenile

Atlantic salmon in a stream polluted by agricultural pesticides," *J. Fish. Res. Board Can.*, **26**(3), 695–699.

Schulz-Baldes, M. (1974). "Lead uptake from sea water and food, and lead loss in the common mussel *Mytilus edulis*," *Marine Biol.*, **25**, 177–193.

Scott, T. G., Willis, Y. L., and Ellis, J. A. (1959). "Some effects of a field application of dieldrin on wildlife," *J. Wildl. Manage.*, **23**(4), 409–427.

Scudder, C. L., and Richardson, D. (1970). "Effect of DDT on isolation-induced aggression in *Mus*," *Environ. Res.*, **3**, 460–462.

Sherburne, J. A., and Dimond, J. B. (1969), "DDT persistence in wild hares and mink," *J. Wildl. Manage.*, **33**(4), 944–948.

Smith, R. M., and Cole, C. F. (1973). "Effects of egg concentrations of DDT and dieldrin on development in winter flounder (*Pseudopleuronectes americanus*)," *J. Fish. Res. Board Can.*, **30**(12), 1894–1898.

Smith, R. D., and Glasgow, L. L. (1965). "Effects of heptachlor on wildlife in Louisiana," *Proc. 17th Annual Conf. Southeast. Assoc. Game and Fish Comm.*, 140–154.

Smyth, H. F., Jr. (1967). "Sufficient challenge," *Food Cosmet. Toxicol.*, **5**, 51–58.

Snyder, N. F. R., Snyder, H. A., Lincer, J. L., and Reynolds, R. T. (1973). "Organochlorines, heavy metals, and the biology of North American accipiters," *BioScience*, **23**(5), 300–305.

Sprague, J. B. (1970). "Measurement of pollutant toxicity to fish. II. Utilizing and applying bioassay results," *Water Res.*, **4**, 3–32.

Spyker, J. M., Sparber, S. B., and Goldberg, A. M. (1972). "Subtle consequences of methylmercury exposure: behavioral deviations in offspring of treated mothers," *Science*, **177**, 621–623.

Stickel, L. F. (1973). "Pesticide residues in birds and mammals," in *Environmental Pollution by Pesticides* (ed. Edwards, C. A.), p. 254, Plenum Press, New York.

Stickel, W. H., Galyen, J. A., Dyrland, R. A., and Hughes, D. L. (1973). "Toxicity and persistence of mirex in birds," in *Pesticides and the Environment: A Continuing Controversy* (ed. Deichmann, W. B.), p. 437, Intercontinental Medical Book Corp., New York.

Thompson, A. R. (1971). "Effects of nine insecticides on the numbers and biomass of earthworms in pasture," *Bull. Environ. Contam. Toxicol.*, **5**(6), 577–586.

Tillander, M., Miettinen, J. K., and Koivisto, I. (1970). "Excretion rate of methylmercury in the seal (*Pusa hispida*)," *FAO Tech. Conf. Mar. Pollut. and Its Effect on Living Resour. and Fishing*, Rome.

Tumasonis, C. F., Bush, B., and Baker, F. D. (1973). "PCB levels in egg yolks associated with embryonic mortality and deformity of hatched chicks," *Arch. Environ. Contam. Toxicol.*, **1**(4), 312–324.

van Klingeren, B., Koeman, J. H., and van Haaften, J. L. (1966). "A study on the hare (*Lepus europeus*) in relation to the use of pesticides in a polder in the Netherlands," *J. Appl. Ecol. Suppl.*, **3**, 125–131.

van Rhee, J. A. (1969). "Effects of biocides and their residues on earthworms," *Meded. Rijksfac. Landbouwwetensch. Gent.*, **34**(3), 682–689.

Van Velzen, A. C., Stiles, W. B., and Stickel, L. F. (1972). "Lethal mobilization of DDT by cowbirds," *J. Wildl. Manage.*, **36**(3), 733–739.

Veith, G. D., and Lee, F. F. (1971). "PCBs in fish from the Milwaukee region," *Proc. 14th Conf. Great Lakes Res.*, 157–169.

Vos, J. G., and Koeman, J. H. (1970). "Comparative toxicologic study with polychlorinated biphenyls in chickens with special reference to porphyria, edema formation, liver necrosis, and tissue residues," *Toxicol. Appl. Pharmacol.*, **17**, 656–668.

Walker, A. I. T., Neill, C. H., Stevenson, D. E., and Robinson, J. (1969). "The toxicity of dieldrin (HEOD) to Japanese quail (*Coturnix coturnix japonica*)," *Toxicol. Appl. Pharmacol.*, **15**, 69-73.

Wallace, G. J., Nickell, W. P., and Bernard, R. F. (1961). "Bird mortality in the Dutch elm disease program in Michigan," *Cranbrook Inst. Sci., Bull.*, **41**, 1-44.

Ware, G. W., and Good, E. E. (1967). "Effects of insecticides on reproduction in the laboratory mouse. II. Mirex, telodrin, and DDT," *Toxicol. Appl. Pharmacol.*, **10**, 54-61.

Warner, R. E., Peterson, K. K., and Borgman, L. (1966). "Behavioral pathology in fish: a quantitative study of sublethal pesticide toxication," *J. Appl. Ecol. Suppl.*, **3**, 223-247.

Webb, R. E., Hartgrove, R. W., Randolph, W. C., Petrella, V. J., and Horsfall, F., Jr. (1973). "Toxicity studies in endrin-susceptible and resistant strains of pine mice," *Toxicol. Appl. Pharmacol.*, **25**, 42-47.

Wiemeyer, S. N., and Porter, R. D. (1970). "DDE thins eggshells of captive American kestrels," *Nature (Lond.)*, **227**, 737-738.

Wiemeyer, S. N., Mulhern, B. M., Ligas, F. J., Hensel, R. J., Mathisen, J. E., Robards, F. C., and Postupalsky, S. (1972). "Residues of organochlorine pesticides, polychlorinated biphenyls, and mercury in bald eagle eggs and changes in shell thickness—1969 and 1970," *Pestic. Monit. J.*, **6**(1), 50-55.

Wiese, I. H., Basson, N. C. J., van der Vyver, J. H., and van der Merwe, J. H. (1969). "Toxicology and dynamics of dieldrin in the crowned guinea-fowl *Numida meleagris* (L)," *Phytophylactica*, **1**, 161-176.

Wiese, I. H., Basson, N. C. J., Basson, P. A., Naude, T. W., and Maartens, B. P. (1973). "The toxicology and pathology of dieldrin and photodieldrin poisoning in two antelope species," *Onderstepoort J. Vet. Res.*, **40**(1), 31-40.

Wilson, V. J. (1972). "Observations on the effect of dieldrin on wildlife during tsetse fly *Glossina morsitans* control operations in eastern Zambia," *Arnoldia (Rhodesia)*, **5**(34), 1-12.

Woodwell, G. M. (1970). "Effects of pollution on the structure and physiology of ecosystems," *Science*, **168**, 429-433.

Note added in proof: Interference is *not* with carbonic anhydrase, but with calcium ATPase. See Miller, D. S., Peakall, D. B., and Kinter, W. B. (1975). "Biochemical basis for DDE-induced eggshell thinning in ducks," *Fed. Proc. Fed. Am. Soc. Exp. Biol.* **34**(3), 811.

3

Aspects of Heavy Metal and Organohalogen Pollution in Aquatic Ecosystems

BOSTWICK H. KETCHUM, V. ZITKO, AND D. SAWARD

The pollutants of major concern in aquatic ecosystems are those which are produced and reach the environment in large amounts, are toxic to aquatic organisms, or are concentrated within organisms to a level greater than that in the environment and which persist for long periods of time so that the environmental concentrations can gradually increase. Toxic heavy metals and organohalogen compounds are among the materials of concern. The toxicity of pollutants is generally determined by short-term, acute bioassay tests which are useful in determining a dangerous concentration, but not necessarily for the determination of a "safe" concentration in the environment. Sometimes acceptable concentrations can be evaluated in the natural environment by comparative studies of polluted and unpolluted ecosystems. Long-term laboratory tests to evaluate chronic toxicity are also desirable to evaluate sublethal effects such as changes in feeding behavior or decrease of breeding capability. Some chronic studies should involve a full generation or more of a given species so that all stages of the life cycle are exposed to the pollutant. The three contributions which follow set forth some of the complexities of aquatic ecosystems and discuss some of the problems involved in their study.

BOSTWICK H. KETCHUM • Woods Hole Oceanographic Institution, Woods Hole, Massachusetts 02543.   V. ZITKO • Fisheries Research Board of Canada, Biological Station, St. Andrews, New Brunswick E0G 2X0, Canada.   D. SAWARD • Department of Agriculture and Fisheries for Scotland, Marine Laboratory, Aberdeen, Scotland.

I

Problems in Aquatic Ecosystems, with Special Reference to Heavy Metal Pollution of the Marine Environment

BOSTWICK H. KETCHUM

Toxicologists are concerned primarily with adverse responses in individual human subjects or in individuals of domesticated species of animal. In contrast, the ecologist is more concerned with the survival of a population. This difference in viewpoints between toxicologists and ecologists is further complicated by the hierarchy of biological organization and structure, each level of which has its own unique complexities. The molecular biologist, whether he is working with a microorganism, with a liver extract, or with some other biological system, is often hopeful that studies of a particular reaction may have general relevance to a wide range of living organisms. Proceeding from *in vitro* extracts through cellular constituents to tissues, organs, and the complete organism, complexity increases at each level of organization. Superimposed upon this increasing complexity are species differences in metabolic pathways and in the response to toxic compounds, as is well illustrated by differences in liver function among mammalian species.

The ecologist starts with the organism, and with all the complexities that are inherent in the structure of an organism, and studies populations and population dynamics (my definition of population is a coherent group of a single species of organisms). He then looks at the combinations of populations which make up communities, and finally at the overall ecosystem which contains many populations and communities, and which encompasses all the reactions among all the components.

Figure 3.1 (from NAS, 1973a) illustrates the essential relationships of the many aspects of this problem. It is supposed to be a generalized pattern applicable to any pollutant that may enter the aquatic ecosystem. The left part of the diagram shows the imports to the system, the central parts shows determinant

76

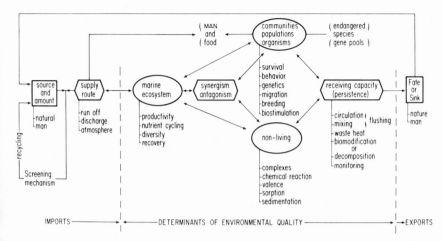

FIG. 3.1. Conceptual framework for water quality evaluation, showing the various parts of the ecosystem and processes which determine the importance of pollutants in the marine environment.

of environmental quality, and the right part shows the exports from the system. Until a few years ago the complexity of the marine ecosystem defeated all attempts to study it in its entirety. The accompanying paper by Saward describes an attempt to simplify a marine ecosystem so that it can be studied by direct measurements which yield information at the food chain level.

In the part of Fig. 3.1 showing impacts on communities, populations, and organisms, acute toxicity affects survival of individuals, but there are also many chronic, sublethal effects of pollution. A pollutant may affect the genetics of a population or the behavior of organisms, such as their migration or their breeding behavior. Some pollutants may be biostimulatory at low concentrations or inhibitory at high concentrations.

Sea water is a highly complex mixture of all the elements known, and there are consequently a number of chemical problems which must be understood in order to evaluate the impact of pollutants. Anything added may form complexes, may undergo chemical reactions, may suffer alteration of valence states, may be sorbed onto particulate matter, or may be sedimented to the bottom, where, although removed from the aqueous phase, it may still have impacts on the sea bed populations. These physical or chemical processes can greatly modify the direct effect of the pollutant on the ecosystem.

Interconnecting all these parts of the ecosystem are the problems of synergism and antagonism. Two different pollutants added to the system may augment each other's action on living organisms or may be mutually antagonistic and thus have less effect.

Ultimately, any aquatic system has a finite receiving capacity for a given pollutant. By receiving capacity I mean the amount of a pollutant which may be added without serious deleterious effects upon the organisms living in the environment. To determine this, one must first know the strictly physical process of circulation and mixing. Waste heat and its exchange with the atmosphere is an example of a pollutant modified only by these physical processes. The receiving capacity of this system depends more upon surface area than volume for waste heat. Other factors influencing receiving capacity are changes imposed by biological, geological, or chemical processes, such as biomodification or decomposition. If we accept the concept of receiving capacity there follows the problems of monitoring, which is required in order to make sure that predictions are correct. A pollutant added to the sea may move from one part of the system to another, but the ultimate fate will be export from the system, and these movements must be determined by monitoring.

Table 3.1 presents estimates of the rate of mobilization of various toxic heavy metals whether produced by the combustion of fossil fuels and reaching the sea via the atmosphere, or reaching the sea in river transport. These figures include natural weathering and any additions to river water by man. When the estimate for the mobilization of each metal is divided by the concentration of that metal considered to pose minimal risk of deleterious effect, a Relative Critical Index is derived. This index gives the volume of water which would receive an annual increment of the element equal to the concentration shown in column D (toxicity) at the given rates of mobilization. The unit, 10^{12} liters, is equal to a cubic kilometer of water. Thousands of cubic kilometers of ocean water are being contaminated by these elements annually. Most of the input results from natural geochemical cycling, but for the elements listed, man's contribution is also significant. Since the total water volume of the oceans is about 1.4×10^{21} liters, the time to raise the concentrations of the whole ocean to toxic levels could also be calculated, giving times, in each case, of many thousands of years. This computation must be treated with some reserve because the oceans are not uniformly mixed, and the concentration at the locality where the pollutant is introduced will invariably increase more rapidly than the average for the whole ocean. On this basis, the eleven elements listed appear to be the most critical toxic metal pollutants. However, adequate data are not available to evaluate all elements in this way, and some others—transuranic elements for example—might be equally important, in some localities at least.

Table 3.2 compares the toxicity of these eleven elements with available estimates of the concentration found in sea water. The ratio of concentration divided by toxicity shows how close the sea water concentration is to the amount considered to pose a risk, though minimal, of deleterious effects. For mercury, for example, one estimate of current sea water concentration suggests that sea water already contains twice as much mercury (the other half as much)

TABLE 3.1. Toxic Elements of Importance in Marine Pollution Based on Potential Supply and Toxicity, Listed in Order of Decreasing Toxicity (from Ketchum, 1975)

Element	Rate of mobilization (10^9 g/yr)*			Toxicity‡ D (μg/liter)	Relative Critical Index (10^{12} l/yr)§	
	A (man) fossil fuels	B (natural) river flow	C total		A/D	C/D
Mercury	1.6	2.5	4.1	0.1	16,000	41,000
Cadmium	0.35†	?	3.0†	0.2	1,750	15,000
Silver	0.07	11	11.1	1	70	11,100
Nickel	3.7	160	164	2	1,350	82,000
Selenium	0.45	7.2	7.7	5	90	1,540
Lead	3.6	110	113.6	10	360	11,360
Copper	2.1	250	252.1	10	210	25,210
Chromium	1.5	200	201.5	10	150	20,150
Arsenic	0.7	72	72.7	10	70	7,270
Zinc	7	720	727	20	330	36,350
Manganese	7.0	250	257	20	350	12,850

*After Bertine and Goldberg (1971), except for fossil fuel production of cadmium.

†Values from *Third Annual Report of the Council on Environmental Quality* (CEQ, 1972); the total includes other sources which are not necessarily included for the other elements.

‡Water quality criteria: concentration considered to pose minimal risk of deleterious effect (NAS, 1973b).

§For definition of Relative Critical Index, see text.

as should be permitted. Nickel appears from these data to be even more of a problem, with sea water concentrations being equal to (or up to three times greater than) the acceptable toxic level. It is well known that methyl mercury is more toxic than the ionic form. Both Goldberg et al. (1971) and Riley and Chester (1971) list mercuric chloride or a chloride complex ($HgCl_2$ or $HgCl_4^{2-}$) and ionic nickel (Ni^{2+}) as the most probable species of these elements in sea water. Recent studies (Brewer and Spencer, 1970) have shown that considerable variation exists in results of different analysts or analytical methods for heavy metals in sea water. *It is clear that we need to know much more about concentrations, distributions, speciation, and toxicity of these elements before final conclusions can be reached about the hazard they represent to the marine ecosystem.*

On the basis of the data in Tables 3.1 and 3.2, which appear to be the best available at present, four different rankings of relative hazard have been

TABLE 3.2. Toxic Heavy Metals of Importance in Marine Pollution Based
on Their Sea Water Concentration and Toxicity

Element	Seawater concentration (μg/liter)		Toxicity (μg/liter) C	Ratios	
	A	B		A/C	B/C
Mercury	0.2*	0.05*	0.1	2	0.5
Cadmium	0.1	0.05	0.2	0.5	0.25
Silver	0.3*	0.1	1	0.3	0.1
Nickel	7*	2	2	3.5	1
Selenium	0.09*	0.45	5	0.018	0.09
Lead	0.03*	0.03*	10	0.003	0.003
Copper	3*	3*	10	0.3	0.3
Chromium	0.5	0.6*	10	0.05	0.06
Arsenic	2.6	2.3	10	0.26	0.23
Zinc	10*	5	20	0.5	0.25
Manganese	2*	2*	20	0.1	0.1

A:Goldberg et al. (1971).
B:Riley and Chester (1971).
C:As in Table 3.1.
*Variations occur; some not related to salinity, depth or ocean basin.

derived, and these are presented in Table 3.3. Most of the priorities suggested by
this ranking are not surprising. For example, the five elements most frequently
ranked in Table 3.3 as being of high potential hazard include (in order of
toxicity) mercury, cadmium, nickel, copper, and zinc. All of these, with the
possible exception of nickel, have already received considerable attention.
Nickel ranks high because of its relatively high toxicity and its considerable
abundance in the environment. At the lower rankings for potential hazard, it
is surprising that lead, which has also been extensively studied, appears to constitute a lesser threat of damage to the marine environment than might be expected.
Toxic effects of lead have been demonstrated for the terrestrial environment,
but there is no evidence that its presence in sea water has been deleterious to
any marine organism.

All the rankings shown in Table 3.3, and the ratios in Tables 3.1 and 3.2,
upon which these rankings are based, depend upon the assessment of toxicity
which is used in each ratio. If any one of the values given for toxicity is in
error, the ranking for the element would be changed. These toxicity values
(NAS, 1973b) were based upon an extensive literature search, but in some cases
adequate data for marine organisms were lacking. In such cases the best avail-

TABLE 3.3. Ranking of Relative Hazards Offered by
Toxic Elements of Importance in Marine Pollution

| Element | Rank order based on: | | | |
| | Table 3.1 | | Table 3.2 | |
	A/D	C/D	A/C	B/C
Mercury	1	2	2	2
Cadmium	2	6	3	4
Silver	10	9	4	6
Nickel	3	1	1	1
Selenium	9	11	8	8
Lead	4	8	9	9
Copper	7	4	4	3
Chromium	8	5	7	7
Arsenic	10	10	5	5
Zinc	6	3	3	3
Manganese	5	7	6	6

able data for fresh-water organisms were used. Application factors ranging from 0.2 to 0.02 were applied to the results of bioassay tests to derive the "concentration considered to pose minimal risk of deleterious effect." The more stringent application factors were used wherever there was evidence of bioaccumulation, with the consequent prolonged effect on the marine ecosystem. Clearly, however, more long-term evaluations are needed before the order of potential hazard of these elements to the marine ecosystem can be accurately evaluated.

In conclusion, there is no doubt that many heavy metals are toxic to marine organisms, and that man's introduction of some of these has already produced unfortunate effects in some local situations. The elements discussed here should certainly be included in any global assessment of potential hazard and in any standards designed to protect the marine environment from damage. Some other elements, such as fission products and particularly the transuranic elements, should also be given consideration, but these have not been discussed since adequate data are not available for the type of analysis used.

II

Organochlorines in the Aquatic Environment

V. ZITKO

The following remarks deal with organochlorine compounds, defined here as chlorinated hydrocarbons, in some cases containing oxygen. Organochlorine compounds containing other heteroatoms, such as phosphorus, are not considered.

Some organochlorine compounds are used as pesticides and are introduced intentionally into the environment. Another group of these compounds consists of industrial chemicals and is introduced into the environment unintentionally. They are used in a variety of technical products or processes and as a result of these applications leak into the environment. Polychlorinated biphenyls (PCB), polychlorinated terphenyls (PCT), chlorinated naphthalenes, and both low- and high-molecular-weight chlorinated paraffins are examples of organochlorine compounds employed as industrial chemicals. Additional compounds of this class are listed elsewhere in this volume. A third group of organochlorine compounds consists of by-products generated in some industrial processes, e.g., chlorinated aliphatic hydrocarbons, formed during the electrolytic production of chlorine and sodium hydroxide. Another example is the family of chlorinated dibenzofurans and chlorinated dibenzodioxins, which are generated as by-products during the production of chlorinated phenols and which then may be carried over into all products based on chlorinated phenols.

The entry of organochlorine compounds into the environment has been studied, and data are accumulating on the aerial fallout of DDT, aldrin, dieldrin, and PCB. However, the less chlorinated PCBs are quite volatile, and the relative proportion of PCB transported on particulate matter and PCB present in the air in the form of vapors is not known and would make an important study. The fallout may reach either land or water surface, and evaporation from water surfaces may take place quite easily. Recent theoretical calculations of PCB evaporation rates are available (MacKay and Wolkoff, 1973), and it is surprising how large quantities of PCB can be codistilled with water. A correlation between the levels of PCB in zooplankton in the Gulf of St. Lawrence and the amount of rainfall in the St. Lawrence River basin a few days earlier has been described (Ware and Addison, 1973), and this is probably the first direct evidence of atmospheric fallout of PCBs and their subsequent accumulation into the biomass.

The organochlorine compounds, as defined above, have generally very low solubility in water, usually in the 0.1–20 μg/liter range, and most of these compounds are adsorbed with strong affinity by suspended solids. Little is known about the bioavailability of adsorbed organochlorines. Our own experiments indicate, for example, that PCB can be taken up by fish from suspended solids. Certainly this area deserves more research attention.

The situation is complicated further by regional variations in the use of pesticides and industrial chemicals. For example, European wildlife samples almost always contain higher levels of hexachlorobenzene (C_6Cl_6) than samples from North America. European samples may also contain more polychlorinated terphenyls than samples from North America. This may be a reflection of a larger-scale use of PCT in Europe than in the United States and Canada.

Considering the problems of organochlorine compounds in aquatic food chains, there is some controversy whether the main route of uptake is from water or from food. Either or both routes can be important, depending on the circumstances. The results of an experiment in which a PCB-contaminated diet was fed to fish are described in a recent paper (Zitko and Hutzinger, 1972). An interesting feature of that experiment was that there was not much accumulation, and certainly no magnification, of the PCB concentration going from contaminated fish food to fish.

Among the other factors affecting the absorption of organochlorines by aquatic animals may be their molecular weight. For example, while fish readily take up PCB, they take up very little, if any, high-molecular-weight chlorinated paraffins. The molecular weight of these compounds is about twice as high as the molecular weight of Aroclor 1254, and chlorinated paraffins may not be able to penetrate biological membranes. Diet composition probably has an influence on the degree of uptake of these compounds. It is possible that the higher the lipid content of the diet is, the lower the degree of uptake. It is probably the partitioning between the lipid phase, represented by aquatic animals, and the water that primarily determines the uptake or absorption of these compounds (see particularly Kenaga, 1972).

Although the metabolism of organochlorine compounds is the subject of papers by Williams and Gillette in this volume, it is important to emphasize here that fish do not extensively metabolize PCB. It was found during the PCB-feeding experiment already referred to that only one peak of Aroclor 1254, containing tetrachlorobiphenyls, disappeared very slowly after a long time.

The metabolites of PCB, hydroxychlorobiphenyls, or, according to the *Chemical Abstracts* nomenclature, chlorobiphenylols, are more toxic than the parent chlorobiphenyls. The same toxicity relationships exist between, for example, hexachlorobenzene and pentachlorophenol. Hexachlorobenzene is several orders of magnitude less toxic than pentachlorophenol, and the same thing can be seen for chlorobiphenyls and chlorobiphenylols, where the latter are more toxic. The fact that fish do not metabolize, or only slowly metabolize chlorobiphenyls may thus be a blessing in disguise.

The detailed mechanism of the toxic action of organochlorine compounds is not known. The main problem with them is that living matter cannot easily handle the carbon-chlorine bond and cannot split off the chlorine atoms unless these are rendered reactive by virtue of the chemical structure of the molecule. However, most of the applications of industrial organochlorine compounds require that these compounds be quite stable.

Studies of dose-effect relationships are urgently needed so that a large number of data on environmental levels of these compounds can be assessed in terms of their toxicological significance. For fish there are only about six papers based on laboratory experiments which give some information on dose-effect relationships. Some other dose-effect relationships have been indicated by field surveys, such as the data obtained by the Canadian Wildlife Service correlating levels of PCB and DDE in cormorant eggs from Lake Ontario and Lake Erie with breeding success. PCB levels in eggs from the Lake Ontario area are about 23 ppm on wet weight basis as compared to 13 ppm in the Lake Erie region. The reproductive success of cormorants is low in Lake Ontario and normal in Lake Erie. In New Brunswick the levels are 5-10 ppm, but data on reproduction are not available. Results of monitoring in this area indicate that the levels have probably been decreasing during the last three years.

A survey of herring gull eggs gives a similar picture. The levels of PCB in Lake Ontario are generally higher than in Lake Erie, and a number of abnormal herring gull chicks were reported from the Lake Ontario area.

The study of toxicity in aquatic animals is complicated by the fact that, generally speaking, aquatic animals have more different stages in their life cycle than terrestrial animals—eggs, larvae, fry, etc.—which may inhabit different parts of the aquatic environment and may also have different susceptibilities to organochlorine compounds. Physical factors may indirectly influence the toxicity of organochlorine compounds. Temperature, sunlight, precipitation, runoff, and climatic variations may affect the amount of available food, fish may be feeding less at low temperature and may accumulate less lipid, etc. All these factors may change the rate of uptake and the level and toxicity of organochlorine compounds.

Limitations in the chemical analysis and determination of organochlorine compounds may further complicate the problem by making it difficult to obtain a true picture of the extent of contamination. It is very difficult positively to confirm the presence of many of the organochlorine compounds at levels normally seen in the environment. In most cases it is impossible to detect a compound at a level of 0.1 μg/g, and it is very difficult to determine a small amount of one compound in the presence of a large amount of another with similar properties. For example, tetrachlorodibenzofurans have been implicated in PCB poisoning in Japan, but their presence was never confirmed either in the PCB preparation liberated into the environment or in the contaminated rice oil. In many cases, suitable methods for the determination of transformation and degradation products of organochlorine compounds are not developed and analytical standards are not available. Many unidentified peaks can be seen in gas chromatograms of environmental samples, and unexpected compounds could easily escape detection. This is an area which deserves much additional research. The problem is further complicated by the fact that many technical organochlorine materials are very complex mixtures of structurally similar compounds, extremely difficult to analyze. PCBs are an example of such a complex mixture. Techniques are now available to separate very many individual chlorobiphenyls, but on the other hand this makes the analysis very time-consuming. Chlorinated paraffins are another technical product which contains a mixture of compounds not only varying in the length of the paraffin chain from C_{16} to C_{28} but also in the degree of chlorination. In addition, depending on the feed stock used for chlorination, these compounds may contain chlorinated straight-chain paraffins, branched-chain paraffins, alicyclic hydrocarbons, and some aromatics.

There is a great deal of variability between individual specimens, even in carefully collected samples. The OECD program on toxic chemicals in the environment involves the sampling of fish and requires the collection of 25 male fish of the same age each year. The samples are taken at the same time of the year, and fish are analyzed individually. Sex and age variations are eliminated and still the variations in the concentration of organochlorine compounds between individual fish are very high. Standard deviations of the order of 30–40% of the mean are not uncommon. The statistical distribution is usually not normal, but skewed to the high values, and often may be approximated by a log-normal distribution. In addition, in some cases it may not be possible to sample equally old fish for several consecutive years, because the fishery may be based on one very abundant year-class. For example, if the conditions were particularly good in 1968, the fishery may be based almost exclusively on this year-class and may remain in this state for the next five or six years. Three-year-old fish may then be plentiful in 1971, but practically unavailable in 1972. In spite of these problems, the data are encouraging, at least in the sense that there is no increase in PCB, DDE, DDT, and DDD levels in fish and in eggs of herring gulls and double-crested cormorants. Most of our data indicate a decrease, or the existence of a steady state, and a similar situation is reported from Europe.

III

An Experimental Approach to the Study of Pollution Effects in Aquatic Ecosystems

D. SAWARD

Many pollution studies in the aquatic environment are short-term investigations, considering for example the effects of acute concentrations of pollutants on isolated species, or how the hydrography of an area will influence the dispersion of known or predicted discharges. Although they provide a basis for control legislation, such studies do not enable us to evaluate more long-term and general effects.

Survey programs can determine the levels of persistent pollutants (e.g., heavy metals and organochlorines) in the water, sediment, flora, and fauna and provide essential information for the identification of areas showing a gradual trend of increasing pollution, and can also indicate levels in food species which may constitute a human health hazard.

Field study programs can indicate long- and short-term effects of existing polluted conditions, and by monitoring aquatic flora and fauna we can identify specific effects, but it is difficult to determine whether all effects are adverse. Changes in species diversity and relative abundance often reveal gradual changes and it is not easy to differentiate between effects attributable to pollutants and those arising from natural population fluctuations. Major changes can sometimes be more confidently attributed to the effects of pollution, but such observations made in retrospect highlight the problem only after the damage has occurred.

There thus seems to be a need for long-term studies of the effects of pollutants upon organisms under experimental conditions and thus for an environmental bioassay which will determine effects upon food chains rather than individual species.

The aquatic environment supports a complex food web, and simple food chains are difficult to isolate and maintain under controlled conditions. The

Marine Laboratory, Aberdeen, has been studying marine food chains since 1964, and some of the work has been adapted to study the effects of pollutants upon parts of the food web.

Shortly after metamorphosis, young flatfish (*Pleuronectes platessa* L.) in the natural environment graze the siphons of a bivalve mollusk (*Tellina tenuis* Da Costa). The siphons are subsequently regenerated. The bivalves were installed in a sand substrate in large fiberglass tanks 3.7 X 1.8 X 1.2 m, provided with an adequate phytoplankton food supply, and young plaice were introduced to feed on the siphons of the mollusks. An intensive study has been undertaken of this simplified three-stage food chain from phytoplankton to bivalve mollusk to fish.

Many factors must be considered in the experimental investigation of the possible adverse effects of a pollutant upon a food chain and upon individual members of this chain. Failure to achieve realistic interrelationships between different trophic levels in the control (unpolluted) system, failure to consider physicochemical interactions between the low concentration of pollutant and the containers in which the experimental system is housed, and neglect of possible relationships between nutrient supply and the magnitude of toxic effects of the pollutant, all reduce the validity of the conclusion of such studies.

In our experiments the density of *Tellina* was kept comparable with natural densities. After initial feasibility studies a density of $450/m^2$ was chosen. To provide an adequate phytoplankton food supply, 40% of the tank water was exchanged daily. Despite settlement and filtration of the circulating water it was impossible to prevent a number of zooplankton species colonizing the tanks. These provided an additional food source for the plaice. In the natural environment the bivalve siphons become progressively less important in the plaice diet as the fish grow older. Experiments were undertaken to determine the optimal age and stocking density for the plaice. The youngest fish achieved the greatest increases in biomass, and with a stocking density of 40 fish per tank, significant increases in biomass were observed. There was adequate biological tissue for chemical and biochemical analyses, and *Tellina* siphon regeneration played a significant role in the dynamics of the food chain.

The system was adapted to study the effects of pollutants. The aims of the experiments are twofold, firstly to study the distribution of added pollutants in the physical and biological components of the tank ecosystem, and secondly to determine metabolic effects of the pollutant upon the three main stages of the food chain—the phytoplankton, *Tellina*, and fish.

Pollutant conditions in the normal environment are very complex. A single specific discharge may contain many potentially toxic chemicals and the receiving water may contain a complex of organochlorines, heavy metals, and essential nutrients such as phosphate and nitrate. Analytical and sampling problems prevented a study being made of such mixed conditions. It was necessary to study a single chemical type, the synergistic effect of two commonly associated pollutants, and the possible antagonistic effects of a pollutant and nutrient enrichment. This necessary simplification made it more difficult to interpret our results in the context of the marine environment.

Separate studies were made of the effects of copper, mercury, cadmium, and lead on the *Tellina* fish food chain. Results were compared with the levels of these pollutants found in an industrialized bay in the outer part of a large Scottish estuary. The bay (Irvine Bay in the Clyde) is a major flatfish nursery area and *Tellina* siphons are important in the fish diet. Pollutant dose concentrations were chosen, after determination of open sea concentrations, of acutely toxic levels for all stages of the food chain and, in the case of copper, of predicted extreme levels associated with a discharge from a coastal factory.

Each pollutant chosen had different physical properties and had to be carefully considered. Ionic copper levels recorded during the experiments were much lower than the administered dose concentrations. This was caused by the formation of natural chelates, adsorption onto particulate material in the water and onto other components of the tank ecosystem, and, in the case of the highest dose level (100 μg/liter), precipitation at the site of dosing. The exact speciation of the copper in the water was very important. The direct toxic action of copper depends upon the concentration of cupric ions in the water, but from the food chain aspect the particulate-bound copper may be of importance, particularly for the herbivore bivalve. It was not possible to determine whether particulate-bound copper was associated with material of the correct size for ingestion by the *Tellina*. All these problems must be solved before the situation can be fully understood and many of them are common to all the metals studied. In addition there were added losses of mercury caused by its evaporation. For example, during dosing, the level of mercury in the air above the tanks rose to 5-6 times the normal background air concentration. Recorded mercury water levels were often as low as 10% of the calculated addition. Water levels of lead were also lower than predicted. Major losses were due to adsorption onto particulate material in the water, the low solubility of some lead compounds, and the association of this element with a surface film at the water–air interface. Concentrations of cadmium in the water were very constant and reflected the dose levels.

Major adsorption of pollutants occurred in the sand substrate, but the degree of adsorption was different for each metal studied. In natural systems the sediment is very important. It often contains a pool of adsorbed metals and can be involved in their recycling into the environment.

The tank walls, an artificial feature of the ecosystem, were an important site of adsorption of added metals. The amount adsorbed depended on the nature of the material colonizing the tank walls and on the metal concerned. For example, copper at a dose concentration of 100 μg/liter had a significant effect on algal colonization of the tank walls. Levels of copper adsorbed in this case were very low, indicating that the fiberglass substrate was comparatively inert. In tanks dosed with lower concentrations of copper the levels observed were much greater. The algae on the tank walls were the important site of adsorption. In contrast, for other chemicals such as oils and organochlorine the glass fiber itself can be of prime importance.

Accumulation in the bivalve and the fish followed the normal pattern for heavy metals. The majority accumulated in the hepatopancreas of the bivalve and the liver of the fish. The fish were assumed to have accumulated very little indirectly via the food chain, as the muscular siphon tissue of the bivalve accumulated very little heavy metal. The highest levels were found in the herbivore *Tellina*. The experiments did not provide information on the mode of entry and uptake of the metals, their metabolism, and their subsequent excretion. These are all very important when considering the overall toxic action.

A regular sampling program made it possible to determine the effects of the heavy metals studied on the carbon fixation of the phytoplankton and the growth and biochemical composition of the *Tellina* and the fish. It was also possible to determine accumulated concentrations of the pollutants in the physical and biological components of the ecosystem. How can we relate such results to the natural environment?

Experiments with copper showed that copper additions calculated to produce concentrations of 10 μg/liter had adverse effects on the food chain, reducing photosynthetic primary production and affecting the growth and condition of both *Tellina* and fish. These levels refer to concentrations of copper only two or three times higher than have been measured in the Clyde, and it is perhaps significant that levels of copper in *Tellina* collected from Irvine Bay are similar to those found in specimens in the tanks after 100 days of exposure to 10 μg copper/liter. It would seem reasonable to conclude that some effects on the natural food web are possible. It also emphasizes the importance of including nonfood species in a survey program, as baseline studies which concentrate on edible tissue analyses because of the relevance to human consumption may be inadequate for some food chain considerations.

These experiments and other food chain studies being undertaken all pose large management problems and do not provide immediate results. Nevertheless, the approach is fully justified as we are able to combine results with survey and monitoring programs and advise on safer levels of acceptability than those indicated by more short-term studies.

References

Bertine, K. K., and Goldberg, E. D. (1971). "Fossil fuel combustion and the major sedimentary cycle," *Science*, **173**, 233–235.

Brewer, P. G., and Spencer, D. W. (1970). *Trace Element Intercalibration Study*, WHOI Tech. Rep., No. 70-62.

CEQ (1972). *Third Annual Report of the Council on Environmental Quality,* U.S. Government Printing Office, Washington, D.C.

Goldberg, E. D., Broecker, W. G., Gross, M. G., and Turekian, K. K. (1971). "Marine chemistry," in *Radioactivity in the Marine Environment*, National Research Council–National Academy of Sciences, Washington, D.C., pp. 137–146.

Kenaga, E. E. (1972). "Guidelines for environmental study of pesticides: Determination of bioconcentration potential," *Residue Reviews*, 44, 73–113.

Ketchum, B. H. (1975). "Biological implications of global marine pollution," in *The Changing Global Environment* (ed. Singer, S. F.), Reidel, Dordrecht, pp. 311–328.

MacKay, D., and Wolkoff, A. W. (1973). "Rate of evaporation of low solubility contaminants from water bodies to atmosphere," *Envir. Sci. Tech.,* 7, 611–614.

NAS (1973a). *Research Needs in Water Quality Criteria 1972*, National Academy of Sciences–National Academy of Engineering, Washington, D.C.

NAS (1973b). *Water Quality Criteria*, EPA-R3-73-033, March 1973, National Academy of Sciences, Washington, D.C.

Riley, J. P., and Chester, R. (1971). *Introduction to Marine Chemistry*, Academic Press, London.

Ware, D. M., and Addison, R. F. (1973). "PCB residues in plankton from the Gulf of St. Lawrence," *Nature (Lond.)*, 246, 519–521.

Zitko, V., and Hutzinger, O. (1972). "Sources, levels and toxicological significance of PCB in hatchery-reared Atlantic salmon," *Am. Chem. Soc. Div. Water, Air, and Waste Chem.*, 12(2), 157–160.

4

Species Variation in the Metabolism of Some Organic Halogen Compounds

R. T. WILLIAMS, P. C. HIROM, AND A. G. RENWICK

4.1. Introduction

Various aspects of the species differences in the metabolism of drugs and other compounds foreign to the body have been reviewed on several occasions (see Williams, 1964, 1967a, b, 1969, 1971a, b, 1974a, b; Williams and Smith, 1965), and some general patterns have emerged. It appears that the basic pattern of xenobiotic metabolism is the same in most species, but within this pattern there are tremendous species variations. The basic pattern of metabolism is simply that a compound usually undergoes transformation in the body in two phases. In the first phase (I) the compound undergoes reactions which can be classified as oxidations, reductions, and hydrolyses and groups such as OH, COOH, NH_2, and SH are introduced into the molecule, and then the products of

R. T. WILLIAMS, P. C. HIROM, and A. G. RENWICK • Department of Biochemistry, St. Mary's Hospital Medical School, London W2 1PG, England.

this phase undergo reactions (II), which are synthetic in nature and result in polar water-soluble products, usually referred to as conjugates:

$$\text{Xenobiotic} \xrightarrow{\text{I}} \begin{bmatrix} \text{Oxidation,} \\ \text{reduction, or} \\ \text{hydrolysis} \\ \text{products} \end{bmatrix} \xrightarrow{\text{II}} \begin{array}{l} \text{Synthetic} \\ \text{products} \\ \text{or} \\ \text{conjugates} \end{array}$$

The reactions of each phase are controlled by enzymes, which occur mainly in the liver but also are found, usually to a lesser extent, in several other tissues, including the intestine, kidney, lung, etc. Species variations in xenobiotic metabolism are often the result of variations in the occurrence and the amounts of the enzymes which carry out the first and second phases. Apart from variations in the route and rate of these molecular biotransformations, there can be variations in absorption, distribution, and excretion of a xenobiotic and its metabolites. These variations often—but not always—can profoundly influence the biological activity and toxicity of a foreign compound.

Let us now try to examine the fate of halogenated compounds in various species from this point of view. The data on these compounds suitable for comparing different species are at present rather sparse because most of the definitive studies have been carried out mainly on one species, the rat.

4.2. Types of Halogenated Compounds in the Environment

Most of the halogenated compounds used in industry, agriculture, and medicine are those containing chlorine, and therefore for present purposes we shall deal with chlorinated compounds. These include chlorinated benzenes, naphthalenes, and biphenyls, the DDT group, the aldrin–dieldrin group, chlorinated cyclohexanes (BHC), chlorinated phenoxyacetic acids, and chlorinated alkanes (see Fig. 4.1). Several of these compounds are characterized biochemically by their slow rate of metabolism and their tendency to remain in the environment and in animals for prolonged periods. Only the more important members of these groups of compounds have been selected for the discussion in the succeeding paragraphs of this brief review.

4.3. Metabolic Reactions of Chlorinated Hydrocarbons

The reactions of chlorinated compounds in the animal body which can be enzyme-catalyzed include the phase I reactions of hydroxylation, epoxidation,

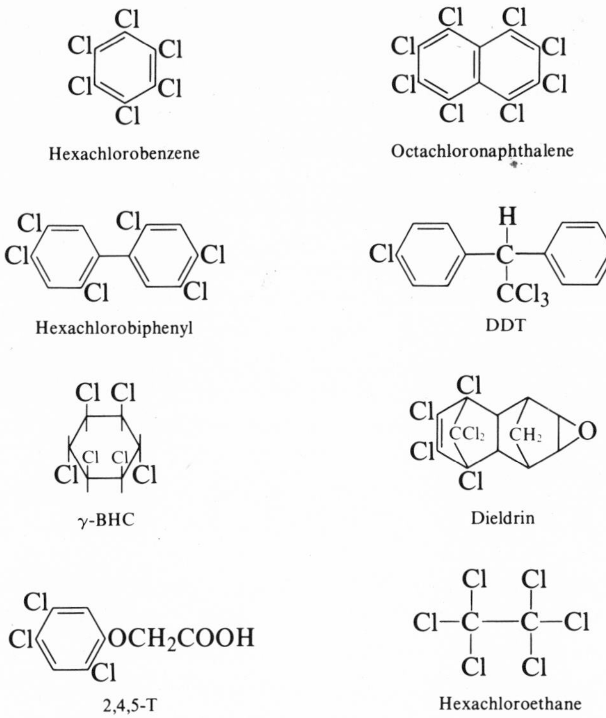

FIG. 4.1. Examples of chlorinated compounds.

hydration of epoxides, dehydrochlorination, and dechlorination and the phase II reactions of glucuronic acid conjugation and mercapturic acid synthesis. The extent to which any of these reactions occurs can depend upon the structure of the chlorinated compound, upon the extent of chlorination, and upon the species, although other factors may also be involved.

It is not possible to consider in this brief review all the groups of chlorinated compounds mentioned above, and in any case data for different species are not always available.

4.4. Chlorinated Benzenes

The chlorinated benzenes, of which there are 12 (three each of di-, tri-, and tetra-, and one each of mono-, penta-, and hexachlorobenzene), are widely used; for example, 1,4-dichlorobenzene is used as a deodorant and hexachlorobenzene as a fungicide. Observations on the metabolism of all these compounds have been made in my laboratory (Williams, 1959), but only in one species, the rabbit, except in the case of monochlorobenzene. The reactions of the chlorobenzenes include hydroxylation to mono- and dihydric phenols followed by the conjugation of these with glucuronic acid and sulfate, and the formation of mercapturic acid. These reactions tend to diminish in extent as the number of chlorine atoms in the molecule increases, although the position of substitution is also important.

For monochlorobenzene, the main routes of metabolism would be expected to be the following:

The extents of these reactions in 13 species using ^{14}C-chlorobenzene, expressed as percentages of the 24-hour excretion of ^{14}C, are shown in Table 4.1. It is to be noted that the basic pattern is quantitatively similar in all species. The main comment that can be made is that mercapturic acid formation is high in the hedgehog and low in the guinea pig. Man appears to be like the guinea pig in this respect, but the other species are fairly similar to one another. It appears that, for chlorobenzene, once the epoxide is formed about 20% follows path (b), 30–40% path (d) to (e), and 40–50% path (c), except in the case of man and the guinea pig, and possibly the ferret and rabbit, in which path (c) is only about 20% and the pathways to the phenol (b) and catechol (d, e) are all about 30% each.

There appear to be no species data on the other chlorinated benzenes, although all 12 compounds have been studied in the rabbit. In this animal, monophenol formation is high in the three dichlorobenzenes (Azouz et al., 1955; Parke and Williams, 1955), in two trichlorobenzenes (1,2,3- and 1,2,4-) (Jondorf et al., 1955), and in one tetrachlorobenzene (1,2,3,4-) (Jondorf et al., 1958), and relatively low in one trichlorobenzene (1,3,5-), two tetrachloro-

TABLE 4.1. Metabolism of ^{14}C-Chlorobenzene in Different Species (from French, 1970)

Species	% of 24-hour excretion of ^{14}C as:		
	4-Chlorophenol	4-Chlorocatechol	4-Chlorophenyl mercapturic acid
Man	33	31	19
Rhesus monkey	19	37	40
Squirrel monkey	14	37	50
Capuchin monkey	19	36	41
Dog	14	45	42
Ferret	33	31	24
Hedgehog	20	12	65
Rabbit	29	38	26
Rat	23	22	49
Mouse	20	31	42
Gerbil	13	26	51
Hamster	15	23	43
Guinea pig	27	35	21

benzenes (1,2,3,5- and 1,2,4,5-), and pentachlorobenzene (Parke and Williams, 1960). Hexachlorobenzene is hardly metabolized at all (Parke and Williams, 1960). With most chlorinated benzenes except monochlorobenzene, mercapturic acid formation is either at a low level or does not occur. An examination of the structures of these chlorinated benzenes shows that metabolism occurs when the molecule contains two unsubstituted vicinal carbon atoms which can presumably be epoxidized (see Table 4.2). In fact, the orientations of the known metabolites of the chlorinated benzenes are those which one would expect from an appropriate epoxide intermediate which can isomerize spontaneously to a phenol, and react with water or glutathione catalyzed by an epoxide hydrase or GSH epoxide transferase, respectively.

4.5. Chlorinated Naphthalenes and Biphenyls (PCB)

Polychlorinated naphthalenes containing five or more chlorine atoms are toxic to animals, while tetrachloronaphthalene produces mild symptoms and the di- and tri- compounds are of low toxicity. These toxic effects seem to be correlated with inability to be metabolized. Presumably the pattern of metabolism (Cornish and Block, 1958) would be similar to that of the chlorinated benzenes, metabolizability being dependent upon an initial epoxidation which

TABLE 4.2. The Extent of Metabolism of Chlorinated Benzenes and Potential Epoxide Formation

Chlorinated benzene	Free vicinal positions	Possibility of epoxide formation	Extent of metabolism
Mono	2,3,4,5,6	+	High
1,2-Di	3,4,5,6	+	High
1,3-Di	4,5,6	+	High
1,4-Di	2,3,5,6	+	High
1,2,3-Tri	4,5,6	+	High
1,2,4-Tri	5,6	+	High
1,3,5-Tri	None	–	Low
1,2,3,4-Tetra	5,6	+	High
1,2,3,5-Tetra	None	–	Low
1,2,4,5-Tetra	None	–	Low
Penta	None	–	Very Low
Hexa	None	–	Very Low

requires vicinal unsubstituted carbons. Species data do not seem to be available on chlorinated naphthalenes.

The metabolic pathways of polychlorinated biphenyls (PCB) are probably similar to those of polychlorobenzenes. Chlorinated biphenyls which contain free vicinal carbon atoms are metabolized by rats, rabbits, and pigeons. This has been shown to be the case with mono-, 4,4'-di-, 2,5,2',5'-tetra-, 3,4,3',4'-tetra-, 2,4,3',4'-tetra-, and 2,4,5,2',5'-pentachlorobiphenyl (Cornish and Block, 1958; Hutzinger et al., 1972; Gardner et al., 1973; Yoshimura and Yamamoto, 1973a, b; Yoshimura et al., 1973; Chen and Matthews, 1974). Trout, however, did not metabolize mono-, 4,4'-di-, or 2,5,2',5'-tetrachlorobiphenyl (Hutzinger et al., 1972). 2,4,5,2',4',5'-Hexachlorobiphenyl (see below), which has no free vicinal carbons, is not metabolized by rats, pigeons, or trout (Hutzinger et al., 1972). The lower polychlorinated biphenyls are also metabolized by Japanese quail

2,4,5,2',5'-penta
metabolized

2,4,5,2',4',5'-hexa
not metabolized

(Bailey and Bunyan, 1972). 5-Hydroxy-2,4,3',4'-tetrachlorobiphenyl is acutely more toxic than the parent 2,4,3',4'-tetrachlorobiphenyl (Yamamoto and

Yoshimura, 1973), and it is suggested that the toxicity of the latter is due to its metabolism to the former. It is also known that several of the chlorinated phenols are more toxic than the corresponding chlorobenzene (Irish, 1962; Deichmann and Keplinger, 1962). It is not clear at present whether the long-term toxicity of polychlorinated benzenes and biphenyls can be ascribed to metabolism to toxic phenols or to their inability to be metabolized. Metabolism to a phenol could result in detoxication, since a phenol is potentially capable of being conjugated with glucuronic acid or sulfate and eliminated from the body.

4.6. 2,2-bis(4′-Chlorophenyl)-1,1,1-trichloroethane (DDT)

It has been shown in various organisms that there are two main initial attacks on the dichlorodiphenyltrichloroethane or DDT molecule. These are reductive dechlorination to DDD (1) and dehydrochlorination to DDE (2). A third minor reaction, namely, aliphatic hydroxylation (3), has been observed in some species (Menzie, 1969). These reactions are confined to the trichloroethane portion of the DDT molecule, the 4-chlorophenyl residues ($R = 4\text{-}ClC_6H_4\text{-}$ in the formulas below) apparently being unattacked. DDD is further metabolized in a series of steps to bis(4-chlorophenyl)acetic acid, DDA, while the hydroxylation product, DDT-OH (kelthane or dicofol), can be metabolized to 4,4′-dichlorobenzophenone. An outline of the metabolism of DDT is as follows:

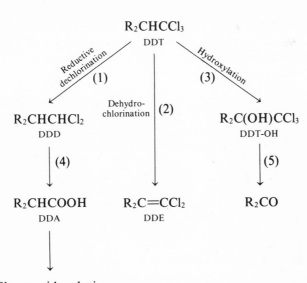

A survey of the literature suggests that the main pathways of DDT metabolism in vertebrates are

$$\text{DDT} \xrightarrow{(1)} \text{DDD} \xrightarrow{(4)} \text{DDA}$$
$$\text{DDT} \xrightarrow{(2)} \text{DDE}$$

But in invertebrates dehydrochlorination (pathway 2) seems to predominate, although variations from one species to another within this pattern occur, as shown in Table 4.3. This table is an attempt to simplify the confusing data which are found in the literature, by simply stating what is the main material found in the feces and urine of some species and in the tissues or excreta of others. The variation in this main pattern is illustrated by the studies of Gingell and Wallcave (1973) and Wallcave et al. (1973) on Swiss mice and Syrian hamsters. The mouse is more susceptible to the acute and subacute toxic effects of DDT than the hamster. Furthermore, DDT is a weak carcinogen in mice, but not in hamsters. The principal urinary metabolite was DDA and the principal fecal

TABLE 4.3. Some Main Metabolites of DDT in Different Species (O'Brien, 1967; Menzie, 1969)

Species	Main metabolites
Rat	DDA (feces, urine)
	DDT (urine)
Mouse*	DDT, DDD (feces)
	DDA, DDE (urine)
Hamster*	DDT, DDD (feces)
	DDA (urine)
Rabbit	DDT, DDA (feces)
	DDA (urine)
Man	DDA (urine)
Monkey	DDA (urine)
Pigeon	DDD, DDE (excreta)
Quail	DDE (excreta)
Blackbird	DDD (excreta)
Chicken	DDA (excreta)
Salmon	DDD
Northern anchovy	DDD
Trout	DDD
Goldfish	DDE
Insects (many species)	DDE
Fruit fly	DDT-OH (Dicofol)

*Gingell and Wallcave (1973).

metabolite was DDD in both species, but the tissue levels of DDT and the liver levels of DDE were much higher in mice than in hamsters.

In fish it is claimed that most of the metabolism of DDT is carried out by intestinal microflora which can convert DDT to DDE and/or DDD (Wedemeyer, 1968).

In insects, DDT is converted mainly to DDE, but in the fruit fly (*Drosophila melanogaster*) it is reported to be converted mainly to the miticide, kelthane or dicofol:

$$R_2CHCCl_3 \xrightarrow{(3)} R_2C(OH)CCl_3$$

4.7. The Aldrin–Dieldrin Group

Aldrin (I) and dieldrin (II) are chlorinated insecticides which are slowly metabolized and persist in the environment. Aldrin can be converted spontaneously to dieldrin, but the conversion also occurs enzymically in all species examined. Table 4.4 shows that the liver microsomes of birds are much less active than those of rats and rabbits in epoxidizing aldrin to dieldrin. This reaction is not a detoxication, since in some species dieldrin is more toxic than aldrin.

TABLE 4.4. Conversion of Aldrin to Dieldrin by Liver Microsomes (from Walker et al., 1973)

Species	Epoxidase activity (mμmole dieldrin formed/min in 30 min)	
	per mg microsomal protein	per g liver
Rat	0.30	4.1
Rabbit	0.34	–
Pigeon	0.078	0.35
Quail	0.20	0.59
Shag	0.06	0.27
Rook	0.31*	0.89*
Fulmar	–	0.81*

*Incubated three times longer than for other species.

Further metabolism of dieldrin probably results in detoxication and there are apparently three pathways whereby this can occur. These include hydration to a diol (III), hydroxylation of the 5,8-methylene bridge to V, and a process equivalent to dehydrochlorination and oxidation to IV.

The main metabolite of dieldrin in female rat urine appears to be dihydro-dihydroxyaldrin (III), in male rat urine, the ketone (IV), and in male and female rat feces, C-12-*syn*-hydroxydieldrin (V) (Matthews et al., 1971; McKinney et al., 1972).

However, there is a paucity of *in vivo* data on species differences in aldrin and dieldrin metabolism (Brooks, 1969). It is known that the main urinary metabolite of dieldrin in rabbits is the dihydrodiol (III) (Korte and Arent, 1965). From *in vitro* studies evidence has been obtained of species differences in the hydration reaction. Dieldrin itself is not readily converted to the diol *in vitro*, but it has been shown to occur slowly in pig and rabbit liver preparations and in certain microorganisms (Brooks et al., 1970). A compound related to dieldrin (HEOD) is HEOM, which lacks the 5,8-methylene bridge of dieldrin. It is nontoxic to the housefly and is readily hydrated by housefly microsomes to a *trans*-dihydrodiol thus:

HEOM

This reaction, when studied *in vitro*, exhibits species variations, and Table 4.5 shows that the livers of some birds are much less active than those of the rat and

TABLE 4.5. Species Variations in the Hydration of HEOM by Liver Microsomes (from El Zorgani et al., 1970)

Species	% hydration by microsomes
Rabbit	98
Rat	94
Rook	92
Jackdaw	90
Fowl	65
Quail	16
Fulmar	13
Pigeon	4

rabbit. This reaction might be used as an indication of the sensitivity of species to cyclodiene epoxides, which might be more toxic to species less able to carry out the reaction.

4.8. Chlorophenoxyacetic Acids

Chlorinated phenoxyacetic acids are extensively used as herbicides and defoliants and therefore become widely dispersed in the environment. They include CPA (4-chloro-), 2,4-D (2,4-dichloro-), MCPA (4-chloro-2-methyl-), and 2,4,5-T (2,4,5-trichlorophenoxyacetic acid). In the soil these compounds are degraded in a few weeks by microorganisms to relatively simple nontoxic substances by

processes involving removal of the acetic acid group, dechlorination, and oxidation and fission of the aromatic ring. Degradation of CPA, 2,4-D, and MCPA by soil pseudomonads has been demonstrated by Evans et al. (1971a, b) and Gaunt and Evans (1971).

The above compounds are strong organic acids, and therefore in animals they could be expected to be excreted mainly in the unchanged state by most animal species. 2,4-D (pKa 2.64) has been reported to be excreted unchanged in the urine by man, dog, rabbit, rat, and sheep. Recent studies of the fate of the defoliant 2,4,5-T in rats, dogs (Piper et al., 1973), and man (Gehring et al., 1973) show that this compound is largely excreted unchanged in these species. The glycine conjugate has been reported as a minor urinary metabolite of 2,4,5-T in the rat (Grunow et al., 1971). There is, however, a species difference in the half-life for the elimination of 2,4,5-T from the body. For an oral dose of 5 mg/kg, this half-life is about 5 h in the rat, 23 h in man, and 87 h in the dog (Piper et al. 1973; Gehring et al., 1973). 2,4,5-T thus takes longer to clear from the dog than from man or the rat, and this may partly explain why it is more toxic to the dog (single oral LD_{50} 100 mg/kg) than to the rat (single oral LD_{50} 300 mg/kg). 2,4,5-T has been suspected of being teratogenic, but it has now been shown to be nonteratogenic in rats and rabbits, although it may still be teratogenic to certain strains of mice (Courtney and Moore, 1971). The teratogenicity of commercial 2,4,5-T has been shown to be due to a chlorinated impurity, 2,3,7,8-tetrachlorodibenzo-p-dioxin:

4.9. Hexachlorocyclohexane

In animals, γ-hexachlorocyclohexane (lindane) is probably broken down relatively rapidly and there is fairly extensive dechlorination, since much of the radioactivity of administered ^{36}Cl-lindane appeared in the urine in the inorganic form (O'Brien, 1967). In insects, e.g., houseflies and grass grubs, the main metabolite appears to be 2,4-dichlorophenylglutathione (Clark et al., 1969), and it has been suggested that lindane may first form a pentachlorocyclohexylglutathione, which then undergoes dehydrochlorination to 2,4-dichlorophenylglutathione. The latter may yield some 2,4-dichlorophenylcysteine by hydrolysis. *In vitro* studies have shown considerable species variations in the degradation of

SR is the glutathione residue, SCH₂CHCONHCH₂COOH
                                       |
                              NHCOCH₂CH₂CHCOOH
                                                |
                                               NH₂

lindane, for Ishida and Dahm (1965) found it to be degraded by homogenates of houseflies and American cockroaches but not by homogenates of German cockroaches, corn borers, honey bees, and rat and rabbit liver.

4.10. Excretion of Organic Chlorinated Compounds in Different Species

During their metabolism in the body, lipid-soluble foreign organic compounds are usually converted into polar, relatively water-soluble metabolites which are readily excreted in the urine and bile. If a compound is already polar it tends to be excreted largely unchanged, as already mentioned in the case of 2,4,5-T, where species differences in the rate of excretion have been found.

Highly chlorinated benzenes, naphthalenes, and biphenyls, DDT, and the dieldrin type of compound are lipid-soluble but are only slowly eliminated from the body. Thus the half-life of dieldrin in man is estimated to be 3-4 months (Brooks, 1969). This slow elimination can be correlated with slow metabolism to polar water-soluble metabolites. Species differences in the rate of elimination have been found. For example, Gingell and Wallcave (1974) found that with oral doses (25 mg/kg) of DDT and DDD the hamster excreted in two days more of the dose in the urine as DDA and its conjugates than mice (see Table 4.6). There was a tendency for the tissue (liver, perirenal fat) levels of DDT and its metabo-

TABLE 4.6. Urinary Excretion and Tissue Concentrations in Mice and Hamsters after Feeding DDT or Its Metabolites (from Gingell and Wallcave, 1974)

Compound fed (25 mg/kg)	% of dose excreted as DDA in two days	
	Mouse	Hamster
DDT	5	10
DDD	13	53
DDE	0	0
DDA	47	60

Tissue*	Total (DDT + DDD + DDE), in ppm	
	Mouse	Hamster
Liver	56	8
Perirenal fat	2390	310

*Examined after six weeks on a diet containing 250 ppm DDT.

lites DDD and DDE to be much higher in mice than in hamsters on chronic feeding of DDT (Table 4.6). Fecal excretion was similar (about 60% of high doses in three days) in both species.

When a compound persists in the body, it could stimulate the activity of drug metabolizing enzymes. This could result in an increased metabolism of the compound itself and of other foreign compounds. Since these highly chlorinated lipid-soluble compounds tend to get stored in fatty tissues it is possible that if their metabolism were stimulated, their concentration in fat would fall. Thus it has been shown that the storage of γ-chlordane in the fat of rats is reduced by feeding DDT (Brooks, 1969). It has also been shown that mice bred from survivors of near-toxic doses of DDT gradually get resistant, the LD_{50} nearly doubling in the ninth generation (Ozburn and Morrison, 1962). However, species differences in these effects can occur. Thus, Gingell and Wallcave (1974) have shown that the urinary excretion of ^{14}C after a single dose of ^{14}C-DDT (25 mg/kg) is increased in hamsters which have been kept on a diet containing 250 ppm of DDT for six weeks, compared with control hamsters not receiving the DDT diet before the dose of ^{14}C-DDT, whereas in mice this did not occur. This species difference was also seen in the effect of DDT on the hexobarbitone sleeping time. DDT in the diet at 250 ppm for six weeks diminished this sleeping time in hamsters but not in mice, yet phenobarbitone (1 mg/ml sodium phenobarbitone in drinking water for five days) diminished the sleeping time in both species.

In various animals, including man, on a fixed dietary intake of DDT and aldrin, the concentration in the tissues increases with time and eventually reaches a maximum or plateau. This may indicate the activation of microsomal enzymes and consequently the stimulation of the metabolism of the compound. The time taken to reach this plateau is dose dependent and there is evidence that this time may vary also with species and, in rats, with sex. In rats on a diet of 0.2 ppm aldrin the plateau storage level (aldrin + dieldrin) was reached in 53 days in male rats and 200 days in females (Ludwig et al., 1964). In man, the plateau was reached in about nine months, when the dose was 211 μg of dieldrin per day (Hunter and Robinson, 1967). With dogs receiving daily 0.1 mg dieldrin/kg, a maximum was approached in 114–121 days, but with endrin there was no accumulation (Richardson et al., 1967). Direct comparison of species, however, is difficult on the basis of the data available.

In reviewing the literature on species differences in the metabolism of organic halogen compounds difficulties arise in the interpretation of data because only rarely has the fate of a compound been investigated in more than a single species by any one group of workers. The various laboratories have used different doses, routes of administration, and analytical methods, and different biological materials both *in vitro*, using tissue homogenates, and *in vivo*, using blood, excreta, and tissues. In many cases, direct comparison of data is not possible since often only one metabolic pathway has been investigated.

The species pattern for the metabolic fate of organochlorines is only vaguely discernible for some compounds at present, since the rate of elimination and the extent of the major metabolic pathways *in vivo* have not been established in a comparable manner for each group of compounds in a number of animal species.

References

Azouz, W. M., Parke, D. V., and Williams, R. T. (1955). *Biochem. J.*, 59, 410-415.
Bailey, S., and Bunyan, P. J. (1972). *Nature (London)*, 236, 34.
Brooks, G. T. (1969). "The metabolism of diene-organochlorine (cyclodiene) insecticides," in *Residue Reviews*, 27, 81-138 (ed. Gunther, F. A.), Springer-Verlag, Berlin.
Brooks, G. T., Harrison, A., and Lewis, S. E. (1970). *Biochem. Pharmacol.*, 19, 255.
Chen, P. R., and Matthews, H. B. (1974). *Soc. Toxicol. Abstracts 13th Ann. Meeting*, Washington, D.C., p. 27.
Clark, A. G., Murphy, S., and Smith, J. N. (1969). *Biochem. J.*, 113, 89-96.
Cornish, H. H., and Block, W. D. (1958). *J. Biol. Chem.*, 231, 583.
Courtney, K. D., and Moore, J. A. (1971). *Toxicol. Appl. Pharmacol.*, 20, 396-403.
Deichmann, W. B., and Keplinger, M. L. (1962). In *Industrial Hygiene and Toxicology*, 2, 2nd. ed., p. 1402. (ed. Patty, F. A.), Interscience, New York.
El Zorgani, G. A., Walker, C. H., and Hassall, K. A. (1970). *Life Sci.*, 9, 415.
Evans, W. C., Smith, B. S. W., Fernley, H. N., and Davies, J. I. (1971a). *Biochem. J.*, 122, 543-551.
Evans, W. C., Smith, B. S. W., Moss, P., and Fernley, H. N. (1971b). *Biochem. J.*, 122, 509-517.
French, M. R. (1970). Ph.D. Thesis, University of London.
Gardner, A. M., Chen. J. T., Roach, J. A. G., and Ragelis, E. P. (1973). *Biochem. Biophys. Commun.*, 55, 1377-1384.
Gaunt, J. K., and Evans, W. C. (1971). *Biochem. J.*, 122, 519-526.
Gehring, P. J., Kramer, C. G., Schwetz, B. A., Rose, J. Q., and Rowe, V. K. (1973). *Toxicol. Appl. Pharmacol.*, 26, 352-361.
Gingell, R., and Wallcave, L. (1973). *Toxicol. Appl. Pharmacol.*, 25, 472.
Gingell, R., and Wallcave, L. (1974). *Toxicol. Appl. Pharmacol.* 28, 385.
Grunow, W., Böhme, C., and Budczies, B. (1971). *Food Cosmet. Toxicol.*, 9, 667-670.
Hunter, C. G., and Robinson, J. (1967). *Arch Environ. Hlth.*, 15, 614.
Hutzinger, O., Nash, D. M., Safe, S., Detreites, A. S. W., Norstrom, R. J., Wildish, D. J., and Zitko, V. (1972). *Science*, 178, 312-314.
Irish, D. D. (1962). In *Industrial Hygiene and Toxicology*, 2, 2nd ed., pp. 1333-1361 (ed. Patty, F. A.), Interscience, New York.
Ishida, M., and Dahm, P. A. (1965). *J. Econ. Entomol.*, 58, 383-392.
Jondorf, W. R., Parke, D. V., and Williams, R. T. (1955). *Biochem. J.*, 61, 512-521.
Jondorf, W. R., Parke, D. V., and Williams, R. T. (1958). *Biochem. J.*, 69, 181-189.
Korte, F., and Arent, J. (1965). *Life Sci.*, 4, 2017.
Ludwig, G., Weis, J., and Korte, F. (1964). *Life Sci.*, 3, 123.
McKinney, J. D., Matthews, H. B., and Fishbein, L. (1972). *J. Agr. Food Chem.*, 20, 597-600.
Matthews, H. B., McKinney, J. D., and Lucier, G. W. (1971). *J. Agr. Food Chem.*, 19, 1244-1248.

Menzie, C. N. (1969). *Metabolism of Pesticides*, Special Scientific Report—Wildlife, No. 127, pp. 128-134, Washington, D.C.

O'Brien, R. D. (1967). *Insecticides: Action and Metabolism*, p. 187, Academic Press, New York and London.

Ozburn, G. W., and Morrison, F. O. (1962). *Nature (London)*, 196, 1009-1010.

Parke, D. V., and Williams, R. T. (1955). *Biochem. J.*, 59, 415-422.

Parke, D. V., and Williams, R. T. (1960). *Biochem. J.*, 74, 5-9.

Piper, W. N., Rose, J. Q., Leng, M. L., and Gehring, P. T. (1973). *Toxicol. Appl. Pharmacol.*, 26, 339-351.

Richardson, A., Lane, J. R., Gardner, W. S., Peeler, J. T., and Campbell, J. E. (1967). *Bull. Environ. Contamination Toxicol.*, 2, 207.

Walker, C. H., El Zorgani, G. A., Craven, A. C. C., Kenney, J. D. R., and Kurukgy, M. (1973). In *Proc. Symp. on Nuclear Techniques in Comparative Studies of Food and Environmental Contamination*, WHO/FAO/IAEA, Helsinki.

Wallcave, L., Gingell, R., and Bronczyk, S. (1973). *Toxicol. Appl. Pharmacol.*, 25, 472.

Wedemeyer, G. (1968). *Life Sci.*, 7(1), 219-223.

Williams, R. T. (1959). *Detoxication Mechanisms*, 2nd ed., Chapman and Hall, London.

Williams, R. T. (1964). "Drug metabolism in man as compared with laboratory animals," *Proc. Eur. Soc. Drug Toxicity*, 4, 9-21.

Williams, R. T. (1967a). "Patterns of excretion of drugs in man and other species," in *Drug Responses in Man*, pp. 77-82 (ed. Wolstenholme, G., and Porter, R.), Churchill Ltd, London.

Williams, R. T. (1967b). *Fed. Proc.*, 26, 1029-1039.

Williams, R. T. (1969). *Pure Appl. Chem.*, 18, 129-141.

Williams, R. T. (1971a). *Ann. N.Y. Acad. Sci.*, 179, 141-154.

Williams, R. T. (1971b) "Species variations in drug biotransformations," in *Fundamentals of Drug Metabolism and Drug Disposition*, Ch. 11, pp. 187-205 (ed. La Du, B. N., Mandel, H. G., and Way, E. L.), Williams & Wilkins, Baltimore.

Williams, R. T. (1974a). "Interspecies scaling," in *Pharmacology and Pharmacokinetics*, pp. 105-113 (ed. Teorell, T., Dedrick, R., and Condiffe, P.), Plenum, New York.

Williams, R. T. (1974b). "Inter-species variations in the metabolism of xenobiotics" (8th CIBA Medal Lecture), *Biochem. Soc. Trans.*, 2, 1-19.

Williams, R. T., and Smith, R. L. (1965). "Biochemistry of rodenticides," in *Drugs and Enzymes, Proc. 2nd Int. Pharmacolog. Meeting, Prague, 1963*, Vol. 4, pp. 331-341, (ed. Brodie, B. B., and Gillette, J. R.), Pergamon, Oxford.

Yamamoto, H., and Yoshimura, H. (1973a). *Chem. Pharm. Bull. (Tokyo)*, 21, 2237-2242.

Yoshimura, H., and Yamamoto, H. (1973b). *Chem. Pharm. Bull. (Tokyo)*, 21, 1168-1169.

Yoshimura, H., Yamamoto, H., and Saeki, S. (1973). *Chem. Pharm. Bull. (Tokyo)*, 21, 2231-2236.

5

Reactive Metabolites of Organohalogen Compounds

JAMES R. GILLETTE

As pointed out by Williams (1959), the reactions by which most foreign compounds, including organohalogen compounds, are metabolized by vertebrate animals can be classified according to two phases. Phase I reactions includes those that either convert one functional group into another (as in the oxidation of alcohol to acetaldehyde and acetic acid) or introduce polar groups into nonpolar compounds (as in the hydroxylation of aromatic compounds, the reduction of nitro compounds, and the hydrolysis of esters). Phase II reactions includes those that conjugate polar groups with glucuronate, sulfate, glycine, glutamine, glutathione, or methyl groups.

Most of the oxidative phase I reactions occur in liver endoplasmic reticulum and are catalyzed by mixed-function oxidases consisting of NADPH cytochrome c reductase and carbon-monoxide-sensitive hemoproteins, collectively called cytochrome P-450 (Gillette, 1966; Gillette et al., 1972).

In the current view of the mechanisms of these enzymes, equivalent amounts of toxicant or drug, oxygen, and NADPH are utilized during the oxidative reactions. The drug substrates combine with the oxidized state of cytochrome P-450 to form complexes that are reduced by an electron from NADPH cytochrome c reductase. Until recently it was generally accepted that the reduced cytochrome P-450 substrate complexes then reacted with oxygen to form oxygenated com-

---

JAMES R. GILLETTE ● Laboratory of Chemical Pharmacology, National Heart and Lung Institute, National Institutes of Health, Bethesda, Maryland 20014.

plexes that then accept a second electron to form "activated oxygen" complexes (Gillette, 1966; Gillette et al., 1972). But the evidence now suggests that in mammalian systems the reduced cytochrome P-450 substrate complexes can accept the second electron before they react with oxygen (Ballou et al., 1974). The source of the second electron has also been debated in the past (Baron et al., 1973). But it now appears that it can originate either from NADPH by way of NADPH cytochrome c reductase or from NADH by way of NADH cytochrome b_5 reductase and cytochrome b_5, which are also present in liver microsomes (Sasame et al., 1973). However the "activated oxygen" cytochrome P-450 substrate complexes may be formed, they rearrange to form oxidized cytochrome P-450 and oxidized products.

Various substrates and inhibitors combine with the oxidized form of cytochrome P-450 and thereby cause small but significant changes in its absorbance spectrum (Gillette et al., 1972; Peterson, 1971; Schenkman et al., 1973). Some substances, such as hexobarbital, aminopyrine, and ethylmorphine, cause a decrease in the spectrum at about 417 nm and an increase at about 391 nm: such substances are called type I compounds. Other substances, such as nicotinamide and aniline, cause a decrease in the spectrum at about 418 nm and an increase at about 423 nm and are called type II compounds. Still other substances cause both kinds of spectral changes, and some cause an intensification of the maximum at about 417 nm. Because of the complexities of these spectral changes and because several endogenous substances including steroids and fatty acids can also alter the absorbance spectrum of cytochrome P-450, the interpretation of the apparent affinity constants and maximal values for the spectral changes is frequently difficult, if not impossible. Nevertheless, it is usually found that type I compounds are metabolized more rapidly than type II compounds because the oxidized cytochrome P-450 complexes with type I compounds are reduced by NADPH more rapidly than are those with type II compounds (Gigon et al., 1969).

The cytochrome P-450 enzyme systems can be inhibited in several different ways (Gillette et al., 1973). For example, various substances can combine reversibly with the oxidized form of cytochrome P-450 and thereby competitively inhibit the metabolism of a given substrate (Mannering, 1971). Other substances, such as piperonyl butoxide, are converted to a metabolite which combines with cytochrome P-450 in a way that prevents the conversion of reduced cytochrome P-450 to its oxygenated form (Franklin, 1971). In addition, some electron acceptors, such as cytochrome c and menadione, can inhibit the metabolism of drugs by competing with cytochrome P-450 for the electrons from NADPH cytochrome c reductase (Gillette, 1966; Gillette et al., 1972, 1973). In fact, there is evidence that cytochrome b_5-mediated reactions in liver microsomes may also inhibit drug metabolism by channeling the electrons of NADPH cytochrome c reductase away from cytochrome P-450 (Correia and Mannering, 1973; West et al., 1974). In accord with this view the rate of drug metabolism may sometimes be greater in the presence of both NADH and NADPH than the sum of the rates in the presence of NADH or NADPH alone. The activities of the cytochrome P-450 enzymes may also be impaired by the prior administration of large doses of certain cations such as Co^{2+} which inhibit ferrochelatase and thereby cause a decrease in the synthesis of cytochrome P-450 heme (Tephley et al., 1973), or by the prior administration of carbon tetrachloride (Smuckler et al., 1967; Castro et al., 1968) or certain allylic compounds (De Matteis, 1973; Levin et al., 1973) which lead to the destruction of cytochrome P-450.

Repetitive administration of a wide variety of substances can accelerate drug metabolism by increasing the activity of cytochrome P-450 systems in liver (Conney, 1967; Conney and Burns, 1972). Indeed, more than 200 substances, including barbiturates, polycyclic hydrocarbons, steroids, polychlorinated insecticides, and biphenyls and even the aromatic oils found in pine, cedar, eucalyptus, and perhaps certain other trees (Ferguson, 1966; Vesell, 1967), enhance the metabolism of drugs by the cytochrome P-450 systems. These substances, however, increase the activity of the enzyme systems in different ways. Pretreatment of animals with phenobarbital causes increases in the amounts of both cytochrome P-450 and NADPH cytochrome c reductase, whereas pretreatment of rats with spironolactone causes very little change in the amount of cytochrome P-450 but increases the activity of NADPH cytochrome c reductase (Gillette et al., 1972). By contrast, pretreatment of animals with 3-methylcholanthrene results in the formation of a variant of cytochrome P-450 called cytochrome P-448, but has little or no effect on the activity of NADPH cytochrome c reductase. Not only does the absorbance spectrum of the carbon monoxide complex of this variant differ from that of the normal kind of cytochrome P-450, but the substrate specificity of the variant differs markedly from that of the normal form.

The reactions catalyzed by these cytochrome P-450 mixed-function oxidases are quite diverse (Brodie et al., 1958; Gillette, 1963; Brodie and Gillette, 1971). For example, compounds that have aliphatic side chains (such as certain barbiturates) or saturated rings (such as steroids) are hydroxylated to form alcohols. Compounds that are either tertiary or secondary amines are oxidatively dealkylated to form aldehydes and either secondary or primary amines. Alkyl-aryl ethers, such as phenacetin, are oxidatively dealkylated to form aldehydes and phenols. Thioethers, such as chlorpromazine, are converted to sulfoxides. Phosphorothionates, such as parathion, phosphonothionates, such as EPN, and phosphorodithionates, such as malathion, undergo oxidative desulfuration to form their respective $P{=}O$ derivatives. Certain primary aromatic amines and their acetylated derivatives, such as p-chloroaniline and N-acetyl-p-chloroanilide, undergo N-hydroxylation to form their hydroxylamino derivatives. Some halogenated aromatic amines, such as p-fluoroaniline, and many halogenated alkanes undergo dehalogenation reactions. Aromatic amines, such as aniline, and aromatic hydrocarbons are converted to phenols either directly or indirectly through the formation of epoxides. Indeed, these enzymes are so versatile that we have begun to believe that there are few low-molecular-weight foreign organic compounds that cannot serve as their substrates. As pointed out by Williams et al. (1974), even the polyhalogenated biphenyls and insecticides that persist in animals for many years are slowly metabolized by these enzymes.

Because the substrate specificity of the cytochrome P-450 enzymes in liver is so broad, there should be little wonder that they also catalyze the oxidation of vitally important substances including various steroid hormones such as cortisone, corticosterone, estrogens, and androgens synthesized in the body (Conney, 1967) and various lipid soluble vitamins such as vitamin D (Richens and Rowe, 1970; Latham et al., 1973). Indeed, several studies have raised the possibility that inducers of these enzymes might cause toxicities by decreasing the concentrations of certain steroid hormones in the body. In most instances, however, the stimulation of metabolism of the steroid hormones brings into play physiological control mechanisms that stimulate the synthesis of the hormone. For example, phenobarbital treatment of rats does not alter the plasma level of corticosterone even though it shortens the half-life of steroids (Bogdanski et al., 1971). Nevertheless, it is possible that in certain animal species or under certain conditions, inducers of cytochrome P-450 enzymes might stimulate the metabolism of endogenous substances to such an extent that the physiological control mechanisms can no longer compensate for their increased metabolism.

Most metabolites formed by cytochrome P-450 enzymes are chemically inert, but they may interact reversibly with various physiological and biochemical processes in the body and thereby cause pharmacological and toxicological responses. By identifying the various metabolites and administering them to animals, investigators are frequently able to determine which of the responses are mediated by the parent drug and which are mediated by the various metabolites. Investigators are also frequently able to determine whether a response is mediated by an active metabolite by using inhibitors and inducers of cytochrome P-450 systems that alter either the rate or the pattern of drug metabolism. For example, when the response is enhanced by inducers and diminished by inhibitors of these systems, it may be inferred that the response is mediated by an active metabolite. Unfortunately, when the response is diminished by inducers and enhanced by inhibitors, investigators cannot reject the possibility that the response is mediated by an active metabolite, because an inducer may increase the metabolism of an active metabolite more than it increases the metabolism of the parent compound, whereas inhibitors may decrease the metabolism of the active metabolite more than they decrease the metabolism of the parent compound. Moreover, it is even more difficult to interpret the effects of various substances on chronically administered drugs and toxicants, because many substances that inhibit cytochrome P-450 enzymes may also be inducers. By following the effects of the inducers and inhibitors on the plasma levels of the metabolites as well as the parent foreign compound, however, investigators are frequently able to resolve many of these difficulties in interpretation.

Occasionally, the cytochrome P-450 enzymes convert foreign compounds to chemically reactive metabolites that either uncouple integrated biochemical processes in cells or combine covalently with various cellular components including proteins, glycogen, lipids, DNA, and RNA. Since the pioneering work of the Millers in Wisconsin (1966, 1970) and of Magee and coworkers in England (Magee and Barnes, 1967), it has become evident that many of these reactive metabolites may account for the carcinogenic effects of certain foreign compounds. Moreover, various investigators have also suggested that chemically reactive metabolites may mediate other kinds of toxicity including mutagenesis, cellular necrosis, hypersensitivity reactions, methemoglobinemia, hemolytic anemia, blood dyscrasias, and fetotoxicities (Brodie, 1967; Judah et al., 1970; Recknagel, 1967; Slater, 1966; Gillette et al., 1974). However, not all chemically reactive metabolites necessarily result in toxicities and not all these kinds of toxicities are necessarily mediated by chemically reactive metabolites. It, therefore, became important to determine which toxicities caused by a given foreign compound may be mediated by chemically reactive metabolites and which are not.

In previous studies of the mechanisms of toxicities mediated by chemically reactive metabolites, various laboratories have assumed that the toxicity results from the covalent binding of the metabolite with a single kind of target substance. They have, therefore, expended considerable effort in attempts to identify the target substance that mediates the toxicity. However, the target substance would obviously depend on the toxicity being studied. Some toxicities may be mediated by the covalent binding of the reactive metabolite to nuclear DNA, others may be mediated by the covalent binding to lipids or to certain enzymes. Moreover, in some kinds of toxicity, such as tissue necrosis and hypersensitivity reactions, the target substance may be any one of a number of different intracellular components and indeed may differ with the reactive metabolite. For example, many investigators believe that the chemically reactive metabolite of carbon tetrachloride causes liver necrosis by combining with phospholipids in the endoplasmic reticulum and thereby promoting lipid peroxidation (Judah et al., 1970; Recknagel 1967; Slater, 1966). But many other substances that also cause centrilobular liver necrosis, such as bromobenzene, do not promote lipid peroxidation (Reynolds, 1972) and therefore cannot cause liver necrosis by this mechanism. Furthermore, the specificity of covalent binding of reactive metabolites to macromolecules can vary markedly with the reactive metabolite being studied. At one extreme of the spectrum, some reactive metabolites, particularly those having relatively low chemical reactivities, may become preferentially bound to certain macromolecules in tissues by first combining reversibly with active centers on a specific macromolecule to form a complex that rearranges to form a covalently bound conjugate. Indeed, this mechanism is the basis of affinity labeling of receptor sites by chemically reactive analogs of endogenous chemical mediators (Singer, 1970), and of the preferential inhibition of choline esterases by organophosphate insecticides and their precursors (O'Brien, 1960). In these situations where relatively few macromolecules are covalently bound to the metabolite or where the toxicity mimics well-characterized pharmacologic actions, the identification of the target substance is relatively easy. At the other extreme, however, highly reactive metabolites of foreign compounds combine indiscriminately with many different kinds of intracellular components including protein, lipids, glycogen, DNA, and RNA (Miller and Miller, 1966; Miller, 1970; Magee and Barnes, 1967; Weisburger and Weisburger, 1973). In most instances, however, the relative rates of covalent binding to different kinds of macromolecules vary with the reactive metabolite and the tissue. Thus, the identification of the target substance can be very difficult. Indeed, when a reactive metabolite interacts with a number of biochemical systems simultaneously, it is difficult to determine whether changes in cell function results from a sequence of changes originating from a single biochemical alteration or from the concerted action of a number of different initial biochemical alterations.

Because highly reactive metabolites can react with so many different kinds of macromolecules in tissues, and because so little is known about the mechanisms by which a given metabolite–macromolecular conjugate might lead to diverse toxicities and much less is known about how combinations of metabolite–macromolecular conjugates might evoke toxicities, there seems to be little reason for assuming that the covalent binding of reactive metabolites to any given type of macromolecule accounts for the toxicity mediated by the reactive metabolites. It also seems evident that the finding of covalently bound radiolabel to tissue macromolecules after the administration of a radiolabeled foreign compound would not be sufficient proof that a reactive metabolite mediated the toxicity under investigation or any other toxicity.

Nevertheless, the incidence and severity of any toxicity mediated by a chemically reactive metabolite should be roughly proportional to the number of target macromolecule–metabolite conjugates formed in the tissue after the administration of the foreign compound. Moreover, changes in the concentration of the reactive metabolite within a given tissue should alter not only the rate of covalent binding of the reactive metabolite to the target macromolecule but also its rate of covalent binding to other macromolecules. Thus, treatments of animals that alter the amount of covalent binding to both the target macromolecules and other macromolecules should cause parallel changes in the incidence and severity of the toxicity. According to this view, it should not be necessary to identify either the reactive metabolite or the target macromolecule in order to determine whether the toxicity was mediated by a chemically reactive metabolite, an inert drug, or inert metabolites. Indeed, with highly reactive metabolites it may not even be necessary that the target substance be present in the sample being assayed for covalent binding.

In order to evaluate our approach for determining whether a toxicity caused by a foreign compound is mediated by a chemically reactive metabolite, studies were carried out on the centrilobular liver necrosis caused by large doses of bromobenzene (Koch-Weser et al., 1952, 1953). Although the urinary metabolites of bromobenzene had been identified many years ago (Azouz et al., 1953; Knight and Young, 1958), a series of recent studies revealed that nearly all of the bromobenzene administered to animals is rapidly converted to a chemically reactive arene oxide, bromobenzene-3,4-epoxide, by a cytochrome P-450 enzyme in liver microsomes (Brodie et al., 1971; Zampaglione et al., 1973; Jollow et al., 1974 a, b). Indeed, as pointed out by Williams et al. (1974), the formation of epoxides presumably accounts for the requirement of two unsubstituted vicinal carbon atoms for the rapid metabolism of halogenated benzenes and biphenyls. Once formed, the bromobenzene-3,4-epoxide may rearrange nonenzymatically to form p-bromophenol, or undergo a hydration catalyzed by an epoxide hydrolase in liver microsomes to form a dihydrodiol which in turn may be dehydrogenated to form a catechol. But about 70% of the epoxide formed in rats receiving a nontoxic dose of bromobenzene is converted to a glutathione conjugate by a glutathionyl transferase in the soluble fraction of liver (Table 5.1). The glutathione conjugate is then hydrolyzed to form the cysteine derivative, which in turn is

TABLE 5.1 Bromobenzene Metabolites in Rat Urine
(from Zampaglione et al., 1973)

Treatment and dose	% of total urinary metabolites				
	Bromophenyl mercapturic acid	4-Bromo-phenol	Bromo-catechol	Bromophenyl dihydrodiol	2-Bromo-phenol
None					
nontoxic dose					
(0.05 mmol/kg)	70	18	4	4	3
toxic dose					
(10 mmol/kg)	48	37	6	4	4
Phenobarbital					
toxic dose					
(1.5 mmol/kg)	46	37	9	7	1
3-Methyl-cholanthrene					
high dose					
(10 mmol/kg)	31	20	10	17	21

acetylated and excreted into urine as a mercapturic acid. The steady-state concentration of the epoxide within hepatocytes thus depends on the relative rates at which it is formed and inactivated by the various enzymatic and nonenzymatic reactions and the rate at which it escapes from the cells and enters the blood.

Initial chemical and radioautographic studies with radiolabeled bromobenzene revealed not only that a metabolite of bromobenzene became covalently bound to liver macromolecules but also that the covalently bound metabolite was localized preferentially in the centrilobular necrotic areas of liver (Brodie et al., 1971). However, studies on the covalent binding of different doses of bromobenzene revealed that the proportion of the dose that became covalently bound remained relatively low until a critical dose between 1.2 and 2.15 nmoles/kg was used (Reid and Krishna, 1973). Above this critical dose the proportion that became covalently bound was nearly doubled and the liver necrosis became manifest (Table 5.2).

The reason for the threshold dose became clear when it was realized that the levels of glutathione in liver are decreased after the administration of toxic doses of bromobenzene until the rate of formation of the glutathione conjugate was limited by the availability of this cosubstrate. This view was confirmed by Jollow et al. (1974a), who showed that the rate of covalent binding of bromobenzene metabolites to liver macromolecules was markedly increased after the glutathione levels were depleted. Moreover, the proportion of the dose excreted into urine as bromobenzene mercapturic acid was significantly smaller after a toxic dose of bromobenzene than it was after a nontoxic dose (Zampaglione et al., 1973).

Although the results of these experiments were consistent with the view that the liver necrosis was mediated by bromobenzene-3,4-epoxide, we did not consider them conclusive. For this purpose, studies were carried out to determine whether various treatments would cause parallel changes in the severity of the necrosis and in the concentration of covalently bound metabolite. For example, the prior administration of diethyl maleate, which depletes the glutathione in

TABLE 5.2. Dose Dependence of Covalent Binding
(from Reid and Krishna, 1973)

Dose (mmol/kg)	Covalent binding (mmol/g protein)	Binding/dose
0.24	0.082	0.34
0.74	0.184	0.26
1.20	0.335	0.28
2.15	1.180	0.55
4.06	2.528	0.62

liver to about the same extent as bromobenzene but does not cause liver necrosis, increased not only the covalent binding of radiolabeled bromobenzene but also the severity of the necrosis (Reid and Krishna, 1973). Moreover, pretreatment of the animals with phenobarbital, which increases the activity of cytochrome P-450 enzymes, also increased both the hepatic necrosis and the amount of covalently bound bromobenzene metabolites (Brodie et al., 1971, Reid and Krishna, 1973). On the other hand, the prior administration of SKF 525-A (β-diethylaminoethyl-2,2-diphenylvalerate), which inhibits the cytochrome P-450 enzymes in liver microsomes (Brodie et al., 1958; Gillette, 1963, 1966), decreases both the severity of the hepatic necrosis and the amount of covalently bound metabolite (Brodie et al., 1971; Reid and Krishna, 1973). Since the changes in the covalent binding of the reactive bromobenzene metabolite paralleled changes in the severity of the toxicity caused by bromobenzene, we conclude that the toxicity was mediated by the reactive metabolite.

The centrilobular liver necrosis caused by other halogenated benzene derivatives is also probably caused by their arene oxide derivatives (Reid and Krishna, 1973). Centrilobular necrosis and large amounts of covalently bound metabolites occur in rat liver after the administration of large doses of iodobenzene or o-dichlorobenzene, but not after the administration of fluorobenzene or p-dichlorobenzene. Moreover, pretreatment of rats with phenobarbital increases the covalent binding of the radiolabel and the severity of the hepatic necrosis of iodobenzene and o-dichlorobenzene, but has little effect on the covalent binding of fluorobenzene and p-dichlorobenzene.

Although SKF 525-A decreased the covalent binding of the reactive metabolite of bromobenzene to liver protein and pretreatment of animsls with phenobarbital increased it, the reason for these results was not evident to us at first. When the rates of formation of the reactive metabolite and the rates of elimination of the parent compound by other routes are directly proportional to the concentration of the parent compound, and when the rates of inactivation of the reactive metabolite along various pathways are directly proportional to concentration of the reactive metabolite (that is, all the processes by which the parent compound and the reactive metabolite are formed or eliminated follow first-order kinetics), the amount of covalently bound metabolite in any given tissue should accumulate until all of the foreign compound in the body is metabolized. Thus, treatments that alter the rates of formation and inactivation of the reactive metabolite should not affect the amount of reactive metabolite that ultimately becomes covalently bound, unless they also cause changes in either the proportion of the dose of foreign compound that is converted to the reactive metabolite or the proportion of the reactive metabolite that becomes covalently bound to tissue macromolecules (Gillette, 1973). Since virtually all of the bromobenzene administered to rats and mice is converted to bromobenzene-3,4-epoxide, phenobarbital pretreatment and SKF 525-A administration would not be expected to affect the proportion of the dose that is converted to the reactive metabolite. Thus, the pretreatment with phenobarbital or SKF 525-A can alter the covalent binding only by changing the proportion of the epoxide that becomes covalently bound. In fact, the pretreatment with phenobarbital should decrease the covalent binding instead of increasing it, because phenobarbital induces the epoxide hydrolase that inactivates bromobenzene-3,4-epoxide (Daly et al., 1972). Moreover, SKF 525-A should have had no effect on the covalent binding, because it presumably has no effect on either the epoxide hydrolase or the glutathione transferase. The reason for the increase in covalent binding became clear when it was found that the pretreatment with phenobarbital increases the covalent binding of the reactive metabolite only after the administration of toxic doses of bromobenzene that deplete the liver of glutathione (Jollow et al., 1974a). After glutathione is depleted, the rate of formation of the glutathione conjugate is no longer directly proportional to the concentration of the epoxide but depends on the synthesis of glutathione or on the mobilization of cysteine. Thus, the proportion of the epoxide that becomes covalently bound depends on the relative rates at which bromobenzene-3,4-epoxide and glutathione are formed. By contrast, phenobarbital pretreatment decreases the covalent binding of low, nontoxic doses of bromobenzene (Table 5.3) (Reid and Krishna, 1973).

Pretreatment of animals with other inducers, however, does not always result in increased covalent binding and toxicity of bromobenzene. For example, the pretreatment of rats with 3-methylcholanthrene decreases both the covalent binding of bromobenzene to liver protein and the severity of liver necrosis (Zampaglione et al., 1973; Reid et al., 1973) by a number of interdependent mechanisms. Since the pretreatment does not alter the biological half-life of bromobenzene in rats, and actually increased the rate of bromobenzene metabolism by liver microsomes, the protective effect must have occurred by a marked alteration in the pattern of metabolism of bromobenzene. Studies on the pattern of urinary metabolites of rats receiving a toxic dose of bromobenzene revealed that the 3-methylcholanthrene treatment resulted in a decrease in mercapturic acid and 4-bromophenol but an increase in bromocatechol, bromophenyldihydrodiol,

TABLE 5.3. Effect of Phenobarbital on the
Covalent Binding of Bromobenzene to
Mouse Liver Proteins *in Vivo*
(from Reid and Krishna, 1973)

Dose	Control	Phenobarbital
0.13	0.074	0.027
1.50	0.794	0.989
4.85	0.443	9.83

and 2-bromophenol (Table 5.1) (Zampaglione et al., 1973). Since 2-bromophenol cannot be formed from the nonenzymatic rearrangement of bromobenzene-3,4-epoxide, it seems likely that 3-methylcholanthrene induces the formation of a different epoxide, presumably bromobenzene-2,3-epoxide. Moreover, the increase in the bromocatechol and the bromophenyldihydrodiol fractions at the expense of mercapturic acids in the urine of 3-methylcholanthrene-treated rats implies that the epoxide hydrase, as well as the cytochrome P-450 enzyme, was induced (Zampaglione et al., 1973; Daly et al., 1972). Increasing the formation of the bromobenzene-2,3-epoxide thus decreases the proportion of the dose of bromobenzene that is converted to bromobenzene-3,4-epoxide, which may be the more reactive arylating intermediate. At the same time, increasing the activity of epoxide hydrase decreases the dependence of hepatic cells on the glutathione transferase in the inactivation of the epoxides, and hence decreases the rate of utilization of glutathione. By decreasing the rate of formation of glutathione conjugates, the concentration of glutathione in liver cells is more easily maintained at relatively high levels by the synthesis of glutathione and the mobilization of nucleophilic substances, such as cysteine from body stores. The net effect is thus a decrease not only in the proportion of the dose that is converted to the more potent reactive metabolite, but also in the proportion of the reactive metabolite that becomes covalently bound.

The covalent binding of bromobenzene is not restricted to liver but also occurs in lung and kidney and to a lesser extent in a number of other tissues (Reid and Krishna, 1973). The source of the reactive metabolite, however, was obscure. If the metabolite were so chemically reactive that it could not leave the tissue in which it was formed, then the covalent binding should be restricted to the tissues containing cytochrome P-450. On the other hand, if the metabolite were relatively stable, it might be able to leave hepatocytes and be carried by the blood to the lungs and kidney. At first it seemed possible that covalent binding of the bromobenzene-3,4-epoxide might be restricted to tissues in which it was formed, because *in vitro* experiments revealed that lung contained cytochrome P-450 enzymes that catalyzed the formation of a reactive metabolite of bromobenzene (Reid et al., 1973; Reid, 1973). But the pretreatment of mice with phenobarbital increased the covalent binding of the reactive metabolite to proteins in lung and kidney after the administration of a toxic dose of bromobenzene, even though the pretreatment with phenobarbital did not increase the activity of cytochrome P-450 in lung. Thus, most of the reactive metabolite that combined with proteins in lung was formed in the liver, even though the lung was also able to synthesize the reactive metabolite.

Although the reactive metabolites of halogenated benzenes and perhaps halogenated biphenyls are mainly epoxides, the reactive metabolites of halogenated alkanes and alkenes are apparently formed by a variety of reactions. The reactive metabolite of carbon tetrachloride and trichloromonobromomethane is presumably trichloromethyl free radical. However, the mechanisms by which the free radical is synthesized from these toxicants may differ. We believe that carbon tetrachloride is converted to the free radical by reductive cleavage catalyzed by a cytochrome P-450 in liver microsomes. In support of this view, the covalent binding of the reactive metabolite of carbon tetrachloride to liver microsomes *in vitro* requires NADPH, occurs more rapidly under anaerobic conditions than in air, and is inhibited by carbon monoxide (Sipes et al., 1972; Uehleke et al., 1973). On the other hand, the covalent binding of the reactive metabolite of trichloromonobromomethane to liver microsomes also re-requires NADPH, but occurs slightly more rapidly in air than in nitrogen (Krishna et al., 1973). Moreover, the anaerobic reaction is not inhibited by carbon monoxide even though pretreatment of the animals with allyl isopropyl-acetamide, which selectively destroys cytochrome P-450 in liver, impairs the covalent binding. The reactive metabolite of chloroform is also formed more rapidly in air than in nitrogen but carbon monoxide blocks the covalent binding of the metabolite under anaerobic conditions. Whatever the mechanism for the formation of these reactive metabolites, it is evident that NADPH cytochrome P-450 reductase is required because an antibody against this enzyme will block the covalent binding of all three toxicants (Krishna et al., 1973). Moreover, the cytochrome P-450 which apparently catalyzes the formation of the reactive metabolites of carbon tetrachloride and chloroform differs from that which metabolizes the metabolism of most drugs. Pretreatment of rats or mice with isopropyl alcohol, which markedly potentiates the toxicity of the toxicants (Traiger and Plaa, 1971), markedly increases their covalent binding to liver lipids and proteins both *in vivo* and *in vitro*, but does not significantly alter the activity of NADPH cytochrome c reductase, the concentration of cytochrome P-450, or the N-demethylation of ethylmorphine (Sipes et al., 1973; Maling et al., 1974).

It is also noteworthy that chloroform but not carbon tetrachloride decreases the concentration of glutathione in liver of rats pretreated with phenobarbital (Sipes et al., 1974), even though carbon tetrachloride is more toxic than chloroform. Although the reason for this difference is obscure, it suggests that the reactive metabolites formed from the two toxicants may have remarkably different properties.

Although acetaminophen (paracetamol) is not a halogenated organic compound, our studies on the formation of its toxic metabolite illustrate other principles that are important in studying the toxicity of reactive metabolites. In both mice and hamsters receiving low doses of the drug, most of it is eliminated in urine as its glucuronide and sulfate conjugates, but about 10–15% of the dose is converted to a reactive metabolite that combines with glutathione and is ultimately excreted in urine as its mercapturic acid (Jollow et al., 1974b). After the administration of high doses of the drug, the glutathione in liver is depleted and the covalent binding of the reactive metabolite is markedly increased, resulting in centrilobular necrosis of the liver (Mitchell et al., 1973a, 1973b; Jollow et al., 1973; Potter et al., 1973; Davis et al., 1974). After these high doses, however, the proportion of the dose that is excreted into urine decreases to values (about 5%) which are similar to those found in rats. But rats convert the drug to the reactive metabolite so slowly that they rarely deplete the liver of glutathione and rarely develop centrilobular necrosis. Thus, the pattern of urinary metabolites of a foreign compound may appear to be virtually identical in two different animal species, but the compound may be toxic in one species and not in the other.

It is also important to realize that a given inducer may cause opposite results in different animal species. In mice, phenobarbital increases the cytochrome P-450 enzyme that converts acetaminophen to its reactive metabolite but has little effect on either the UDP-glucuronyl transferase or PAPS transferase which catalyzes the formation of the glucuronide and sulfate conjugates of acetaminophen. Thus, in mice, phenobarbital exerts little if any effect on the biological half-life of the drug (Jollow et al., 1974b), but it markedly increases both the covalent binding of the reactive metabolite to liver protein and the severity of the liver necrosis, because it increases the proportion of the dose that is converted to the reactive metabolite. By contrast, in hamsters, phenobarbital only slightly increases the liver cytochrome P-450 enzyme that catalyzes the formation of the reactive metabolite but markedly induces UDP-glucuronyl transferase. Thus, in hamsters, phenobarbital shortens the biological half-life of acetaminophen, but decreases both the covalent binding of the reactive metabolite to liver protein and the severity of the liver necrosis, because it decreases the proportion of the dose that is converted to the reactive metabolite.

Summary

In addition to determining whether a compound or a mixture of compounds causes various toxicities, it is important to discover whether the compound causes toxicities by combining reversibly with active sites, by altering the metabolism of endogenous substrates or exogenous vitamins, by being converted to metabolites that combine reversibly with active sites, or by being converted to chemically reactive metabolites. Such knowledge may provide clues to ways by which the toxicity of environmental pollutants may be prevented in endangered species or ways by which the pollutants may be decreased in the food chain. In some situations, induction of enzymes that hasten the elimination of toxicants may effectively prevent the toxicity. But in other situations, induction of these enzymes may potentiate toxicities.

In the present paper, I have attempted to illustrate a number of situations in which broad generalizations should be accepted with caution.

1. Studies with several halogenated benzenes and other foreign compounds indicate that severe toxicities such as liver necrosis may occur only when a threshold dose is exceeded. At low doses, these foreign compounds may be innocuous but at high doses they may cause serious toxicities. At these high doses either a greater proportion of the dose is converted to a reactive metabolite or a greater proportion of the reactive metabolite combines with tissue components and thereby causes the toxicity.

2. Which of these situations predominates may be influenced by prior administration of inducers or inhibitors of drug-metabolizing enzymes. The effects of the pretreatment may depend on the dose. At low doses of bromobenzene, phenobarbital pretreatment decreases the covalent binding of the reactive metabolites, whereas at high doses the pretreatment increases the covalent binding of the reactive metabolite. Thus, any toxicity that is caused by low levels of the reactive metabolite would be decreased by pretreatment of animals after low doses of the toxicants are administered, but would be increased after high doses are given.

3. The administration of certain inducers may affect the severity of toxicities by altering the proportion of the toxicant that is converted to reactive metabolites. Thus, the pretreatment of animals with 3-methylcholanthrene decreases the proportion of bromobenzene that is converted to bromobenzene-3,4-epoxide and thereby decreases its covalent binding and toxicity.

4. Even though enzyme systems that form reactive metabolites are present in extrahepatic tissues, it cannot be automatically assumed that all of the reactive metabolite that reacts with components of extrahepatic tissues is formed in those tissues. However, when a major portion of the covalently bound reactive metabolite in extrahepatic tissues is produced in those tissues, various treatments may decrease toxicities in some tissues but enhance them in others.

5. A given inducer may cause opposite effects in different species. For example, in mice, pretreatment with phenobarbital potentiates the liver necrosis caused by acetaminophen but in hamsters it decreases the toxicity.

6. Seemingly trivial differences in the structure of halogenated organic compounds may result in marked differences in toxicity and in the mechanism of reactive metabolite formation. For example, o-dichlorobenzene is more toxic than p-dichlorobenzene, presumably because o-dichlorobenzene may form an epoxide analogous to bromobenzene-3,4-epoxide, whereas p-dichlorobenzene cannot. Moreover, the formation of free radicals from CCl_4 and CCl_3Br may occur by different enzymatic pathways in liver microsomes and the reactive metabolite of chloroform may not be a free radical. Thus, it may be a mistake to extrapolate data from one compound to another, even when they appear to be structurally similar.

References

Azouz, W. M., Parke, D. V., and Williams, R. T. (1953). *Biochem. J.,* **55**, 146.

Ballou, D. P., Veeger, C., van der Hoeven, T. A., and Coon, M. J. (1974). *FEBS Letters,* **38**, 337.

Baron, J., Hildebrandt, A. G., Peterson, J. A., and Estabrook, R. W. (1973). *Drug Metabol. Dispos.,* **1**, 129.

Bogdanski, D. F., Blaszkowski, T. P., and Brodie, B. B. (1971). *J. Pharmacol. Exptl. Therap.* **179**, 372.

Brodie, B. B. (1967). "Idiosyncrasy and intolerance," in *Ciba Foundation Symposium on Drug Response in Man* (ed. Wolstenholme, G. E. W., and Porter, R.), J & A. Churchill Ltd., London, pp. 188–213.

Brodie, B. B., and Gillette, J. R. (1971). *Handbook of Experimental Pharmacology,* Vol. 28: *Concepts in Biochemical Pharmacology,* Pt 2 (ed. Brodie, B. B., and Gillette, J. R.), Springer-Verlag, Berlin.

Brodie, B. B., Gillette, J. R., and La Du, B. N. (1958). *Ann. Rev. Biochem.,* **27**, 427.

Brodie, B. B., Reid, W. D., Cho, A. K., Sipes, G., Krishna, G., and Gillette, J. R. (1971). *Proc. Nat. Acad. Sci.,* **68**, 160.

Castro, J. A., Sasame, H., and Gillette, J. R. (1968). *Life Sci.,* **7**, 129.

Conney, A. H. (1967). *Pharmacol. Rev.,* **19**, 317.

Conney, A. H., and Burns, J. J. (1972). *Science,* **178**, 576.

Correia, M. A., and Mannering, G. J. (1973). *Mol. Pharmacol.* **9**, 455.

Daly, J. W., Jerina, D. M., and Witkop, B. (1972). *Experientia,* **28**, 1129.

Davis, D. C., Potter, W. Z., Jollow, D. J., and Mitchell, J. R. (1974). *Life Sci. Sci.,* **14**, 2099.

De Matteis, F. (1973). *Drug Metabol. Dispos.* **1**, 267.

Ferguson, H. C. (1966). *J. Pharm. Sci.,* **55**, 1142.

Franklin, M. R. (1971). *Xenobiotica,* **1**, 181.

Gigon, P. L., Gram, T. E., and Gillette, J. R. (1969). *Molec. Pharmacol.,* **5**, 109.

Gillette, J. R. (1963). *Prog. Drug Res.,* **6**, 11.

Gillette, J. R. (1966). *Adv. Pharmacol.,* **4**, 219.

Gillette, J. R. (1973). *Proc. 5th Int. Congr. Pharmacol.,* **2**, 187.

Gillette, J. R., Davis, D. C., and Sasame, H. A. (1972). *Ann. Rev. Pharmacol.,* **12**, 57.

Gillette, J., Sasame, H., and Stripp, B. (1973). *Drug Metabol. Dispos.,* **1**, 164.

Gillette, J. R., Mitchell, J. R., and Brodie, B. B. (1974). *Ann Rev. Pharmacol.,* **14**, 271.

Jollow, D. J., Mitchell, J. R., Potter, W. Z., Davis, D. C., Gillette, J. R., and Brodie, B. B. (1973). *J. Pharmacol. Exp. Therap.,* **187**, 195.

Jollow, D. J., Mitchell, J. R., Zampaglione, N., and Gillette, J. R. (1974a). *Pharmacology,* **11**, 151.

Jollow, D. J., Thorgeirsson, S. S., Potter, W. Z., Hashimoto, M., and Mitchell, J. R. (1974b). *Pharmacology,* **12**, 251.

Judah, J. D., McLean, A. E. M., and McLean, E. K. (1970). *Amer. J. Med.,* **49**, 609.

Knight, R. H., and Young, L. (1958). *Biochem. J.,* **70**, 111.

Koch-Weser, D., De la Huerga, J., and Popper, H. (1952). *Proc. Soc. Exp. Biol. Med.,* **79**, 196.

Koch-Weser, D., De la Huerga, J., Yesinick, C., and Popper, H. (1953). *Metabolism,* **2**, 248.

Krishna, G., Sipes, I. G., and Gillette, J. R. (1973). *The Pharmacologist,* **21**, 158.

Latham, A. N., Millbank, L., and Richens, A. (1973). *J. Clin. Pharmacol.,* **13**, 337.

Levin, W., Jacobson, M., Sernatinger, E., and Kuntzman, R. (1973). *Drug Metabol. Dispos.* **1**, 275.

Magee, P. N., and Barnes, J. M. (1967). *Adv. Cancer Res.,* **10,** 163.

Maling, H. M., Eichelbaum, F. M., Saul, W., Sipes, I. G., Brown, E. A. B., and Gillette, J. R. (1974). *Biochem. Pharmacol.,* **23,** 1479.

Mannering, G. J. (1971). In *Handbook of Experimental Pharmacology,* Vol. 28: *Concepts in Biochemical Pharmacology,* Pt 2, p. 452 (ed. Brodie, B. B., and Gillette, J. R.), Springer-Verlag, Berlin.

Miller, E. C., and Miller, J. A. (1966). *Pharmacol. Rev.,* **18,** 805.

Miller, J. A. (1970). *Canc. Res.,* **30,** 559.

Mitchell, J. R., Jollow, D. J., Potter, W. Z., Davis, D. C., Gillette, J. R., and Brodie, B. B. (1973a). *J. Pharmacol. Exp. Therap.,* **187,** 185.

Mitchell, J. R., Jollow, D. J., Potter, W. Z., Davis, D. C., Gillette, J. R., and Brodie, B. B. (1973b). *J. Pharmacol. Exp. Therap.,* **187,** 211.

O'Brien, R. D. (1960). In *Toxic Phosphorous Esters,* Chap. III, Academic Press, New York.

Peterson, J. A. (1971). *Arch. Biochem. Biophys.,* **144,** 678.

Potter, W. Z., Davis, D. C., Mitchell, J. R., Jollow, D. J., Gillette, J. R., and Brodie, B. B. (1973). *J. Pharmacol. Exp. Therap.,* **187,** 203.

Recknagel, R. O. (1967). *Pharmacol. Rev.,* **19,** 145.

Reid, W. D. (1973). *Exp. Molec. Pathol.,* **19,** 197.

Reid, W. D., and Krishna, G. (1973). *Exp. Molec. Pathol.,* **18,** 80.

Reid, W. D., Ilett, K. E., Glick, J. M., and Krishna, G. (1973). *Ann. Rev. Respir. Dis.,* **107,** 539.

Reynolds, E. S. (1972). *Biochem. Pharmacol.,* **21,** 2555.

Richens, A., and Rowe, D. J. F. (1970). *Br. Med. J.,* **4,** 73.

Sasame, H. A., Mitchell, J. R., Thorgeirsson, S., and Gillette, J. R. (1973). *Drug Metabol. Dispos.,* **1,** 150.

Schenkman, J. B., Cinti, D. L., Moldeus, P. W., and Orrenius, S. (1973). *Drug Metabol. Dispos.,* **1,** 111.

Singer, S. J. (1970). In *Molecular Properties of Drug Receptors,* p. 229, Churchill, London.

Sipes, I. G., Corsini, G., Krishna, G., and Gillette, J. R. (1972). *5th Intern. Congr. Pharmacol. Volunteer Papers,* p. 86.

Sipes, I. G., Stripp, B., Krishna, G., Maling, H. M., and Gillette, J. R. (1973). *Proc. Soc. Exp. Biol. Med.,* **142,** 237.

Sipes, I. G., Sagalyn, A., and Brown, B. R. (1974). *Fed. Proc.,* **33,** 219.

Slater, T. F. (1966). *Nature (Lond.),* **209,** 36.

Smuckler, E., Arrhenius, E., and Hultin, T. (1967). *Biochem. J.,* **103,** 55.

Tephley, T. R., Webb, C., Trussler, P., Kniffen, F., Hasegawa, E., and Piper, W. (1973). *Drug Metabol. Dispos.,* **1,** 259.

Traiger, G. L., and Plaa, G. L. (1971). *Toxicol. Appl. Pharmacol.,* **20,** 105.

Uehleke, H., Hellmer, K. H., and Tabarelli, S. (1973). *Xenobiotica,* **3,** 1.

Vesell, E. S. (1967). *Science,* **157,** 1057.

Weisburger, J. H., and Weisburger, E. K. (1973). *Pharmacology Rev.,* **25,** 1.

West, S. B., Levin, W., and Lu, A. Y. H. (1974). *Fed. Proc.,* **33,** 587.

Williams, R. T. (1959). *Detoxication Mechanisms,* Wiley, New York.

Williams, R. T., Hirom, P. C., and Renwick, A. G. (1975). Chapter 4 of this volume.

Zampaglione, N., Jollow, D. J., Mitchell, J. R., Stripp, B., Hamrick, M., and Gillette, J. R. (1973). *J. Pharmacol. Exp. Therap.,* **187,** 218.

6

Active Sites of Biological Macromolecules and Their Interaction with Heavy Metals

G. L. EICHHORN

6.1. Introduction

Metal ions are required for many biological processes in which biomacromolecules are engaged. These molecules frequently contain metal ions on the active site, e.g., in carboxypeptidase, alkaline phosphatase, carbonic anhydrase, cytochrome c, hemoglobin, ferredoxins, etc. The metal ions in such substances are directly involved in the mechanism of the biological process which the macromolecules are designed to mediate.

Biologically active metal ions can sometimes be displaced from the active site by other metal ions. Thus the active site of a macromolecule is a potential locus for the interaction of toxic metals. In considering the chemical basis for the action of toxic metal ions, however, one must take into account not only the active site, but every electron donor group on the macromolecule that can be used to bind metal ions, whether or not it is a part of the active site. Among such

G. L. EICHHORN ● Laboratory of Molecular Aging, National Institutes of Health, National Institute of Aging, Gerontology Research Center, Baltimore City Hospitals, Baltimore, Maryland 21224.

functional groups are the imidazole, sulfhydryl, hydroxyl, carboxyl, amino, guanidinium, and peptide groups on proteins, and the heterocyclic bases, ribose hydroxyls, and phosphate groups on nucleic acids.

It must be recognized that toxicity is a relative term. Metal ions that are essential for biological activity at one concentration become toxic at a different concentration. Diseases that result from an excess of essential elements are well known; examples are Wilson's disease (Scheinberg and Sternlieb, 1960) from an overload of copper, and hemochromatosis (Dreyfus and Schapira, 1964) from an overload of iron.

Since the molecular basis of the toxic behavior of metals is not well understood at present, it is instructive to speculate on the ways in which toxicity can result from reactions of metal ions with macromolecules.

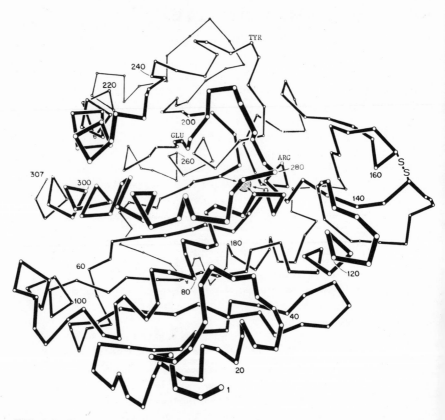

FIG. 6.1. Structure of carboxypeptidase A (from Lipscomb, 1970). Amino acids are numbered from the amino-terminal to the carboxyl-terminal residue. The zinc is shown as a centrally located shaded area. Some of the amino acids thought to be active, according to the mechanism of Fig. 6.2, are specified by the conventional three-letter abbreviation.

6.2. Metal Ions and Active Sites

Possibly the most extensively studied metal-containing biomacromolecule, and the first to be characterized crystallographically, is the zinc enzyme bovine pancreatic carboxypeptidase A (Ludwig and Lipscomb, 1973), whose function is to cleave the carboxyl-terminal amino acid of a protein. The structure of this enzyme is shown in Fig. 6.1. A mechanism (Lipscomb, 1970) proposed for the action of the enzyme upon tyrosyl-glycine substrate is demonstrated in Fig. 6.2. According to this mechanism, the zinc binds to the carbonyl oxygen of the terminal peptide, and draws electrons in its direction and away from the peptide linkage, which is therefore weakened and made more susceptible to hydrolysis. Evidently, zinc is only a part of the active site, which involves also certain amino acids that act upon the peptide linkage simultaneously with the zinc. Coleman and Vallee (1961) demonstrated some time ago that the zinc can be replaced by other metal ions, as shown in Table 6.1. When the zinc is replaced by cobalt, the activity actually increases. There is also activity with nickel, very little with manganese, and zero activity with copper, mercury, cadmium, and lead. Thus one could speculate that the reason for the toxicity of mercury and cadmium, for example, is that they can displace the zinc required for activity in carboxypeptidase. Unfortunately no one has shown that these metals actually get to the carboxypeptidase in a living organism. The difficulty with crediting any potentially toxic reaction with responsibility for toxicity in organisms is that there is such a large number of such reactions that it is difficult to determine which of them is the culprit.

Another example of an enzyme in which the displacement of active zinc by other metal ions leads to inactivation is carbonic anhydrase (Coleman, 1967,

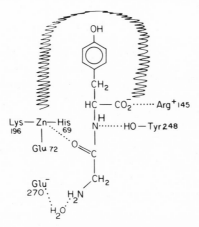

FIG. 6.2. Postulated mechanism of action of carboxypeptidase, according to Lipscomb (1970).

TABLE 6.1 Peptidase Activity* of Metallocarboxypeptidases (from Coleman and Vallee, 1961)

[(CPD)Me]†	Relative activity
[(CPD)Zn]	7.5
[(CPD)Co]	12.0
[(CPD)Ni]	8.0
[(CPD)Mn]	0.6
[(CPD)Cu]	0
[(CPD)Hg]	0
[(CPD)Cd]	0
[(CPD)Pb]	0

*Substrate: carbobenzoxy-glycyl-L-phenylalanine.
†1 g atom metal per mole of apoenzyme; CPD = carboxypeptidase.

1973), the enzyme that catalyzes the interaction of carbon dioxide with water (Table 6.2). Zinc is most active, and cobalt displays activity, but all other metal ions displacing the zinc produce little or no activity.

If the active site of an enzyme, which is usually defined by enzymologists as the part of the molecule into which the substrate fits and is acted upon, were the only kind of site of importance for metal interaction, this presentation could end here, since the principle of a metal at an active site being displaced by other metal ions which inactivate the enzyme has been illustrated, and there is no reason for exhausting the list of examples. Metal toxicity, however, probably involves other types of interactions in addition to those on the active site.

TABLE 6.2. Enzymatic Activities of Metallocarbonic Anhydrase B (from Coleman, 1967)

Metal	Relative activity in hydration of CO_2 *
Apoenzyme	400
Mn(II)	400
Co(II)	5 700
Ni(II)	500
Cu(II)	127
Zn(II)	10 200
Cd(II)	430
Hg(II)	5

*Determined by the method of Wilbur and Anderson.

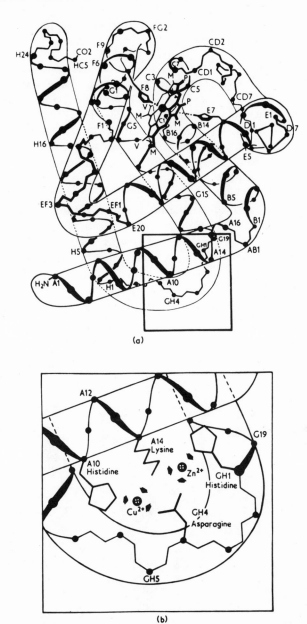

FIG. 6.3. (a) Structure of myoglobin, after Dickerson (1964) (from Banaszak et al., 1965). The iron is placed in the porphyrin structure in the upper center and is bound to the F-8 histidine. (b) Enlargement of the rectangular area in (a) to show the binding sites for Cu^{2+} and Zn^{2+}.

6.3. Reaction of Metal Ions with Sites Other Than the Active Site

The myoglobin molecule (Fig. 6.3), the protein that binds oxygen in muscle, contains an active site in the form of iron porphyrin. When metal ions interact with myoglobin, however, they do not displace the iron, which is very strongly bound, but attack another site instead (Breslow, 1973). Copper ions, for example, bind as shown in Fig. 6.3(b), and are liganded to histidine, lysine, and asparagine. Zinc ions bind to the same lysine and asparagine as copper, but to a different histidine (Banaszak et al., 1965). Thus the active site of a biological macromolecule that contains metal ions is not necessarily the site to which extraneous metal ions will bind.

From this point on, therefore, this paper will involve the interaction of metal ions with binding sites of the macromolecules that are not conventional active sites, although they are certainly active toward interaction with metal ions. Some of the groups on proteins to which metal ions bind have been noted in the introduction. The binding of copper ions to one of the most thoroughly studied proteins—bovine serum albumin—is illustrated in Fig. 6.4 (Peters and Blumenstock, 1967); the copper binds to an amino group and a histidine group as well as to two peptide nitrogens.

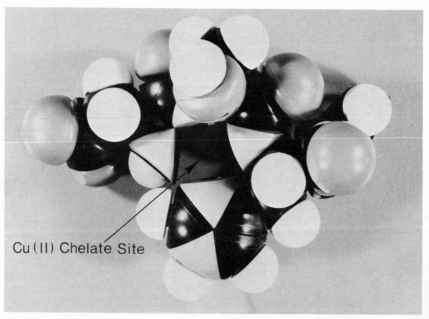

Cu (II) Chelate Site

FIG. 6.4. Cu^{2+} binding site in bovine serum albumin at the terminal Asp-Thr-His sequence (from Peters and Blumenstock, 1967; corrected figure obtained through private communication from Dr. Peters).

6.4. Activation *vs*. Inhibition

Thus metal ions can not only displace an indigenous metal from a biological macromolecule at the active site but can also bind to other sites on such a molecule. It is not surprising, therefore, that the same metal ion, by binding to different sites at various concentrations, can have beneficial and adverse affects on the same substance. Perhaps this is an illustration at the molecular level of Dr. Stickler's statement that substances that are toxic at high levels may be beneficial at low levels.

The effect of metal ions on the enzyme oxalacetate decarboxylase, which catalyzes the cleavage of the carbon dioxide molecule from oxalacetate, illustrates how the same metal ions can both activate and deactivate an enzyme. Speck (1949) demonstrated some time ago how the activity of this enzyme depends on the metal concentration, for a large variety of metal ions (Fig. 6.5). Some strongly binding metal ions like Cu^{2+} and Pb^{2+} produce very low activity at very low concentration, but as the metal ion concentration is increased the

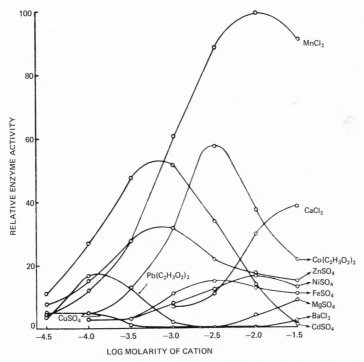

FIG. 6.5. Effect of metal ions on the enzymatic decarboxylation of oxalacetic acid (from Speck, 1949).

activity decreases and becomes zero at somewhat higher concentrations. Other metal ions like Zn^{2+} and Cd^{2+} produce optimal activities at higher concentrations, and they too cause inhibition as the concentration of the metal ions is increased beyond the optimal. With some metal ions like calcium, for example, the activities still rise at the highest metal concentration that can be achieved; possibly, if still higher concentrations were experimentally feasible, these metal ions would also inhibit.

An obvious explanation of this phenomenon is that at low metal concentrations the metal ions are being placed into an active site, or at least into a position in which they have a beneficial effect upon the enzyme, and at high metal ion concentrations the excess metal ions then attach themselves to other binding sites, causing inhibition.

Similar effects are produced by addition of metal ions to an enzyme which does not ordinarily require metal ions at all. The enzyme ribonuclease, whose purpose is to cleave nucleic acids into nucleotide monomers, has an active site involving two histidines and a lysine (Breslow, 1973). Metal ions are not required for the reaction, but they have a profound effect on the enzyme (Eichhorn et al., 1969) (Fig. 6.6). All metal ions that have been studied activate the enzymes at low concentration and inhibit at higher concentration. The explanation is as before; at low concentration the metal presumably binds to an activating site and at high concentration it binds to an inhibiting site.

Thus far we have touched on two possible molecular mechanisms for metal toxicity, namely, (1) the toxic metal displacing a beneficial metal from an active

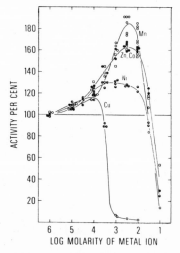

FIG. 6.6. Effect of metal ions on the enzymatic activity of ribonuclease (from Eichhorn et al., 1969).

site and (2) a toxic metal binding to a deactivating site on the molecule. These mechanisms arise from studies of metal ions binding to proteins. Further possible mechanisms for toxicity are suggested by studies of metal binding to nucleic acids.

6.5. Metal Binding to Nucleic Acids

Nucleic acids, like proteins, contain a large number of sites to which metal ions can bind, namely, phosphate, ribose hydroxyl, and heterocyclic bases. The nucleic acids consist of ribose phosphate backbones to which the heterocyclic "bases" are attached (Fig. 6.7). They can be divided into two types, deoxyribonucleic acids (DNA), which do not contain $2'$-hydroxyl groups, and ribonucleic acids (RNA), which do. The monomers of the nucleic acid macromolecules are called nucleosides (base + ribose) and nucleotides (base + ribose + phosphate). The bases, adenine (A), cytosine (C), guanine (G), and uracil (U) in RNA, or thymine (T) in DNA, whose sequence on the ribose phosphate backbone determines the genetic code, also contain a number of electron donor groups which can bind metals, namely, amino groups, heterocyclic nitrogens, and oxygens.

Figure 6.8 presents a very schematic representation of nucleic acid function. The DNA molecule is the primary source of genetic information, and each strand

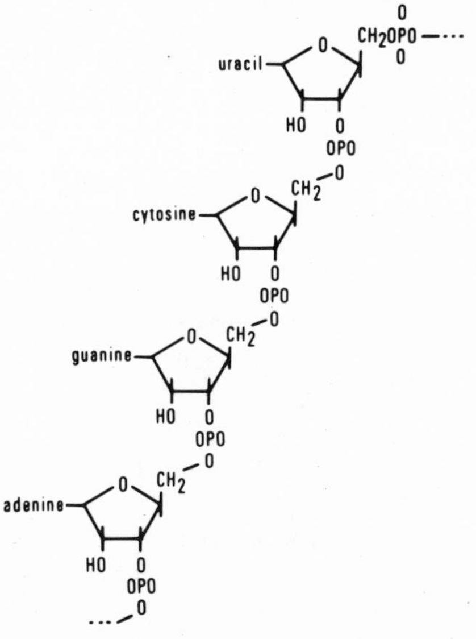

FIG. 6.7. Ribose–phosphate backbone of nucleic acids.

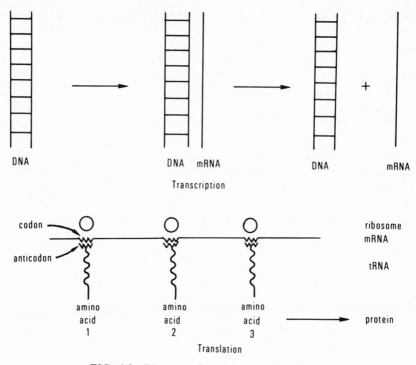

FIG. 6.8. Diagram of nucleic acid functions.

of the double helix contains a sequence of bases that determines the genetic code. The DNA molecule replicates itself in the cell nucleus by an unwinding of the double helix into separate coils. It also serves as a template on which RNA (messenger or mRNA) with a similar sequence of bases is formed. This process is called transcription. The messenger RNA then dissociates from the DNA template in the nucleus and moves into the cytoplasm, where particles called ribosomes foster recognition between the "codons" on the messenger RNA and "anticodons" on transfer RNA molecules, which are the bearers of specific amino acids. Thus a specific codon is "translated" into a specific amino acid. Protein synthesis then involves the formation of peptide linkages between these amino acids.

Metal ions are important in holding together some of the particles required in protein synthesis. For example, in E. coli ribosomes two small particles must be combined into larger particles in order for protein synthesis to take place. 10^{-2} M Mg^{2+} is required for this aggregation process (Goldberg, 1966). Thus metal ions in a biological system can serve as a glue to hold particles together.

6.6. Metal Ions and Crosslinking in Polynucleotides

This property of metal ions can also have deleterious consequences. The DNA molecule (Fig. 6.9) consists of two strands, each of which has as a sugar-phosphate backbone to which the heterocyclic bases are attached. These bases are hydrogen bonded in a complementary fashion, i.e., whenever A is on one strand, T must be on the other, and whenever G is on one strand, C must be on the other. As a consequence, each strand is complementary to the other, and both DNA strands contain a form of the genetic code.

When metal ions bind to the phosphate groups on the surface a very different kind of effect can be expected from that which will occur when the metal ions bind to the bases, because metal ions binding to bases compete with hydrogen bonds and thus can destroy the double helix (Eichhorn, 1973).

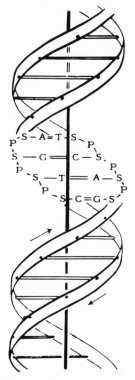

FIG. 6.9. Structure of DNA, showing GC and AT base pairs. P = phosphate, S = sugar (ribose).

.This difference in effects due to phosphate and base binding is dramatically illustrated in Fig. 6.10, which demonstrates the unwinding of the double helix into single strands (Eichhorn, 1962). Since the double helix has a lower ultraviolet absorbance than the separated strands (due to the π-interaction of the bases in the duplex), absorbance changes can be used to study this transition. Curve A demonstrates such a "melting curve" in the absence of divalent metal ions. As DNA is heated, the double helix remains stable until a temperature is reached at which it unwinds and transformation to single strands occurs. Curve B represents the effect of magnesium ions on this melting curve; the transition occurs at a higher temperature because magnesium ions binding to the phosphate groups *stabilize* the DNA helix. Copper ions (curve C), on the other hand, because they bind to the bases and compete with the hydrogen bonding, lower the melting temperature and therefore *destabilize* the DNA helix.

As Fig. 6.10A reveals, when DNA is cooled in the absence of divalent metal ions there is a slight decrease in absorbance; only a total decrease in absorbance to the original level would indicate reformation of the double helix. This partial decrease in absorbance is explained in Fig. 6.11. When the DNA double helix is heated in the absence of divalent metal ions, the two unwound chains become entangled in the solution in such a manner that the complementary bases are out of register. When the solution is cooled down again, the complementary bases simply cannot find each other any more. Hence, the strands remain unasso-

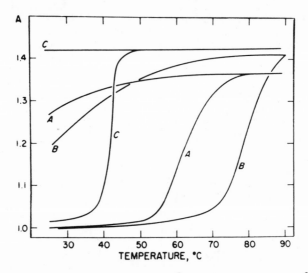

FIG. 6.10. Heating and cooling of 5×10^{-5} M(P) DNA in 5×10^{-3} M NaNO$_3$ and (A) no divalent metal, (B) 10^{-4} M Mg^{2+}, (C) 10^{-4} M Cu^{2+} (from Eichhorn, 1962).

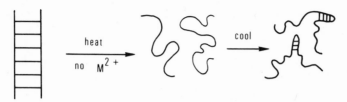

FIG. 6.11. Formation of hairpin loops on cooling DNA in absence of divalent
metal ions (from Eichhorn, 1973).

ciated, but there are a certain number of complementary bases within each
single chain which can form hairpin loops.

Let us now consider the effect of metal ions binding to bases on the unwinding of DNA. Figure 6.12 illustrates what happens when DNA is heated in the
presence of Zn^{2+} ions (Shin and Eichhorn, 1968). The DNA unwinds when the
transition temperature is exceeded, but when the unwound DNA is cooled back
down, the absorbance reverts to its original value, before heating, indicating the
reformation of the double helix. This reversible unwinding and rewinding has
been illustrated with zinc, but occurs, under a variety of conditions, with other
metal ions that bind to the bases (Eichhorn and Clark, 1965; Eichhorn and
Shin, 1968).

Why do metal ions convert the otherwise irreversible unwinding of DNA into
a reversible process? Figure 6.13 contains an explanation. We believe that the
metal ions form cross-links between the strands, thus holding the two chains in
close proximity, so that when the DNA is cooled and the double helix becomes
thermodynamically stable again, the complementary bases can now find each
other. This phenomenon illustrates another possible way in which metals can
produce deleterious effects; they can form cross-links in undesirable ways.
[Mercury ions incidentally form very strong cross-links (Yamane and Davidson,

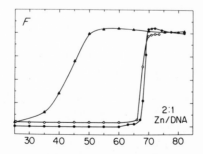

FIG. 6.12. Heating and cooling curve of 5×10^{-5} M(P) DNA in the presence of
10^{-4} M Zn^{2+}. ● heating, ▲ cooling, ○ reheating (from Shin et al., 1968).

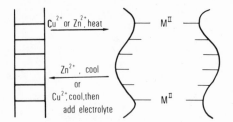

FIG. 6.13. Diagram of unwinding and rewinding of DNA in the presence of divalent metal ions. Temperature reversible reaction with Zn^{2+} is described in the text. With Cu^{2+}, rewinding requires cooling the heated DNA, and the addition of a high concentration of electrolyte.

1961; Katz, 1963).] If metal ions produced such cross-links in DNA in the cell, obviously difficulties would result. Again, I have presented a type of reaction that could be toxic in the cell, but again I want to stress that I do not know whether such a reaction does in fact take place in the cell.

6.7. Stabilization of DNA Double Helix by Metal Ions

Let us now consider the effect of metal ions binding to the phosphate groups. As was noted, magnesium ions, which bind to phosphate, stabilize the DNA double helix. The reason for this stabilization is clear—DNA that is not stabilized by association with positive ions is very unstable. In fact, if solid DNA is dissolved in distilled water, it unwinds (Thomas, 1954) because the negative charges on the phosphates in close proximity to each other on the molecule repel each other to such an extent that the molecules assume conformations which separate the charges further. This tendency to unwind can be countered by neutralizing the charges on the negative phosphate groups by positive ions (Fig. 6.14).

6.8. Mispairing of Nucleotide Bases

This effect of positive charges in stabilizing the DNA double helix can lead, we believe, to other deleterious effects, as I shall now illustrate. Remember that in order for the genetic code to be correctly transmitted the complementary bases (Fig. 6.9) must always hydrogen-bond with each other and not with other bases. Thus, A must react with T (or U), and G must react with C; it must not be any other way.

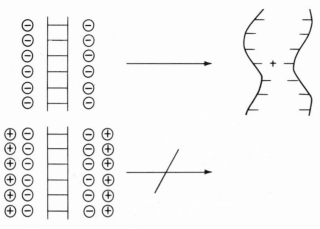

FIG. 6.14. Diagram for stabilization of DNA double helix by metal ions binding to phosphate.

Complementary bases are not so different from noncomplementary bases. Figure 6.15 demonstrates that two complementary bases, U and A, have the same hydrogen bonding scheme as two noncomplementary bases, I and A. If the complementary interaction (U + A) results in proper transmission of the genetic code, then the noncomplementary interaction (I + A) will produce error in the transmission of the genetic code. But the noncomplementary bases do interact, only less strongly than the complementary bases. *Complementary base pairing is*

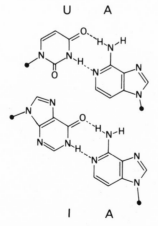

FIG. 6.15. Comparison of complementary bases (U-A) and noncomplementary "mispaired" bases (I-A).

relatively strong, while noncomplementary base pairing, or mispairing, is rela-tively weak.

Complementarity is important not only in the recognition of the bases in the two strands of DNA but also in protein synthesis, which requires that a codon on messenger RNA must be recognized by an anticodon on transfer RNA (see Fig. 6.8). The codon contains a sequence of three bases, and the anticodon contains the three bases complementary to those on the codon. Thus, the codon (CUU) of messenger RNA is designed to recognize the anticodon (GAA) of the particular transfer RNA that specifically binds, and will incorporate, phenylal-anine into protein. Sometimes one of these bases can be replaced by another without changing the amino acid incorporated—in this case C can be replaced by U. If, on the other hand, C is replaced by G or A, the codon becomes that for leucine instead of phenylalanine. Thus a mistake in the recognition of one complementary base pair would cause the incorporation of the wrong amino acid.

Such a mistake in protein synthesis can result from the presence of the wrong concentration of metal ions (Fig. 6.16). Szer and Ochoa (1964) studied the effect of magnesium ion concentration on the incorporation of phenylala-nine into protein under the influence of UUU codons (from polyuridylic acid). There is an optimal magnesium concentration for the incorporation of phenyl-alanine, and at higher Mg^{2+} concentrations, phenylalanine incorporation di-

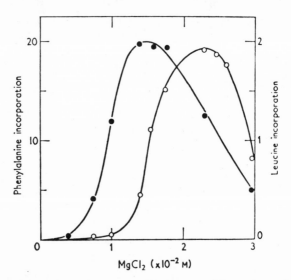

FIG. 6.16. Incorporation of amino acids into protein, using poly(U) as mes-senger RNA, as a function of Mg^{2+} concentration. ● phenylalanine, ○ leucine (from Szer and Ochoa, 1964).

minishes, but the incorporation of leucine is stimulated. Thus, at the high Mg^{2+} concentrations at which the "correct" amino acid incorporation has decreased, the incorporation of an "incorrect" amino acid occurs. Thus high magnesium ion concentrations can produce errors in protein synthesis.

This phenomenon can be explained by the following hypothesis. As was previously indicated, metal ions stabilize the interaction of nucleotide strands. At *low* metal ion concentrations, therefore, strand interaction is relatively unstable and only the strongest base pairs will interact. The strongest base pairs are the complementary base pairs. At *high* metal ion concentrations strand interaction is stabilized. Therefore, not only the most stable base pairs, but also weaker base pairs, will interact, thus leading to mispairing of bases.

This explanation invites experiments to prove that metal ions can indeed induce mispairing (Eichhorn et al., 1973). Such an experiment is illustrated by the reaction of a 1:1 copolymer of U and I with a polymer containing only A. If reaction is restricted by complementarity, the A on the homopolymer should react only with its complementary base U on the copolymer. If mispairing or indiscriminate interaction occurs, A should react not only with U but also with I, as shown in Fig. 6.17. If none of the I bases reacts (complementarity), there should be a 2:1 stoichiometry of interaction between the poly(I,U) and poly(A). If, on the other hand, we get mispairing, there should be a 1:1 interaction. Fig. 6.18 reveals that at low Mg^{2+} ion concentration there is a 2:1 interaction but that as the Mg^{2+} concentration is increased the reaction eventually becomes 1:1. In other words, low metal ion concentrations favor complementary base pairing, while mispairing occurs at high metal ion concentrations. This and other experiments have shown that at high metal ion concentrations errors are produced in the recognition of base pairs, which could lead to errors in many of the processes that are involved in genetic information transfer. It should be emphasized that, although mispairing is induced by metal

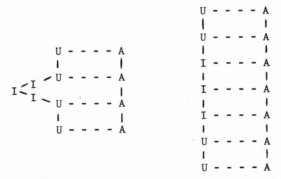

FIG. 6.17. Diagram for complementary interaction (left) and indiscriminate interaction leading to mispairing (right) between poly(A) and poly(I, U).

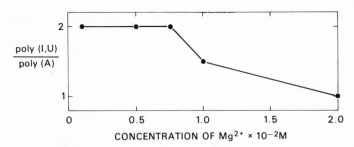

FIG. 6.18. Variation of stoichiometry of reaction of 9×10^{-5} M poly(I, U) and poly(A) with increasing Mg^{2+} concentration.

ions at the same concentrations that result in errors in protein synthesis, a causal relationship has not been established, and explanations other than mispairing can be suggested for the errors in protein synthesis.

6.9. Cleavage of Biomacromolecules by Metal Ions

Metal ions can also depolymerize nucleic acids (Eichhorn and Butzow, 1965). A metal ion binding to a phosphate group can draw electrons away from the phosphodiester linkage in RNA and polyribonucleotides generally, thus making the bond relatively unstable and susceptible to hydrolysis. The macromolecule is then degraded into smaller fragments. Figure 6.19 shows that a large number of metal ions, e.g., manganese, cobalt, nickel, copper, and zinc, will promote such depolymerization (Butzow and Eichhorn, 1965). The depolymerization of macromolecules in a cell would, of course, constitute another possible toxic effect.

Many metal ions are capable of binding to a variety of sites on nucleic acid molecules, and therefore can produce a variety of effects on these substances. Thus Zn^{2+} binding to bases produces reversible unwinding of DNA, while Zn^{2+} binding to phosphate promotes RNA depolymerization. Such multiple reactivity of metal ions is one of the factors that makes it difficult to pinpoint the cause of toxicity.

6.10. Conclusions

I have tried to illustrate a few of the ways in which metal ions can cause deleterious effects in biologically important macromolecules. In summary, the

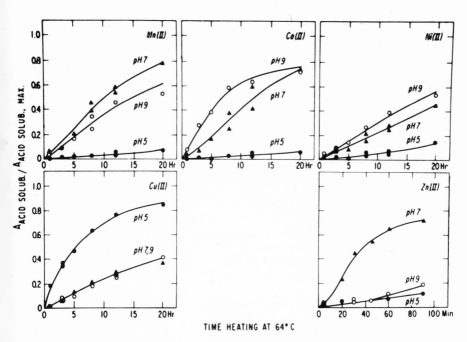

FIG. 6.19. Degradation of 1×10^{-4} M(P) poly(A) by 10^{-4} M concentrations of various metal ions. Ordinate is a function of extent of degradation (from Butzow and Eichhorn, 1965).

possible toxic reactions that have been considered are (1) the displacement of an essential metal from an active site by a "toxic" metal; (2) the binding of metal ions to undesired parts of a macromolecule; (3) cross-linking, which can produce undesired aggregations; (4) errors in protein synthesis, which may be caused by (5) mispairing of nucleotide bases, and (6) the depolymerization of biological macromolecules. At this time it is not possible to assess the importance of any of these potential mechanisms for *in vivo* toxicity.

References

Banaszak, L., Watson, H. C., and Kendrew, J. C. (1965). *J. Mol. Biol.*, **12**, 130.

Breslow, E. (1973). In *Inorganic Biochemistry*, p. 227 (ed. Eichhorn, G. L.), Elsevier, Amsterdam.

Butzow, J. J., and Eichhorn, G. L. (1965). *Biopolymers*, **3**, 95.

Coleman, J. E. (1967). *Nature*, **214**, 193.

Coleman, J. E. (1973). In *Inorganic Biochemistry*, p. 448 (ed. Eichhorn, G. L.), Elsevier, Amsterdam.

Coleman, J. E., and Vallee, B. L. (1961). *J. Biol. Chem.*, **236**, 2244.

Dickerson, R. E. (1964). *The Proteins*, Vol. 2 (ed. Neurath, H.), Academic Press, New York.

Dreyfus, J.-C., and Schapira, G. (1964). In *Iron Metabolism*, p. 296 (ed. Gross, F.), Springer, Berlin.

Eichhorn, G. L. (1962). *Nature, Lond.*, **194**, 174.

Eichhorn, G. L. (1973). In *Inorganic Biochemistry*, Vol. II, p. 1210 (ed. Eichhorn, G. L.), Elsevier, Amsterdam.

Eichhorn, G. L., and Butzow, J. J. (1965). *Biopolymers*, **3**, 79.

Eichhorn, G. L., and Clark, P. (1965). *Proc. Natl. Acad. Sci. U.S.*, **53**, 586.

Eichhorn, G. L., and Shin, Y. A. (1968). *J. Am. Chem. Soc.*, **90**, 7323.

Eichhorn, G. L., Clark, P., and Tarien, E. (1969). *J. Biol. Chem.*, **244**, 937.

Eichhorn, G. L., Pitha, J., Richardson, C., and Tarien, E. (1973). *Abst. Ninth International Congress of Biochemistry*, Stockholm; also (1973). *Argonne Symposium on Metal Ions in Biological Systems*, pp. 43–66 (ed. Dhar, S. K.), Plenum, New York.

Goldberg, A. (1966). *J. Mol. Biol.*, **15**, 663.

Katz, S. (1963). *Biochim. Biophys. Acta.*, **68**, 240.

Lipscomb, W. N. (1970). *Acc. Chem. Res.*, **3**, 81.

Ludwig, M. L., and Lipscomb, W. N. (1973). In *Inorganic Biochemistry*, p. 438 (ed. Eichhorn, G. L.), Elsevier, Amsterdam.

Peters, T., and Blumenstock, F. A. (1967). *J. Biol. Chem.*, **242**, 1574.

Scheinberg, I. H., and Sternlieb, I. (1960). In *Metal Binding in Medicine*, p. 275 (ed. Seven, M. J.), Lippincott, Philadelphia.

Shin, Y. A., and Eichhorn, G. L. (1968). *Biochemistry*, **7**, 1026.

Speck, J. F. (1949). *J. Biol. Chem.*, **178**, 315.

Szer, W., and Ochoa, S. (1964). *J. Mol. Biol.*, **8**, 823.

Thomas, R. (1954). *Trans. Faraday Soc.*, **50**, 304.

Yamane, T., and Davidson, N. (1961). *J. Am. Chem. Soc.*, **83**, 2599.

Part II
INVITED PAPERS

7

Behavior of Mercury in Natural Systems and Its Global Cycle

R. WOLLAST, G. BILLEN, AND F. T. MACKENZIE

Because of the significant use of mercury in man's activities, there has been increased interest in the chemistry of mercury and its compounds in the past decade. Also, because of the known volatility of mercury, there has been a great deal of concern about its sources, sinks, and transfers in the environment. In this paper, we discuss the thermodynamic and kinetic (chemical and biological) aspects of mercury and its compounds in an attempt to explain its behavior in the environment. Based on these chemical principles, which enable us to define pathways of mercury transport in the environment, and on estimates of natural system masses and fluxes between systems, we construct tentative pre-man and present-day models of the global cycle of mercury. Comparison of these two cycles enables us to predict man's contributions to the natural cycle of mercury.

R. WOLLAST and G. BILLEN • Department of Environmental Science, University of Brussels, Brussels, Belgium. F. T. MACKENZIE • Department of Geology, Northwestern University, Evanston, Illinois.

7.1. Chemical Transformations of Mercury in the Aquatic Environment

7.1.1. Introduction

A first step in describing the chemical behavior of an element is to consider an equilibrium model in which the stability and solubility of the various forms of the element are described on the basis of fundamental thermodynamic properties. One method, now in extensive use, of pictorially representing these models is the E_h-pH diagram (Garrels and Christ, 1965). A tentative diagram for inorganic species of mercury was first presented by Symons (1962) and further extended and discussed by Hem (1970). These diagrams may now be further modified and improved by taking into account more recent data and more rigorous treatment.

Stability diagrams generally are sufficient to describe the chemical behavior of solids and aqueous species on a long-term basis. However, they may be misleading in the case of environmental problems, where reaction rates play an important role. Therefore, the theoretical stability diagram of inorganic forms of mercury will be discussed below on the basis of kinetic experiments.

We also know (Hem, 1970) that the known organic species of mercury are thermodynamically unstable with respect to inorganic species in aquatic environments. The chemical transformation rate of an organic into an inorganic compound, however, is commonly extremely slow; therefore, it is also informative to construct a chemical stability diagram in which thermodynamic relations among metastable phases are represented. This form of representation is used for the methylmercury compounds discussed below.

7.1.2. Stability Diagram for Inorganic Mercury Species

As an example of stability relations among solid and dissolved inorganic species of Hg in river water, an E_h-pH diagram was constructed for Hg in the Sambre River of Belgium. This river was selected as an example because of the availability of good analytical data on Hg, and because Hg is being introduced into the river by industrial activities along its banks. We found it necessary to modify the original diagram of Symons (1962) and Hem (1970) because of more recent data on the chemical species of mercury.

The first modification of the diagrams of Symons and Hem is to use a value of 56 ppb for the solubility of liquid mercury (instead of 26 ppb). Our value is based on the work of Cranston and Buckley (1972) and on our own measurements. Also, contradictions exist in the previous diagrams concerning the pos sible occurrence of Hg_2^{2+}, and the fact that the diagrams are independent of total dissolved mercury. It can be demonstrated that the occurrence of Hg_2^{2+} is only possible if the total concentration of mercury in solution exceeds 450 ppm, a concentration which is unusual in natural environments, even those that are heavily polluted. Also the diagrams are not independent of total dissolved mercury.

Furthermore, it can be shown that sulfide complexes of mercury are more numerous than reported in previous diagrams (Barnes et al., 1967). However, the complexes do not modify significantly the general shape of the diagram and rather obscure the graphic representation. They were not taken into account here (Fig. 7.1).

Despite the modifications discussed above, the main conclusions of Hem remain valid and are summarized below:

(1) High solubilities of mercury only occur in well-oxygenated waters.
(2) In moderately oxidizing conditions, the predominant species of mercury is undissociated mercury ($Hg°$).

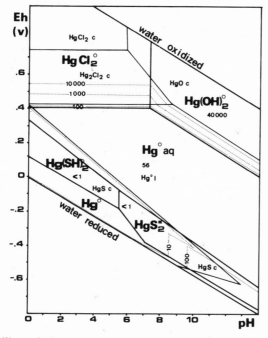

FIG. 7.1. Stability relations among mercury compounds in river water (Sambre River, Belgium) at 25°C and 1 atmosphere total pressure. Solid lines are stable boundaries for dissolved species and solids; dashed lines are contours of mercury dissolved species showing the maximum solubility in the presence of the solid phase.

(3) In more reducing environments, the extremely insoluble cinnabar will precipitate, but its solubility may be increased in very reducing conditions by conversion of mercuric ion to free metal or by the occurrence at high pH of the stable HgS_2^{2-} ion.

The usual presence of relatively large amounts of iron oxides and hydroxides in river suspensions or in sediments may modify markedly the precipitation of cinnabar. If we consider the competitive precipitation of iron and mercury sulfide, it appears that the field of direct precipitation of cinnabar is drastically reduced by the presence of Fe_2O_3 (Fig. 7.2). Presumably, coprecipitation of HgS iron sulfides occurs, but no quantitative data are available for this process.

The E_h-pH diagram describes fairly well the occurrence of dissolved species of mercury. For example, transformation of $Hg°$ to Hg^{2+} and *vice versa* is rapid and is currently used for analytical purposes.

Experiments on the rate of formation of sulfide complexes from $Hg°$ (Fig. 7.3) show that these reactions are slower than those for other inorganic species but again sufficiently rapid to bring the system near equilibrium after a few minutes even for very dilute solutions. Oxidation of sulfide species occurs via a complex rate mechanism depending on the oxidation–reduction potential, pH, and concentration of major ions in solution such as Cl^-. For the composition of

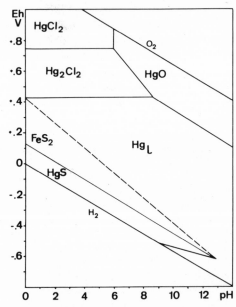

FIG. 7.2. Stability relations of mercury solid phases in equilibrium with Sambre River water and in the presence of Fe_2O_3.

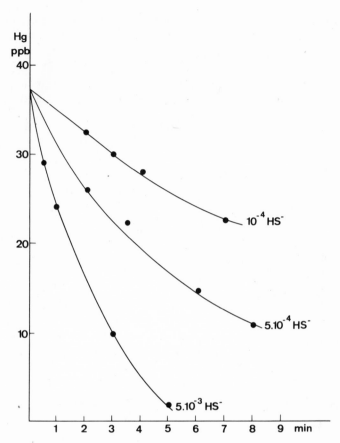

FIG. 7.3. Rate of complexing of Hg° by HS⁻ as a function of the concentration of HS⁻ ion.

Sambre River water, we obtained an experimental oxidation rate of 10–20% mercuric ion produced per hour.

Finally, it is important to consider the possible volatilization of mercury from aqueous solution containing the species Hg°. At saturation concentration (56 ppb), the vapor pressure of gaseous mercury is equal to the vapor pressure of liquid mercury and corresponds at 25°C to a concentration of about 12 mg Hg/m³ of air. The vapor pressure of less concentrated solutions decreases proportionately according to Henry's law. Even in well-aerated water, the air in equilibrium with a solution of 0.001 ppb of Hg° contains 0.2 μg/m³. These values exceed the normal content of mercury in the atmosphere near the land surface (~1 ng/m³); thus, the mercury gradient from water to air favors volatilization.

7.1.3. Stability Diagram for Organic Mercury Species

The thermodynamic constants for organic species of mercury are not known except for dimethylmercury (Wagman et al., 1968). Although this compound may be considered to be one of the most stable organic species of mercury, it is unstable with respect to all the inorganic species appearing in the E_h-pH diagram of Fig. 7.1. Thermodynamically, this compound, and also methylmercury ion, should decompose spontaneously. However, the rate of these reactions in the absence of bacteriological activity is extremely slow. We could not detect any change after one month in the concentration of CH_3HgCl or CH_3HgCH_3 in spiked samples of sterilized and aerated Sambre River water. Thus, it may be useful to consider an E_h-pH diagram for methylmercury species to predict the behavior of these compounds.

Schwarzenbach and Schellenberg (1965) obtained the equilibrium constants of methylmercury ion with various ligands. In river waters and in absence of sulfide ions, two predominant forms may occur depending on pH: CH_3HgCl and CH_3HgOH. Their respective fields of metastability are represented in Fig. 7.4. The behavior of methylmercury in the presence of sulfide ions appears to be

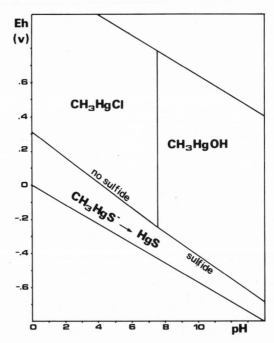

FIG. 7.4. E_h-pH plot of the stability relations among methylmercury compounds in the Sambre River water.

more complicated. Schwarzenbach and Schellenberg measured the association constant for two complexes:

$$2CH_3HgOH + S^{2-} = CH_3HgSHgCH_3 + 2OH^-, \quad K = 10^{18.76}$$

and

$$CH_3HgSHgCH_3 + S^{2-} = 2CH_3HgS^-, \quad K = 10^{4.2}$$

These values were used to calculate the stability field of CH_3HgS^- in Fig. 7.4. Dadič and Grdenič (1960), however, observed that solutions of methylmercury sulfide ion are unstable. They attributed this instability to a photochemical decomposition reaction. Experiments conducted in our laboratory show that the decomposition also occurs in the dark and is due to the formation of a precipitate of colloidal HgS. The reaction is extremely rapid and is completed after a few hours. Two mechanisms may be considered to explain the precipitation of HgS:

$$CH_3HgSHgCH_3 \rightarrow CH_3HgCH_3 + HgS$$

or

$$CH_3HgS^- + H^+ \rightarrow CH_4 + HgS$$

Similar mechanisms have been proposed by Beletskaya et al. (1967, 1970). Work is now in progress to delineate the actual mechanism.

The fact that reactions of this type occur is important when we consider the possible production of methylmercury in reducing environments. If these reactions obtain at sufficiently low E_h values, where sulfate ions may be reduced to sulfide, methylmercury will appear as a labile compound, with the Hg precipitating finally as HgS. As a consequence, in very reducing conditions such as the interstitial waters of organic rich muds, methylation is possible only if the initial sulfate concentration in the interstitial water is low.

7.2. Microbiological Transformations of Mercury in Aquatic Environments

7.2.1. Introduction

During recent years, the idea that microbiological activity may be a major factor in the turnover of mercury in natural environments has become a generally accepted concept. Indeed, many workers have found that some bacteria present in natural and polluted environments can perform the interconversion of mineral and organic (generally more toxic) forms of mercury. On the one hand,

Jensen and Jernelöv (1969) were the first to show that lake sediments incubated with mercuric chloride can produce methylmercury, and that this capacity is lost when the sediments are autoclaved, demonstrating the biological nature of the transformation. Such a methylating activity has also been detected in pure cultures and in enrichments of several bacteria: *Clostridium* (Yamada and Tonomura, 1972), *Methanobacter* (Wood et al., 1968; Billen, 1973), *Neurospora* (Landner, 1971). On the other hand, degradation of organomercuric substances into metallic mercury vapor in soils was described as early as 1944 (Booer, 1944; Kimura and Miller, 1964). The bacterial origin of the degradation was established by Tonomura et al. (1968), who isolated a methylmercury-resistant bacterium *Pseudomonas* able to induce methylmercury decomposition and vaporization. The same bacterial activity involving mineralization of methylmercury into elemental mercury and methane was found to be present in lake and river sediments (Spangler et al., 1973; Billen et al., 1974).

Most of the studies cited above, however, were performed following the established techniques of classical microbiology, in that enrichments of pure cultures were used as starting materials. Thus, these studies may have little application to *in situ* natural conditions because the physiological state and composition of the microbiological communities in these cultures probably bear little relationship to those in natural systems. These studies can demonstrate the presence of a microorganism with a particular potential activity in a natural medium but they cannot predict whether or not the organism will be active in the medium, nor, *a fortiori*, assess the quantitative value of its *in situ* activity.

The facts that almost all types of bacteria have resistant forms and the enrichment techniques of classical microbiology are very efficient prevent us from using as evidence of an effective bacterium activity in a natural environment the simple observation that the bacterium can be isolated in laboratory cultures from that environment.

In this section, we attempt to define the microbiological activities involving mercury transformations that can be significant in natural aquatic systems and the factors that affect these activities. Both the abiotic factors acting on the individual physiology of the organisms and the biotic factors, such as population size and dynamics, that determine *in situ* bacterial activity are discussed below. The discussion is somewhat qualitative because of lack of sufficient empirical and theoretical data.

7.2.2. Influence of Physicochemical Conditions

The redox state of a system is the major physicochemical parameter affecting biological activity in natural waters. It is customary in classical microbiology to distinguish between aerobic and anaerobic systems. Some authors associate oxidizing conditions with the former and the presence of sulfides with the latter. This distinction is too simplistic from the chemical point of view. The absence of a rigorous definition of anaerobiosis has created some confusion in interpretation of the processes of mercury methylation and mineralization in natural environments. The use of oxidation–reduction potential (E_h) and pH parameters characterizing physicochemical conditions for microbial life (Baas-Becking et al., 1960; Stumm, 1966; Berner, 1971) helps to clarify the situation, if we take cognizance of the operational difficulties associated with E_h measurements in natural environments.

On an E_h–pH diagram of the system C–N–O–S–H, constructed for the composition of a representative fresh water (Berner, 1971), and within the limits of natural environments (Baas-Becking et al., 1960), three major zones of biological activity can be distinguished (Fig. 7.5) (Billen and Wollast, 1973):

1. An "aerobic" zone, where E_h is determined to a significant extent by the presence of O_2 and aerobic respiration obtains [see Berner (1971) for discussion of measurement of E_h in aerobic waters].
2. An "oxidizing anaerobic" zone, where oxygen and sulfides are not present at equilibrium and nitrate or iron respiration and various fermentations can occur.
3. A "reducing anaerobic" zone, where sulfides are produced by sulfate respiration.

Construction of E_h–pH diagrams for the systems Hg–S–Cl–H$_2$O and Hg–S–C–H$_2$O (Section 7.1) for mineral and organic forms of mercury shows that dissolved mineral mercury can be present as oxidized species ($Hg(OH)_2$ or $HgCl_2$) in the aerobic zone and in elemental form ($Hg°$) or as organically complexed oxidized species in oxidizing anaerobic conditions. Mineral mercury is precipitated as insoluble HgS in the reducing anaerobic zone; if sufficient iron is present, however, Hg is probably incorporated in pyrite (FeS_2). Methylmercury may be produced in aerobic and oxidizing anaerobic conditions but is spontaneously broken down in the presence of sulfides.

It is now possible to compare these zones with the probable potential activity field of various organisms involved in mercury transformations, either methylating or mineralizing.

The biochemical mechanism of mercury methylation always consists of an interference of mercury with the metabolic reaction involving methyl transfer (Wood et al., 1968; Imura et al., 1971; Landner, 1971, 1972). Methyl transfer reactions are frequently mediated by B_{12}-coenzymes (cobalamin), which are the only biological molecules having a carbon-metal bond, and acting as carbanion carriers (Ingraham, 1964). Carbanion transfer from an organometallic to another metal is a well-known reaction in organometallic chemistry. Methane-producing bacteria and various species of *Clostridia* (effectively recognized as

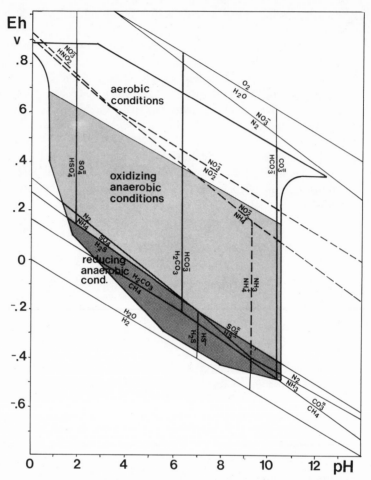

FIG. 7.5. E_h–pH diagram of the system C-N-S-O-H established for a representative fresh water. Limits of the natural environment (Bass Becking et al., 1960), and major fields of metabolic activity are superimposed on the diagram.

methylating species) are known to use extensively the transfer of a methyl group mediated by cobalamin in their energy-yielding metabolism (Stadtman, 1967; Hogenkamp, 1968). Because both organisms are commonly found as active cells in sediments, they are probably the most important microorganisms responsible for the methylation of mercury.

In Fig. 7.6, the E_h–pH regions of potential activity of these microorganisms are shown. The delineation of the regions is based on observations compiled by Baas-Becking et al. (1960), data of Barker (1936) for methane-producing bac-

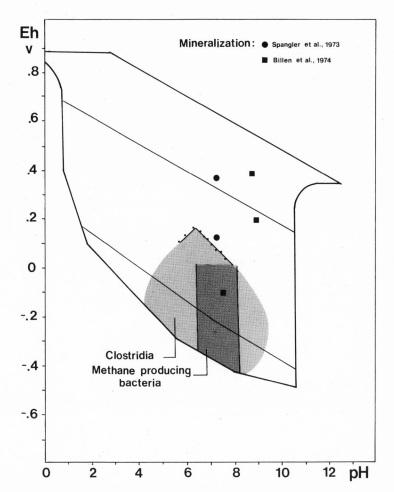

FIG. 7.6. Fields of potential activity of microorganisms involved in mercury methylation and mineralization.

teria, and on the study of Hanke and Bailey (1945) on the upper limit of E_h for growth of various species of *Clostridia*. These zones are potential zones of intense methylation, although the possibility of a weak methylation by other organisms in other conditions cannot be excluded. Comparison of Figs. 7.5 and 7.6 suggests that the most significant methylation should occur in oxidizing anaerobic conditions.

Some authors have stated that mercury methylation obtains mainly in aerobic conditions (Landner, 1972). One of the arguments for such a statement is based on the insolubility of mercuric sulfide, which would make mercury unavailable for biological methylation (Fagerström and Jernelöv, 1971). We have shown above, however, that methylation is most intense in oxidizing anaerobic conditions where HgS is not stable. In a laboratory experiment, Jernelöv (1970) attempted to determine the amount of methylmercury released to water from sediments enriched at different depths with mercuric chloride. He observed the maximum release of methylmercury when mineral mercury was added to the first few centimeters of the sediment. This result is also interpreted as evidence that methylation only occurs in aerobiosis. However, the type of organic rich sediment used by Jernelöv could well be anaerobic below the first few millimeters in depth. Furthermore, the method used (determination of methylmercury accumulated in fishes after 15 days) is not a direct measurement of methylation in the sediments, but depends on the diffusion rate of methylmercury out of the sediment.

As shown in Fig. 7.6, mineralization of organomercury may occur over a broad range of E_h-pH conditions. From lake sediments, Spangler et al. (1973) isolated a large number of bacterial strains able to demethylate methylmercury in aerobic conditions (E_h 330 mV, pH 7.2).* Many of these strains were facultative anaerobes and also degraded methylmercury in oxidizing anaerobic conditions (E_h 100 mV, pH 7.2).* Billen et al. (1974) detected mineralization of methylmercury in cultures from river sediments in the following conditions: E_h 350 mV, pH 8.2; E_h 210 mV, pH 8.0; E_h - 100 mV, pH 7.4.

7.2.3. Dynamics of Bacterial Populations in the Presence of Mercury

Addition of toxic mercury compounds to a medium modifies the bacterial community by selecting resistant organisms. In many cases, the resistance toward a mercury compound seems to be linked with the capacity of the organism to transform it. Therefore, the transformation capacity of a bacterial community can be increased in response to an increased concentration of mercury.

For methylmercury-mineralizing bacteria, which all display some resistance toward methylmercury (Spangler et al., 1973), this phenomenon of "sociological adaptation" was demonstrated in cultures by Billen et al. (1974). Three precultures of the bacterial community of mercury-polluted river sediments containing, respectively, 100, 50, and 0 ng/liter methylmercury were incubated for 7 days and then served as inoculum for three new cultures containing 100 ng/liter. The curves of methylmercury disappearance in the three cultures (Fig. 7.7) show that a modification induced on the bacterial community by prolonged in-

---

*Values obtained by us on a medium of the same composition as that used by Spangler et al. (1973).

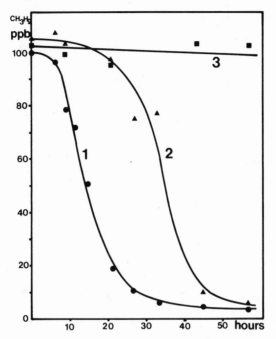

FIG. 7.7. Effect of preincubation of the bacterial community of river sediments in presence of methylmercury on its mineralizing activity. Consumption of methylmercury initially present at 100 ppb in cultures, respectively inoculated with the same number of bacteria from three precultures containing 100 ppb (1), 50 ppb(2), and 0 ppb (3) methylmercury chloride (from Billen et al., 1974).

cubation with mercury caused an increase in the community's mineralizing activity; the lag period necessary before the beginning of the degradation of methylmercury is reduced by pre-incubation in an increasing concentration of this substance.

In another experiment, the methylmercury concentration of two growing cultures of the original bacterial community was increased each 2½ h by the addition of 10 μg/liter and 1.5 μg/liter methylmercury to the respective cultures. Total bacterial numbers, methylmercury-resistant bacteria numbers, and actual methylmercury concentration in the cultures were followed during 50 h (Fig. 7.8). Comparison of the actual methylmercury concentration curve with the rate of addition of methylmercury shows that the community can adapt itself very rapidly to additions. After 35 h (during which a significant modification in the bacterial composition occurs, as suggested by the total bacterial number curve), the mineralizing activity equals the addition of methylmercury and the concentration is maintained at a low value. In an experiment with lake sediments incu-

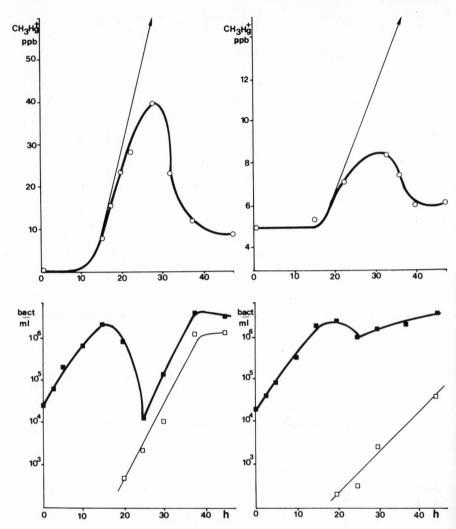

FIG. 7.8. Effect of repeated additions of methylmercury on two cultures of the bacterial community of the Sambre River sediments. (a) and (b), rate of addition of methylmercury (—); actual methylmercury concentration in the cultures (—○—); (c) and (d), total bacterial numbers in the culture (—■—); methylmercury resistant bacteria numbers (—□—).

bated for 100 days with mineral mercury, Spangler et al. (1973) observed exactly the same curve for methylmercury, suggesting that the population of mineralizing bacteria can also adapt itself rapidly enough to equilibrate production of methylmercury by methylating organisms.

For methylating bacteria, the same phenomenon of population adaptation has also been suggested in the case of a response to mineral mercury pollution. At least for some methylating organisms, transformation of mercury corresponds to a detoxification mechanism of complexation of the methylmercury, rendering it inactive (Landner, 1972). Resistant strains of *Neurospora crassa*, obtained by selection on a medium containing $HgCl_2$, were found to have a methylating capacity ten times higher than natural strains of these organisms (Landner, 1971, 1972).

7.2.4. Biological Turnover of Mercury

The previous discussion on the localization of methylating and mineralizing organisms in terms of E_h and pH has shown that both transformations of mercury can occur physiologically in the same physicochemical conditions and particularly in oxidizing anaerobic conditions, i.e., in conditions commonly found in bottom sediments of rivers, lakes, and seas. Moreover, studies on the population dynamics of mineralizing and methylating microorganisms suggest that addition or production of mercury in one form, either mineral or organic, in a natural environment can modify the composition of the bacterial community by favoring organisms able to transform it into the other form. Owing to this mechanism, the activity of both methylating and mineralizing organisms could increase simultaneously, and eventually a steady state could be reached.

Although quantitative measurements of *in situ* organism activities are lacking in the literature, an order of magnitude estimate of the rates of microbial transformations can be deduced from some laboratory experiments in which untreated natural samples rather than cultures were used as starting materials. The experiments of Jensen and Jernelöv (1969) showed net methylation rates of about 40 ng per gram of sediment per day and 15 ng per gram of sediment per day, respectively, for aquarium mud and lake Längsjön sediments enriched with 100 μg $HgCl_2$ per gram of sediment (a concentration commonly attained in polluted areas). An experiment reported by Spangler et al. (1973) gives a net rate of methylmercury mineralization of about 15 ng per gram of sediment per day in Lake St Clair (Michigan, USA) sediments. These estimates suggest that methylation and mineralization of mercury can occur at similar rates in natural environments, and that the rates of biological transformations should not be neglected when considering material fluxes in aquatic systems.

Biological methylation and mineralization of mercury are quantitatively important pathways of mercury transfers in natural environments. A small imbalance between these two processes determines whether the environment acts as a source or sink of methylmercury.

7.3. Cycle of Mercury and Man's Contribution

7.3.1. Introduction

During the past decade increased attention has been paid to development of models of the sedimentary cycle of materials (e.g., Goldberg, 1971; Garrels and Mackenzie, 1971, 1972; Pytkowicz, 1973; Wollast, 1974). The models provide a theoretical framework for the behavior of natural systems such as the ocean, atmosphere, and sedimentary rocks and for the sources, sinks, and pathways of materials migrating through the systems. These models are especially helpful in identifying and evaluating man's contributions owing to industrial activities, fossil fuel combustion, sewage disposal, etc. to natural systems (Garrels et al., 1973).

Perhaps it is premature at this stage of our knowledge of mercury to construct a global model principally because of our scant knowledge of mercury concentrations and distributions in natural systems and mercury transfer rates between systems. For example, about 80% of the total solid entering the ocean each year is transported by rivers draining Southeast Asia. There are no published analyses, however, of the suspended sediment of these rivers.

Despite these problems, we attempted to construct a global model of the cycle of mercury (MacKenzie and Wollast, 1975). Because of the volatility of mercury and its presence in significant concentrations in materials that are combusted, we suspected that man's contributions to the cycle could be important; thus, a model of the cycle, no matter if elementary, is needed to evaluate these contributions.

7.3.2. The Pre-man Cycle

The pre-man cycle (Fig. 7.9) was constructed by solving a series of simultaneous equations representing fluxes among reservoirs and assuming that the system reached a stationary state. The conditions used to solve the simultaneous equations were:

1. Depositional rate = 'uplift' rate = 13×10^8 g Hg/yr.
2. Total flux to atmosphere = 250×10^8 g Hg/yr, based on Greenland ice sheet data (Weiss et al., 1971).
3. One-third of total atmospheric flux returns to land in rain, whereas two-thirds falls on the sea surface.

The reservoir masses are based on estimates of Hg concentrations in individual reservoirs and total mass of reservoir.

It can be seen from Fig. 7.9 that a significant site of mass transfer in the pre-

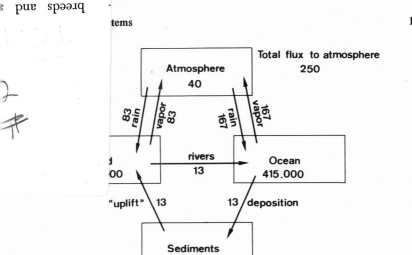

FIG 7.9. Tentative pre-man cycle of mercury (fluxes in units of 10^8 g/yr; reservoir masses in units of 10^8 g).

man sedimentary cycle of Hg is between the atmosphere and the earth's surface. Indeed, the total flux of 250×10^8 g/yr is about 20 times greater than that involving land–ocean–sediment transfer. This result is not unexpected because of the well-known volatility of Hg, discussed in previous sections. This volatility is strikingly demonstrated by the fact that the ratio Hg/Al in atmospheric "particulates" is 200 times greater than the Hg/Al ratio of crystalline rocks. Also, because of the low boiling points and vapor pressures of Hg compounds, there should be more Hg in the atmosphere than is detected in atmospheric "particulates," reflecting the fact that significant transport of Hg through the atmosphere probably is in the vapor state.

The maximum estimate of Weiss et al. (1971) of the degassing flux to the atmosphere of 1.5×10^{11} g Hg/yr probably represents an extreme value because they assume Hg is washed out of the *whole* atmosphere 40 times a year. It is likely that the concentration of Hg in the atmosphere shows an exponential decrease with increasing elevation similar to other gases originating at the earth's surface (CO for example). Thus, significant mass transfer to the earth's surface is limited to the lower portion of the atmosphere. Also, they assume the washout rate represents only the land degassing rate; however, as we show in our models, a significant portion of the total flux to the atmosphere comes from the sea surface.

Indeed, the total flux of mercury to the atmosphere (2.5×10^{10} g/yr) prior to man's activities recorded in the Greenland snow by Weiss et al. may not be explained by considering only degassing in the soil zone. At the present rate of continental denudation ($6.4 \ 10^{-3}$ cm/yr) and for a mean difference between the concentration of Hg in shales and soils of 100 ppb, total volatilization of Hg in soil would represent only 21×10^8 g/yr.

However, rain contains large amounts of mercury, probably as Hg°, which may be easily recycled from soils to the atmosphere. During the methylation-demethylation cycle, owing to the bacterial activity discussed in the previous sections, the volatile Hg° species represents an important intermediary product and may account for release of mercury to the atmosphere from soils, sediments, and surface waters. In the case of sea water, for example, the occurrence of 0.0001 μg Hg per liter as Hg° is enough to assure a transfer of 167×10^8 g Hg/yr from the oceans to the atmosphere, assuming an exchange coefficient across the air-water interface D/Z equal to 7×10^4 cm/yr (Broecker, 1962).

The vapor introduced to the atmosphere from the land and sea surface is washed out during rains. It can be seen from Fig. 7.9 that vapor transport from the land and sea surface to the atmosphere before man was balanced by equal transfers of Hg in rain back to the surfaces.

The residence times of Hg in the four reservoirs are: land, 1000 yr; atmosphere, 60 days; ocean, 32,000 yr; and sediments 2.5×10^8 yr. The relatively short residence times of Hg in the atmospheric and land reservoirs again reflect mainly the volatile character of mercury.

Using the pre-man cycle of Hg as background, we can now discuss the present cycle.

7.3.3. Present Cycle

The most obvious difference between the pre-man and present cycles of Hg (Fig. 7.10) is the increased fluxes between reservoirs of the present cycle. These increased fluxes are principally due to the increased rate of Hg input into the land reservoir owing to mining and utilization of Hg by man and to emissions of Hg to the atmosphere owing to chlor-alkali production, combustion of fossil fuels, cement manufacturing, and roasting of sulfide ores. Our total emission estimate is about 50% greater than that of Weiss et al. (1971). This difference principally reflects the fact that because of the known high volatility of Hg, we conclude that all of the mercury in combustible coal, oil, lignite, and gas will be released as vapor to the atmosphere. The calculation of Weiss et al. is based on release of only a portion of the mercury in coal and lignite. Approximately 2.14×10^{15} g of coal and lignite and 2.29×10^{15} of oil and gas is burned each year. With an average mercury content of 1×10^{-6} g Hg per gram of fuel, we obtain a mercury emission rate owing to combustion of 50×10^8 g Hg/yr. Weiss et al. calculate 16×10^8 for coal and lignite combustion. This value added to annual mercury emissions from chlor-alkali production, cement manufacturing, and roasting of sulfide ores, of 30×10^8 g, 10^8 g, and 20×10^8 g, respectively, gives a total Hg emission of about 100×10^8 g/yr.

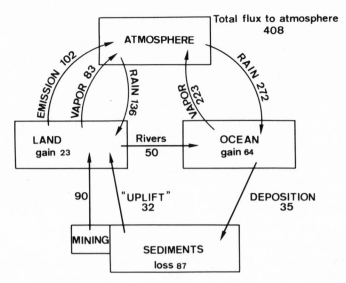

FIG. 7.10. Tentative present-day cycle of mercury (reservoir changes and fluxes in units of 10^8 g/yr).

The estimated total vapor flux of Hg to the atmosphere in the model of the present cycle is 408×10^8 g/yr, an increase of about 60% over the pre-man cycle. This value results from the assumption that the sea surface to atmosphere flux of mercury will be increased by about one-third of the pre-man ocean-atmosphere flux. This assumption is substantiated below. The input to the atmosphere is assumed to be removed in rain over the land and sea in proportion to their surface areas. The residence time of 36 days for Hg in the atmosphere justifies this assumption. Rain over the ocean results in a net input of Hg into the ocean surface of 49×10^8 g/yr; this value plus the addition of Hg to oceans via streams (50×10^8 g/yr) minus the sedimentation rate (35×10^8 g/yr) results in an accumulation of Hg in the ocean of 64×10^8 g/yr. We feel that, although some of this Hg enters living biota, most of it is stored in sea water in dissolved form.

Several factors justify this conclusion. The total mass of Hg in living oceanic biota today is only 7×10^8 g, and the Hg concentrations in the organic and skeletal phases of the biota are only 0.12 and 0.40 ppm, respectively.

The uptake of Hg in the photic zone by the biota is about 58×10^8 g Hg/yr. It would be expected that if a large part of the oceanic gain of Hg each year entered the biota, the total mass of Hg and its concentration in the biota would be greater than observed. Indeed, the calculated gain in the ocean exceeds the uptake rate. A simple calculation further justifies our conclusion: with an ocean surface area of 360×10^{16} cm^2 and a mixed layer depth of the ocean of 200 m, the storage of Hg in this layer would result in an increase of concentration of the order of 0.0001 g Hg per liter per year. This increase in total Hg is large enough to increase Hg° sufficiently in sea water to account for the increased rate of evasion of Hg vapor from the sea surface today as compared to pre-man time (223×10^8 and 167×10^8 g/yr, respectively).

It is interesting to further compare the present total flux of Hg vapor to the atmosphere with the pre-man flux. The present rate is about 1.6 times the pre-man rate. Thus, we would predict that concentrations of Hg in glacial ice formed during recent time would be about two times greater than those of the past. Indeed, Weiss et al. (1971) observed that waters deposited in the Greenland ice sheet prior to 1952 contained 60 ± 17 ng Hg/kg H_2O, whereas waters deposited as ice from 1952 to 1965 contained 125 ± 52 ng Hg/kg H_2O, an observation in good agreement with our prediction and our assumption of an increase of about 30% in the ocean–atmosphere flux.

It appears that the net result of mining and utilization of Hg on land and the increased Hg content of rain over land have resulted in an increase of about 0.02% in the Hg content of the land surface (soil). Such an increase suggests that even the degassing rate of the land's surface during recent times may be greater than that prior to man's interference with the Hg cycle.

Mining, mercury utilization by man, and emissions have increased the total Hg content of rivers about four times. Today's rivers carry about equal masses of Hg in dissolved and solid form to the oceans. This relation is difficult to understand because, generally, suspended sediment in rivers contains 3–4 times more Hg than the water. The problem may be that analyses of "dissolved" Hg in waters include very fine suspended matter and Hg complexed by organic acids. Nevertheless, man's interference with the Hg cycle appears to have increased the total Hg content of rivers.

In summary, man's contributions to the Hg cycle rival the nature fluxes. The major pathways affected are land–atmosphere–ocean and land–ocean. It is likely that Hg is currently being stored on land and in the ocean. Some of the Hg enters the biota of the ocean, but it is not likely that on a global basis there has been a significant increase in the mercury content of organisms. This same conclusion was reached by Weiss et al. (1971). The main impact of Hg on organisms may be on air-breathing terrestrial forms.

References

Baas-Becking, L. G. M., Kaplan, I. R., Moore, D. (1960). "Limits of natural environment in terms of pH and oxidation–reduction potentials," *J. Geol.,* **68,** 243–284.

Barker, H. A. (1936). "Studies upon the methane producing bacteria," *Arch. Mikrobiol.,* **7,** 404–420.

Barnes, H. L., Romberger, S. B., and Stemprok, M. (1967). "Ore solution chemistry. II. Solubility of HgS in sulfide solutions," *Economic Geology,* **62,** 958–982.

Beletskaya, I. P., Kurtis, A. L., and Reutov, O. A. (1967). "Electrophilic substitution at the aromatic carbon atom. VI. Kinetics and mechanism of anion catalyzed protolysis of arylmercuric bromides in dimethylformamide," *Zh. Org. Khim.*, **3**, 1930-1933 (Russ.); *C.A.*, **68**, 48721s.

Beletskaya, I. P., Butin, K. P., and Reutov, O. A. (1970). "Iodide ion catalyzable hydrolysis of organomercuric compounds in dimethylformamide," *Izv. Akad. Nauk SSSR, Ser. Khim.*, **1970**, 1680 (Russ.); *C.A.*, **74**, 12330y.

Beletskaya, I. P., Butin, K. P., and Reutov, O. A. (1971). "The $SE_1(N)$ mechanism in organometallic chemistry," *Organometal. Chem. Rev. (Sect. A)*, **7**, 51-79.

Berner, R. A. (1971). *Principles of Chemical Sedimentology*, Chap. 7, p. 114, McGraw-Hill, New York.

Billen, G. (1973). "Etude de l'ecometabolisme du mercure dans un milieu d'eau douce," *Hydrobiological Bulletin*, **7**, 60-68.

Billen G., and Wollast, R. (1973). "Transformations biologiques du mercure dans les sédiments de la Sambre," *Rapport de synthèse, projet Sambre. Journées d'étude des 27 et 28 novembre, 1972*, pp. 191-232, CIPS.

Billen, G., Joiris, C., and Wollast, R. (1974). "A bacterial methylmercury-mineralizing activity in river sediments," *Water Research*, **8**, 219-225.

Booer, J. R. (1944). "The behaviour of mercury compounds in soil," *Ann. Appl. Biol.*, **31**, 340-359.

Broecker, W. S. (1962). in *The Sea* (ed. Hill, M. H.), Vol. 2, p. 88, Interscience, New York.

Cranston, R. E., and Buckley, D. E. (1972). Mercury pathways in a river and an estuary," *Environ. Sc. Techn.*, **6**, 274-278.

Dadič, M., and Grdenič, D. (1960). "Symmetrical and mixed bisalkylmercuric sulphides," *Croat. Chem. Acta*, **32**, 39.

Fagerström, T., and Jernelöv, A. (1971). *Water Research*, **5**, 121.

Furakawa, K., Suzuki, T., and Tonomura, F. (1969). "Decomposition of organic mercurial compounds by mercury-resistant bacteria," *Agr. Biol. Chem.*, **33**, 128-130.

Garrels, R. M., and Christ, Ch. L. (1965). *Solutions, Minerals and Equilibria*, Harper and Row, New York.

Garrels, R. M., and MacKenzie, F. T. (1971). *Evolution of Sedimentary Rocks*, W. W. Norton, New York.

Garrels, R. M., and MacKenzie, F. T. (1972). "A quantitative model for the sedimentary rock cycle," *J. Marine Chem.*, **1**, 27-40.

Garrels, R. M., MacKenzie, F. T., and Hunt, C. A. (1973). *Man's Contributions to Natural Chemical Cycles*, Northwestern University, Evanston.

Goldberg, E. D. (1971). "Atmospheric dust, the sedimentary cycle and man," *Geophysics*, **1**, 117-132.

Hanke, M. E., and Bailey, J. H. (1945). "Oxidation reduction requirements of *Cl. Welchii* and other *Clostridia*," *Proc. Soc. Exp. Biol. Med.*, **59**, 163.

Hem, J. D. (1970). "Chemical behavior of mercury in aqueous media," *U.S. Geological Survey, Professional Paper 713*, pp. 19-24, Washington.

Hogenkamp, H. P. C. (1968). "Enzymatic reactions involving corrinoids," *Ann. Rev. Biochem.*, **37**, 225.

Imura, N., Sukegawa, E., Pan, S. K., and Nagao, K. (1971). "Chemical methylation of inorganic mercury with methylcobalamin, a vitamin B_{12} analogue," *Science*, **172**, 1248-1249.

Ingraham, L. L. (1964). "Biological Grignard reagents," *Ann. N. Y. Acad. Sci.*, **112**, 713.

Jensen, S., and Jernelöv, A. (1969). "Biological methylation of mercury in aquatic organisms," *Nature (Lond.)*, **223**, 753.

Jernelöv, A. (1970). "Release of methylmercury from sediments with layers containing inorganic mercury at depths," *Limnol. and Oceanogr.*, **15**, 958-960.

Kimura, Y., and Miller, V. L. (1964). "The degradation of organomercury fungicides in soil," *Agr. Food Chem.,* **12,** 253–257.

Landner, L. (1971). "Biochemical model for the biological methylation of mercury suggested from methylation studies *in vivo* with *Neurospora crassa, Nature (Lond.),* **230,** 452–454.

Landner, L. (1972). "The biological alkylation of mercury," *Biochem. J.,* **130,** 67P–69P.

MacKenzie, F. T., and Wollast, R. (1975). "Global physical dispersion models," in *Methods to Protect Man and Ecosystems from Adverse Effects of Pollutants* (ed. WHO, Geneva) (in press).

Miller, M. A., and Harmon, S. A. (1967). "Genetic association of determinants controlling resistance to mercuric chloride, production of penicillinase and synthesis of methionine in *Staphylococcus aureus," Nature (Lond.),* **215,** 531–532.

Pytkowicz, R. M. (1973). "The carbon dioxide system in the oceans," *Swiss J. Hydrol.,* **35,** 8–28.

Schwarzenbach, G., and Schellenberg, M. (1965). "Complex chemistry of the methylmercury cation," *Helv. Chim. Acta,* **48,** 28–46.

Spangler, W. J., Spigarelli, J. L., Rose, J. M., Flippin, R. S., and Miller, H. M. (1973). "Degradation of methylmercury by bacteria isolated from environmental samples," *Appl. Microbiol.,* **25,** 488–493.

Stadtman, T. C. (1967). "Methane fermentation," *Ann. Rev. Microbiol.,* **21,** 121.

Stumm, W. (1966). "Redox potential as an environmental parameter: conceptual significance and operational limitation," *Proc. Int. Water Pollution. Res. Conf. (3rd, Munich),* **1,** 283–308.

Symons, D. (1962). "Stability relations of mercury compounds," in *Equilibrium Diagrams for Minerals at Low Temperature and Pressure* (ed. Schmitt, H. H.), p. 164, Cambridge Geological Club of Harvard.

Tonomura, K., Maeda, K., Futai, F., Nakagami, T., and Yamada, M. (1968). "Stimulative vaporization of phenylmercuric acetate by mercury-resistant bacteria," *Nature (Lond.),* **217,** 644–646.

Tonomura, K., and Kanzaki, F. (1969). "The reductive decomposition of organic mercurials by cell free extract of a mercury-resistant *Pseudomonas," Biochim. Biophys. Acta,* **184,** 227–229.

Wagman, D. D., Evans, W. L., Parker, V. B., Harlow, I., Bailey, S. M., and Schumm, R. H. (1968). "Selected values of chemical thermodynamic properties," *Nat. Bur. Standards. Tech. Note 270-4,* p. 141.

Weiss, H. V., Koide, M., and Goldberg, E. D. (1971). *Science,* **174,** 692–694.

Wollast, R. (1974). "The silica problem," in *The Sea* (ed. Goldberg, E. D.), Vol. 5, Wiley, New York.

Wood, J. M., Kennedy, F. S., and Rosen, C. G. (1968). "Synthesis of methylmercury compounds by extracts of a methanogenic bacterium," *Nature (Lond.),* **220,** 173–174.

Yamada, M., and Tonomura, K. (1972). "Formation of methylmercury compounds from inorganic mercury by *Clostridium cochlearium," J. Ferment. Technol.,* **50,** 159–166.

8

Mobilization of Metals in the Dutch Wadden Sea*

J. C. DUINKER

8.1. Introduction

Approximately 10% of the water and 50% of the suspended matter supplied by the Rhine to the North Sea enter the Dutch Wadden Sea. According to Zimmerman and Rommets (1974), the water in the western part of the Dutch Wadden Sea contains, on an average, 7% Rhine water and 7% fresh water from Lake Yssel, composed mainly of Rhine water supplied by the river Yssel. The west–east transport of water within the Wadden Sea is very limited; on the other hand, fine-grained suspended matter from the North sea is accumulated within the Wadden Sea toward the eastern part (Postma, 1954, 1961; van Straaten and Kuenen, 1957, 1958).

This paper is concerned with tracing the fate of metals in the Dutch Wadden Sea, in both particulate and dissolved forms. Special attention is given to copper and zinc on the basis of their concentrations in North Sea water (Dutton et al., 1973; Duinker et al., 1974), and iron and manganese because of the scaveng-

---

*For further details see Duinker et al. (1974). Recent work of Elderfield and Hepworth (1975) supports the main aspects of the mobilization processes of metals as described there and in the present report.

J. C. DUINKER • Netherlands Institute for Sea Research, P.O. Box 59, den Burg, Texel, Netherlands.

ing properties of their hydrous oxides and the usefulness of managanese as a tracer for sediment transport studies (de Groot 1963, 1966, 1973).

8.2. Methods

Samples of water and suspended matter were obtained by bucket sampling and filtration on board ship. Bottom samples were taken with a van Veen grab. Metal concentrations in solution were obtained according to the concentration-extraction procedure proposed by Brooks et al. (1967). Concentrations in suspended matter and bottom material were determined as a leachable fraction (0.1 N HCl during 18 h) and as total metal content after complete digestion of the sample.

Size distributions of bottom and suspended sediment were determined according to the classical settling methods used in soil science. The usual pretreatment with HCl was replaced by a treatment of the sample suspended in double-distilled water in an ultrasonic bath for 15 min. Thus, individual subsamples could be analyzed for their metal content.

The average mineral composition of Wadden Sea suspended matter samples is

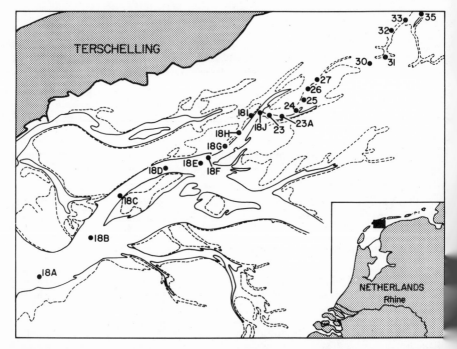

FIG. 8.1. Site of investigation in the Terschelling watershed area. Contours at 0 and 2 m below LLWS.

70-80% quartz, 10% feldspars, and 10-15% clay minerals. The relative contributions of these main groups appeared to vary little, but the relative contributions of the different clay minerals—illite, kaolinite, and smectite—showed considerable variations over the Wadden Sea area. On an average, some 5% of the suspended matter consists of organic carbon. The leaching agent used causes some clay mineral lattice breakdown, probably less than 10%. However, the fractions of copper, zinc, and manganese being leached appear to be well defined and represent 80-90% of the total amounts present.

8.3. Area of Investigation

From 1971 onward, regular sampling surveys have been made throughout the Dutch Wadden Sea. Relatively large variations (with respect to both time and place) in the metal concentrations were found. These variations could not be related to the degree of mixing between the different water masses. Near Terschelling the bottom configuration takes the form of a watershed, and this area (Fig. 8.1) was selected for a closer investigation. From west to east water depth and current velocity in the tidal channel decrease toward the watershed, where small suspended particles can settle, causing accumulation of trace metals.

The results described in this paper pertain to Tidal Stations 18H and 30 (Fig. 8.1) in the period 16-19 April, 1973. A characteristic pattern of the current velocity for one tidal period is given in Fig. 8.2

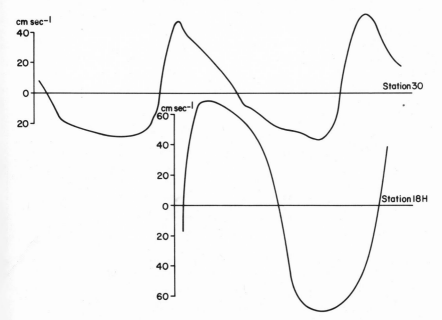

FIG. 8.2. Current velocity characteristics at Tidal Stations 18H and 30.

8.4. Results

8.4.1. Tidal Stations

The relevant data on the tidal stations are presented in Fig. 8.3. It is not obvious how the concentrations of dissolved copper and zinc could readily be correlated with the data on either salinity or the metal content of suspended matter samples. Maxima in the amount of suspended matter in the surface layer occur around slack water, in combination with a minimum in the leachable metal content. At the same time the concentration of dissolved reactive silicate increases. Strong maxima in copper and zinc concentrations in the dissolved state are observed; they appear around maximum current velocity, 1 to 3 h before the maxima in the amount of suspended matter.

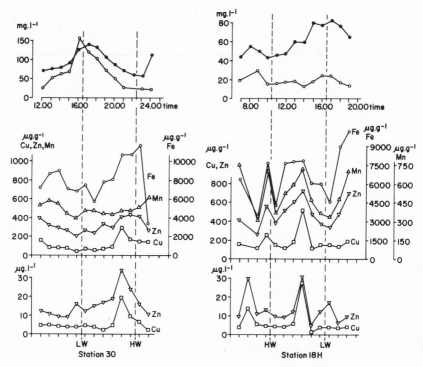

FIG. 8.3. Tidal Stations 18H and 30. Metal concentrations in the water phase (bottom); leachable metal concentrations in suspended matter (middle); suspended matter in milligrams per liter (○) and reactive silicate (●) in relative concentration units (top). Salinity values are within the range 31.055–33.250%.

TABLE 8.1. Metal Contents in Bottom Sediment at Stations in the Terschelling Watershed Area

Station	Particles <16 μm (wt. %)	Metal (μg/g dry weight)							
		Cu		Zn		Mu		Fe	
		(a)	(b)	(a)	(b)	(a)	(b)	(a)	(b)
23	36.0	5	75	80	490	180	350	1,600	17,000
24	6.5	2	50	30	450	95	180	950	5,300
27	35.0	4	50	60	530	150	280	2,300	15,500
30	7.5	4	33	30	350	90	190	900	6,500
32	5.0	2	20	25	–	40	160	625	5,000
33	2.5	1	25	5	350	9	65	215	2,200
30 core	13.0	2	50	15	350	60	200	500	8,500

(a) Leached metal fraction (0.1 N HCl).
(b) Total metal content after complete digestion of the sample. The data on the contribution of the particles smaller than 16 μm (weight %) are included.

8.4.2. Bottom Samples

From Postma (1954, 1961) and van Straaten and Kuenen (1958) it is known that continuous exchange of bottom and suspended sediment takes place in this area. To find an explanation for the behavior of suspended matter, the relevant properties of bottom particles were therefore analyzed (Table 8.1):

de Groot (1963) established a linear relationship between the weight percent fraction of particles smaller than 16 μm and the total metal content (after complete digestion of the sample) for cogenetic freshly deposited bottom samples, usually obtained along the shore. This relation appears to hold (within the limited data available) for the samples of the watershed area as well, both for the total metal contents and for the leached fractions (Table 8.1). The values obtained by extrapolating the relationship toward 100% of the particles smaller than 16 μm are given in Table 8.2. These calculated values compare favorably with the metal concentrations that have been obtained by direct measurement in the < 16 μm size fraction at the different stations.

8.4.3. Suspended Matter

If suspended matter reflected the properties of the corresponding size fractions in the bottom layers, the leachable metal concentrations would be in the following ranges: copper 1–15; zinc 20–225; manganese 25–450; iron 1000–6000 μg/g dried sediment, depending on the fraction of particles smaller than 16

TABLE 8.2. Metal Content of Bottom Sediment Samples in the Terschelling Watershed Area, Extrapolated for 100% of the Sample Being Smaller Than 16 μm

Metal	Weight (μg/g dry weight)	
	(a)	(b)
Cu	15	100
Zn	225	700–900
Mn	450	600
Fe	6,000	30,000–40,000

(a) Leached metal fraction (0.1 N HCl).
(b) Total metal content after complete digestion of sample.

μm. The particle size distributions of suspended matter samples obtained in this area are very similar, 60-70% of the particles having an equivalent diameter smaller than 16 μm. This would imply that metal concentrations in this area would show only small variations for suspended matter at different stations, with values (extrapolated toward 100% smaller than 16 μm) halfway between the lower and upper limits just mentioned.

The values that have been determined throughout the Wadden Sea are much higher, even without correction for the particle size effect. Moreover, they show considerable variations: copper 150-500; zinc 200-600; manganese 350-1000; iron 6000-10,000 μg/g dried sediment, with few exceptions.

The conclusions to be drawn is that the metal content in suspended matter cannot be interpreted by assuming that suspended matter is represented by eroded bottom particles, even if the data have been corrected for the grain size distribution. This aspect should be considered in transport studies of metals by sediment particles.

8.4.4. Continuous Particulate Fraction

The differences between bottom and suspended material may be interpreted in terms of a "fine" fraction of particulate matter, which remains continuously in suspension and carries an important fraction of the metals considered here. A number of arguments support this postulate. First, laboratory experiments showed considerable differences between freshly sedimented and Millipore-filtered identical sea water samples, the latter having both higher weights (10-30%) of particulate matter per unit volume and higher metal contents (up to

TABLE 8.3. Metal Content of Suspended Matter Obtained by
Filtration (b) and Deposition in the Laboratory (a) of Originally
Identical Sea Water Samples

Samples were leached with 0.1 N HCl (18 h)

Station	Metal (μg/g dry weight)							
	Cu		Zn		Mn		Fe	
	a	b	a	b	a	b	a	b
18H	40	150	90	410	130	400	2100	6000
23	70	330	150	890	440	560	5300	7800
25	130	250	220	670	400	630	6600	9000
27	190	430	350	770	450	470	7000	7500
30	70	90	160	310	255	580	4950	8600

500%, depending on the particular samples and the metal considered) (Table
8.3). Second, the fraction that is usually considered to resist settling in the
Dutch Wadden Sea, i.e., that consisting of particles with an equivalent diameter
smaller than 0.5 μm, was found to represent a large percentage (40-60%) of the
fraction <16 μm. The continuous fraction may well consist of colloidal iron and
manganese hydrous oxides, including trace elements.

8.5. Interpretation of Data from Tidal Stations

The relative minima in the leachable metal concentrations in the suspended
matter samples of the tidal stations can now be interpreted. Particles with low
metal content, having been eroded from the bottom, decrease the relative metal
content of suspended matter. The pattern of more or less scattered values of
metal contents in suspended matter samples in the intermediate region of the
tidal stations can be interpreted in terms of a mixing process between the "fine"
continuously suspended fraction with low density and high metal content and
"coarse" bottom particles characterized by low metal values. This can be demonstrated by the relationship that was found to exist between the amount of suspended matter per unit volume and its metal content for surveys through the
area of Fig. 8.1 at low and high tide (Fig. 8.4). The most plausible explanation
for the occurrence of the sharp maxima for the dissolved copper and zinc concentrations is a contribution from the interstitial water to the metal concentration of the overlying water. In fact, during the work described here, values for
the concentrations of copper, zinc, manganese, and iron dissolved in the inter-

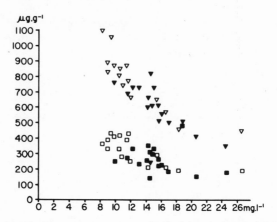

FIG. 8.4. Leachable copper and zinc concentrations in suspended matter at stations sampled during high and low tide (stations of Fig. 8.1). ▽ Zinc at low tide; ▼ zinc at high tide; □ copper at low tide; ■ copper at high tide.

stitial water phase have been found to be roughly one to two orders of magnitude higher than in the overlying water.

8.6. Mobilization Processes

Part of the suspended matter that is introduced from the North Sea will settle in the Wadden Sea. It will lose part of its metal load under reducing conditions and the interstitial water will be enriched in metals by this process. Diffusion of dissolved metals will take place from the interstitial water into the overlying water, where the change in concentration may remain undetected due to the low levels and the low molecular diffusion velocity. As a result of tidal and wind action the interstitial water may lose its metal content to the overlying water, which will result in a sudden and detectable increase in metal concentration of this overlying water. Metals are either taken up in the water phase as soluble complexes or they are attached to suspended matter (a) in colloidal form, (b) by adsorption, or (c) by uptake in marine organisms. The observations show (Fig. 8.4) that for both zinc and copper a linear correlation exists between the amount of suspended matter per unit volume and its metal content. For the low-tide samples, low weights of suspended matter are associated with high metal values; for the high-tide samples, higher weights are associated with lower metal values. Where deviations from the linear relationship occur, they appear to be associated with samples taken at times when maximum metal concentration were appearing in the water phase.

According to these studies it appears probable that suspended matter can im mediately take up part of the dissolved copper and zinc supplied by the interstitial water. The nonconservative character for copper and zinc in this mixing process is further supported by the observation that the maxima in the dissolved concentrations are much sharper than the maxima for the reactive silicate as shown by van Bennekom et al. (1974).

The present investigations took place under severe wind conditions. This may have contributed to obtaining data that would otherwise have remained unrecorded. In a more recent set of observations (at Tidal Station 27, August 1973) obtained during a long period of extremely calm weather, none of the extreme features that characterize the present work has been found. Because of the frequent sampling scheme it is improbable that any maxima would have stayed unobserved.

The processes that have been described take place under natural conditions; they must be of a general character, applicable to any estuarine environment. These processes are responsible for the mobilization of metals under reducing conditions; on the other hand they prevent a net accumulation of metals in the bottom sediments in an area like the Dutch Wadden Sea where net sedimentation takes place. Tidal action and a reducing situation seem to be necessary conditions for the occurrence of these processes. Removal of tidal action from such an area may, if metal supply continues, cause high metal concentrations in interstitial water.

8.7. Summary

The metals copper, zinc, iron, and manganese are mobilized in bottom sediments of the Dutch Wadden Sea into intersitial water, where metal concentrations in solution one to two orders of magnitude higher than in the overlying water have been detected. Exchange of metals between interstitial water and the overlying water can take place under particular hydrographic and meteorological conditions, giving rise to short-term increases in the water phase concentrations. Tidal action and reducing conditions are partly responsible for these mobilization processes; on the other hand they reduce or prevent the net accumulation of metals in the Dutch Wadden Sea. Evidence is given for the existence of a "fine" fraction, probably consisting of colloidal iron and manganese hydrous oxides including trace elements, that resists settling in the natural conditions of the Wadden Sea. This fraction may be responsible, in part, for the removal of the mobilized elements out of the Wadden Sea into the North Sea. This fraction with a relatively high metal content will settle elsewhere, perhaps in the deep ocean. It is suggested that removing the tidal action from an area where these conditions prevail may result in high metal concentrations in interstitial water.

References

Bennekom, A. J. van, Krijgsman-van Hartingsveld, E., van der Veer, G. C. M., and van Voorst, H. F. J. (1974). "The seasonal cycle of reactive silicate and suspended diatoms in the Dutch Wadden Sea," *Neth. J. Sea Res.,* 8(2), 174-207.

Brooks, R. R., Presley, B. J., and Kaplan, I. R. (1967). "APDC-MIBK extraction system for the determination of trace elements in saline waters by atomic absorption spectro-photometry," *Talanta,* 14, 809-816.

Duinker, J. C., van Eck, G. T. M., and Nolting, R. F. (1974). "On the behavior of copper, zinc, iron and manganese and evidence for mobilization processes in the Dutch Wadden Sea," *Neth. J. Sea Res.,* 8(2), 214-239.

Dutton, J. V. R., Jefferies, D. F., Folkard, A. R., and Jones, P. G. W. (1973). "Trace metals in the North Sea," *Mar. Pollut. Bull.,* 4, 135-138.

Elderfield, H., and Hepworth, A. (1975). "Diagenesis, metals and pollution in estuaries," *Mar. Pollut. Bull.,* 6(6), 85-87.

Groot, de A. J. (1963). "Mangaantoestand van Nederlandse en Duitse holocene sedimenten," *Versl. Landbouwk. Onderz. Ned.,* 69, 1-164.

Groot, de A. J. (1966). "Mobility of trace elements in deltas," *1. Trans. Comm. II and IV Int. Soc. Soil Sci., Aberdeen,* pp. 267-279.

Groot, de A. J. (1973). "Occurrence and behavior of heavy metals in river deltas, with special reference to the Rhine and Ems rivers," in *North Sea Science* (ed. Goldberg, E. D.), pp. 308-325, MIT Press.

Postma, H. (1954). "Hydrography of the Dutch Wadden Sea," *Arch. néerl. zool.,* Vol. 10, No. 4, 106 pp.

Postma, H. (1961). "Transport and accumulation of suspended matter in the Dutch Wadden Sea," *Neth. J. Sea Res.,* 1, 148-190.

Straaten, L. M. J. U. van, and Kuenen, Ph. H. (1957). "Accumulation of fine grained sedi-ment in the Dutch Wadden Sea," *Geol. Mijnb.,* 19, 1-110.

Straaten, L. M. J. U. van, and Kuenen, Ph. H. (1958). "Tidal action as a cause of clay accu-mulation," *J. Sedim. Petrol.,* 28, 406-413.

Zimmerman, J. T. F., and Rommets, J. W. (1974). "Natural fluorescence as a tracer in the Dutch Wadden Sea and the adjacent North Sea, *Neth. J. Sea. Res.,* 8(2), 117-125.

9

Metallothionein and the Toxicity of Cadmium

M. WEBB

Cadmium has an extremely long biological half-life and thus, even at low levels of exposure, human beings and domestic animals are liable to accumulate during their lifetimes considerable amounts of the metal, most of which will be stored in the livers and kidneys. Because of this cumulative property of cadmium it is possible to produce in experimental animals, either by feeding or parenteral administration, similar total body burdens and liver and kidney levels in short periods of time.

In these short-term experiments with laboratory animals, as in humans and other mammalian species exposed to the metal in the environment, cadmium accumulates in the livers and kidneys as metallothionein. The name "metallothionein" was given by Vallee and his collaborators to a cadmium-containing protein that was isolated initially from horse kidney (Margoshes and Vallee, 1957; Kägi and Vallee, 1960, 1961) and subsequently from human kidney (Pulido et al., 1966). Later, with the increasing interest in the toxicology of cadmium, proteins of similar properties (low molecular weight, high content—about 30%—of cysteine residues, virtual absence of aromatic amino acids) were isolated from the livers and kidneys of experimental animals [see, e.g., Friberg et al., (1971) for a summary of the literature]. Although these proteins probably are true metallothioneins, and will be referred to as such in the following discussion, it should be stressed that none of them has been characterized as extensively as the horse and human kidney proteins.

M. WEBB • MRC Toxicology Unit, Carshalton, Surrey, England.

From recent research it seems that "metallothioneins" may have a physiological function in the control of the metabolism of certain essential trace metals.
This discovery has led to confusion in the terminology of these proteins, which
is no longer as defined by Kägi and Vallee (1960) and seems in dire need of
clarification. This could be achieved if the term "thionein" were used for the protein moiety and qualified according to the major bound cation, for example,
"zinc-thionein," "cadmium-thionein," etc. In this system the prefix "metallo-
would be used in the same sense as in "metalloprotein."

Because of their high cysteine contents the metallothioneins are an interesting and unusual group of proteins, but are not unique. Neonatal liver, for example, contains an insoluble copper-containing protein, initially thought to be
located in the mitochondria and termed neonatal mitochondrocuprein (Porter,
1970), but later found to be in nonmitochondrial particles, probably heavy
lysosomes, and now renamed cuprocysteinin (Porter and Hills, 1974). This
protein and, particularly, a soluble derivative obtained from it by S-sulfonation
(Porter, 1970), shows many analogies in amino acid composition, particularly
with regard to its high contents of cysteine residues, lysine, glycine, and proline,
with metallothionein. In contrast to metallothionein, however, cuprocysteinin
does not contain free —SH groups, either before or after removal of the bound
metal, and it seems that the insolubility of the latter protein is related to its high
content of disulfide bridges (Porter, 1970).

In the liver of the rat (Shaikh and Lucis, 1970a; Webb 1972a), mouse (Nordberg, Piscator and Lind, 1971), and rabbit (Nordberg et al., 1972), metallothionein
is known to be an inducible protein, which is synthesized in response to the uptake of the toxic cation. With doses of cadmium below a certain critical level the
content of metallothionein in the liver at a given time increases roughly in proportion to the dose (Shaikh and Lucis, 1970b), the metal binding sites seemingly
being fully saturated at all times (Webb 1972b; Bremner and Marshall, 1974).
Although a protein identical to metallothionein, but with zinc as the main
cation component, can be induced in rat liver by administration of excess zinc
(Webb 1972a), in the normal adult animal the content of the metal-containing
thionein is so low that it is barely detectable (e.g., Webb, 1972a; Nordberg et al.,
1972; Piotrowski et al., 1973). Nevertheless, it is possible that thionein has a
normal biological function in the regulation of zinc and—probably—copper
metabolism. Thus, small amounts of zinc-thionein have been found in the liver
of the female but not of the male rat (Webb, 1972a). Also, the observations of
Bremner et al. (1973) suggest that the inducible synthesis of zinc-thionein in
rat liver occurs once the zinc content of the tissue exceeds 30 μg/g wet weight
(a situation achieved by various experimental regimes, including restriction of
food intake) and appears to provide a mechanism whereby zinc is either con-
served or detoxified. Furthermore, from horse liver Kägi (1970) has isolated a
protein very similar to horse kidney metallothionein in amino acid composition
but with zinc as the main cation component.

The liver of the neonatal rat contains much larger quantities of copper than that of the adult animal (Underwood, 1956). Part of this excess copper is associated with the insoluble cuprocysteinin (Porter and Hills, 1974). In the soluble fraction of neonatal rat liver the distribution of copper is similar to that in the corresponding fraction of the liver of the copper-loaded adult rat (Bloomer and Sourkes, 1974) in which, in addition to hepatocuprein (mol. wt. about 35,000–40,000 daltons), the excess cation is bound in a protein of molecular weight of about 11,000–12,000 daltons. This latter protein absorbs strongly at 250 nm, has a high content of (masked) —SH groups, and, although not extensively characterized, is considered to be closely related to, or identical with, metallothionein (Evans et al., 1970). Previously, similar proteins had been isolated from the chick intestine (Starcher, 1969), the duodenum, liver, and kidney of the rat (Evans and Cornatzer, 1970), and bovine liver and duodenum (Evans et al., 1970) and assumed to function in the absorption and/or transport of zinc and copper.

Bremner and Marshall (1974) also have found a soluble protein, very similar to metallothionein, but with zinc and copper as the principal bound cations, in calf and lamb liver, and have shown that the total amount of $Zn^{2+} + Cu^{2+}$ that is present in this protein (and presumably, since the apoprotein alone appeared to be absent from the liver, the protein itself) is determined by the content of liver Zn^{2+}. *In vitro* experiments showed that all of the zinc and part of the copper in this protein was displaced by treatment with a low concentration of cadmium, this displacement being accompanied by an increase in the absorbance at 250 nm, a behavior typical of the Cd^{2+} chromatophore in metallothionein.

It appears therefore that, at least in liver and possibly other organs of various animal species, thionein may play some part in the binding of copper and zinc as well as cadmium. The situation is complicated, however, since crude, cadmium-induced metallothionein (which also contains zinc together with small amounts of copper), appears to be resolved on further fractionation into two or more protein components that contain different relative amounts of the various cations. Nordberg et al. (1972), for example, separated rabbit liver metallothionein by isoelectric focusing into two main protein components of pI 3.9 and 4.5. These were very similar in amino acid composition, but differed greatly in their contents of zinc and cadmium; both forms contained cadmium, but only that of pI of 4.5 contained significant amounts of zinc. Isoelectric focusing, however, is a far from ideal method for the fractionation of crude metallothionein (R. W. Stoddart and M. Webb, in preparation) and, in particular, separation is very dependent upon the ratio of protein to ampholytes. Bremner and Marshall (1974), however, also reported that the copper- and zinc-containing metallothionein-like protein of calf liver was resolved on Biogel P 10 into three fractions. Whereas all of these had high cysteine contents and molar ratios of —SH groups to total metal of 2.8–3.0, the ratio of zinc to copper was 4.8 in one of them and greater than 100 in the other two. Recent research, therefore, seems to have complicated rather than clarified the chemistry and biochemistry of metallothionein, and more work is very necessary to establish whether there is a family of these proteins. It is possible that the partial removal of a metal ion, either *in vivo* or during the isolation of the protein, could lead to intermolecular polymerization through the formation of disulfide bridges. Although studies on the conformation of metallothionein are lacking at present, it appears to be established that three —SH groups are involved in the binding of each metal atom (Kägi and Vallee, 1960, 1961; Nordberg et al. 1972; Bremner and Marshall, 1974). While, spatially, these must be close together, intramolecular disulfide formation at the metal binding site would utilize only two of them.

It has been suggested frequently that the inducible synthesis of metallothionein provides the mammalian organism with a protective mechanism against the immediate toxic effects of cadmium ions (see Friberg et al., 1971). In the normal rat, there is a lag between the administration of cadmium and the appearance of the high-affinity binding protein in the liver cytosol. Although even at the earliest times after dosing the content of cadmium in the cytosol may be quite high, the cation is bound by a protein fraction of high molecular weight. Once synthesis of the specific binding protein has been induced, cadmium is transferred to it from the high-molecular-weight components and appears in the cell sap as metallothionein. At the same time the total content of cadmium in the cytosol increases, while the amounts bound by the particulate cellular components decrease (Webb, 1972c).

Once bound with the apoprotein, thionein, cadmium persists in the liver and kidney for a prolonged period. Cotzias et al. (1961), for example, found that the total body turnover of $^{109}Cd^{2+}$ in the mouse was negligible, even on subsequent challenge with cadmium or zinc. Also, in rats 14 months or more after a single subcutaneous injection of $CdCl_2$ (Webb, 1972a) or $^{109}CdCl_2$ (M. Webb, unpublished observations), metallothionein containing either Cd^{2+} or $^{109}Cd^{2+}$ is still present in the liver. It is probable therefore that a significant amount of this protein-bound cation persists throughout the lifespan of the animal, although, as Shaikh and Lucis (1970c) have shown, there is, apparently, continual turnover of the protein moiety.

At the LD_{50} level the first few hours after intravenous injection of cadmium are critical, and if the animal survives for this period it usually recovers, although the subsequent weight gain remains below normal.* The mechanism of the acute

---

*Although the introduction of LD_{50} values at first may seem outside the scope of this conference, it is likely that the same receptors will interact with cadmium whether or not the dose is lethal. Thus, the reactions that lead to death may differ quantitatively, but not qualitatively, from those responsible for other effects at chronic exposure. Such effects have been reported to include arteriosclerosis, high blood pressure, hypertension, and decreased life expectancy (see, e.g., Schroeder and Vinton, 1962; Schroeder et al., 1966; Fischer and Thind, 1971; Malcolm, 1973).

death has not been defined. The classic autoradiographic study of the distribution, after a single intravenous injection, of $^{109}Cd^{2+}$ in the mouse by Berlin and Ullberg (1963), together with the quantitative measurements of Nordberg and Nishiyama (1972), has shown that although the concentrations in the liver and kidney are much greater than in other organs, significant amounts of the metal are located in the mammary gland, spleen, pancreas, bone marrow, lung, hyperphysis, thyroid, salivary and lymph glands, adrenal, myocardium, and skin, with small, but detectable, quantities in the brain and muscle. Hemorrhagic lesions in sensory ganglia in response to cadmium have been observed by Gabbiani (1966). It seems probable, therefore, that interaction of cadmium with vital processes in tissues or organs other than the liver and kidney will provide the explanation for the lethal action of the metal at acute exposure. In this connection the observations of Jacobs et al. (1956) on the extreme and apparently specific effect of very low concentrations of cadmium on mitochondrial oxidative phosphorylation should not be forgotten.

There can be little doubt that in terms of total body burden of cadmium, metallothionein is protective. It has been shown repeatedly, for example, that experimental animals will tolerate a much higher total dose of cadmium when given as multiple doses at frequent intervals than when administered as a single injection. Under the former conditions, cadmium accumulates in the liver and kidneys as metallothionein, in which form the metal must be less toxic since, at least below certain limits (200 $\mu g/g$ wet weight in the kidney) the total body burden of cadmium is not correlated with toxic manifestations (Nordberg et al., 1971).

With experimental animals it has been known for some time that pretreatment with a low dose of cadmium protects against a subsequent normally lethal dose of the cation. Similarly, protection against cadmium-induced injury to the testis is achieved by pretreatment of the animal with a high dose of zinc (Webb, 1972b). In both instances, protection can be explained by the induction of metallothionein synthesis, the liver being conditioned to the synthesis of this protein, which continues without lag when the animal is challenged with cadmium. Furthermore, the weanling rat is much less susceptible to cadmium than is the adult, the LD_{50} for the former being almost three times that of the latter (R. Verschoyle and M. Webb, unpublished observations). This also can be explained on the protection hypothesis, if it is accepted that the liver of the neonatal rat contains a protein identical with metallothionein, except that zinc and copper are the cation components.

If the metal binding groups of metallothionein are fully saturated, there are two ways in which the protein could be protective against a second dose of cadmium. Either cadmium could displace zinc, which also occurs in significant concentration in the protein already present, or the protein could be synthesized immediately without any lag, since the liver is conditioned to its synthesis. Both of these alternatives may occur. It has been shown, for example, that on administration of cadmium to rats protected by pretreatment with excess zinc, the contents not only of cadmium but also of zinc and protein in the metallothionein fraction increase (Webb, 1972b), although it has not been established whether at the earliest times there is initial substitution of cadmium for zinc. That such substitution can occur is shown by the replacement of cadmium in metallothionein by mercury.

Intravenously administered $^{203}Hg^{2+}$ is known to accumulate in the soluble fractions of rat liver and kidney in two nondialysable protein fractions, one of which has a molecular weight of about 11,000, and appears to be the mercury derivative of thionein (Jakubowski et al., 1970; Wisniewska et al., 1970). *In vivo*, mercury does not seem to be an active inducer of thionein synthesis, but readily replaces other metals in the small amounts of metallo-(zinc ?)-thionein that are present in these tissues (L. Magos and M. Webb, unpublished results). The greater affinity for mercury of the sulfhydryl binding sites of thionein *in vitro* than for cadmium, zinc, and copper is well known, and has been used by Piotrowski et al. (1973) as the basis for a method for the estimation of the metallothionein content of animal tissues. Increased uptake of mercury (with decreased nephrotoxicity) has been observed in the kidneys of male rats that have been pretreated with cadmium (L. Magos and M. Webb, unpublished results). Increased uptake is also observed in the liver and, as in the kidney, is correlated, at least in part, with the ability of mercury to displace cadmium from the presynthesized metallothionein.

There are, however, a number of reasons against the ready acceptance of this protection hypothesis. For example:

1. At least in mice, the protective effect of pretreatment with a low dose of cadmium lasts for little more than three days (Yoshikawa, 1970), whereas the induced synthesis of metallothionein continues for longer than this. Furthermore, other cations, for example, indium and lead, which do not induce the synthesis of a (metallo)thionein, also protect mice against a toxic dose of cadmium when administered in advance of the latter (Yoshikawa, 1970).

2. The restriction of food intake which, in the rat, induces the synthesis of zinc-thionein (Bremner et al., 1973a) does not alter the intravenous LD_{50} of cadmium (R. Verschoyle and M. Webb, unpublished results).

3. If rats are made resistant to cadmium by pretreatment with the unlabeled cation and then are dosed with $^{109}Cd^{2+}$, much greater amounts of the isotope are accumulated in the livers of the pretreated animals than in the livers of the untreated controls, and all of this excess cadmium is bound in metallothionein. In all other tissues that have been examined, however, the levels of $^{109}Cd^{2+}$ are the same in the pretreated group and the normal controls. It seems, therefore, that the pretreated animal accumulates a

greater amount of $^{109}Cd^{2+}$ in the liver, since this is conditioned to the synthesis of metallothionein. This extra binding does not mean that less cadmium is taken up by other organs, but that a greater percentage of the dose is retained in the pretreated animals (R. Verschoyle and M. Webb, unpublished results).

There is much evidence that at chronic low-level exposure, cadmium is an antagonist of the metabolism of both zinc and copper (see, e.g., Bunn and Matrone, 1966; Petering et al., 1971). Although, as Mills et al. (1973) have pointed out, there is no clear evidence that concentrations of cadmium such as those found in the environment are sufficient to induce a metabolic zinc deficiency, many of the effects of low-level exposure to the former cation resemble those of copper deficiency. The significance of these effects is increased by the observations of Anke et al. (1971) that the copper deficiency induced by cadmium in goats is transferred from the dam to the kid. Thus, although at low levels of exposure cadmium does not cross the placenta, its effects do and, for the next generation, these effects may be very dangerous.

An approach to the study of continual exposure to very low levels of cadmium has been made by Mills and his collaborators. It has been shown, for example, that dietary concentrations of 3-4 μg Cd^{2+}/g have marked effects upon copper and, to a lesser extent, zinc metabolism in newborn lambs and, even immediately after birth, some alterations in copper storage are apparent if the maternal diet contains higher levels (12 μg/g) of cadmium (Mills and Dalgano, 1972).

The mechanisms by which cadmium influences the metabolism of zinc and copper is unknown. Both of these essential trace metals are toxic in higher concentrations, and their metabolism normally must be under rigorous homeostatic control (e.g., Cotzias et al., 1962). It is an interesting speculation whether the apparent interaction between either of them and cadmium is related to the accumulation of "unphysiological" concentrations of metallothionein. This protein, after its induction by cadmium, remains in the liver and kidney for prolonged periods and accumulates not only the inducing cation, but also zinc [Webb, 1972b; cf. the transfer of zinc from muscle, bone, and feathers to the liver observed by Anke et al. (1971) in hens on a cadmium-supplemented diet]. In contrast, zinc-thionein, when induced by excess zinc, has a short biological half-life (Webb, 1972a; Davies et al., 1973).

Thus, despite the evidence of Shaikh and Lucis (1970c) that the thionein moiety of metallothionein undergoes continual turnover, there is evidence that the metabolism of the apoprotein is abnormal in the presence of cadmium. In the rat, cadmium supplementation of the diet leads not only to the accumulation of cadmium in the liver and kidney but also to the accumulation of high levels of copper in the latter organ, only part of which is bound in metallothionein (M. Webb, unpublished observations). Since there is a molecular link between iron and copper metabolism (e.g., Frieden, 1973) antagonism of the latter by cadmium could have a secondary effect on, for example, hemoglobin biosynthesis (cf. Bunn and Matrone, 1966).

With regard to the long-term effects of cadmium, metallothionein may not be innocuous. In animals, including humans, the kidney is the critical organ at acute exposure to cadmium, and in all species there seems to be a limit—about 200 μg Cd^{2+}/g wet weight—to the amount that can be stored in the kidney before renal damage occurs (Friberg et al., 1971). Since cadmium is cumulative, the accumulation of a kidney cadmium burden of this level could occur through the daily assimilation of small amounts of cadmium over a number of years. At low levels of exposure there is little doubt that most, if not all, of this cadmium would be present as metallothionein. Piscator (1964, 1966) suggests that cadmium is transported into the kidney by glomerular filtration of metallothionein, which is assumed to be synthesized in the liver. The progressive accumulation of metallothionein in the tubules by reabsorption from the filtrate continues until the kidney is "saturated," when renal damage occurs. At this stage, proteinuria begins, and cadmium, bound to metallothionein, is excreted in the urine. Obviously, this hypothesis needs further investigation and, in the intact animal, for example, it is going to be difficult to show whether there is significant transport of metallothionein from the liver to the kidney. Irrespective of the tissue of origin of the protein, however, it has been established by Nordberg (1971) that, in mice, in which proteinuria—indicative of renal tubular damage—has been induced by repeated subcutaneous injections of cadmium, the cation is excreted in the urine bound to a small protein that appears to be identical with metallothionein.

Nordberg (1971) has also reported some interesting results from experiments in which mice were given a total of 1.1 mg Cd^{2+}/kg body weight as a mixture of ionic Cd^{2+} and cadmium bound to metallothionein, the latter being prepared from the livers of cadmium-exposed rabbits. A dose of 1.1 mg/kg of ionic Cd^{2+} alone produced the expected damage to the testis but had no effect on the kidney, whereas with a combination of 0.6 mg cadmium as metallothionein and 0.5 mg Cd^{2+} as $CdCl_2$, the testes were unaffected but tubular damage occurred immediately in the kidney. It is, perhaps, unfortunate that this work was done with rabbit, not mouse liver metallothionein, and that the effects of metallothionein alone were not reported. Nevertheless, it does appear that cadmium, at least when bound to rabbit liver metallothionein, is not injurious to the testes but can cause immediate damage to the kidney of the mouse. In this connection it seems that studies on the toxicology and metabolism of metallothionein are more than necessary, since it cannot be assumed that the effects observed by Nordberg were due specifically to metallothionein. The simultaneous administration of cysteine with cadmium, for example, causes a significant increase in toxicity (decrease in the LD_{50}), enhances both the deposition of cadmium in the kidney and the selective destruction of the proximal convoluted tubules, but prevents the cadmium-induced injury to the testis (Kennedy, 1968; Gunn et al., 1968). Similarly, penicillamine increases the lethality and nephrotoxicity of cadmium and, at the same time, increases the uptake of the cation by the kidney of the rat (Lyle et al., 1968). It seems, therefore, that cadmium chelates with these simple —SH compounds (cysteine and penicillamine) and is transported more effectively to the kidney. Presumably cadmium must be transferred from these complexes to a storage protein (thionein ?) within the kidney since, at least with penicillamine, neither the urinary nor fecal excretion of the cation is affected.

References

Anke, M., Henning, A., Groppel, B., and Lüdke, H. (1971). *Arch. Exp. Vet. Med.*, **25**, 799.

Berlin, M., and Ullberg, S. (1963). *Arch. Environ. Health.*, **7**, 686.

Bloomer, L. C., and Sourkes, T. L. (1974). In *Trace Element Metabolism in Animals–2, (Proc. 2nd Internat. Cong. Trace Element Metabolism in Animals)*, University Park Press, Baltimore.

Bremner, I., and Marshall, R. B. (1974). *Br. J. Nutr.*, **32**, 283 and 291.

Bremner, I., Davies, N. T., and Mills, C. F. (1973). *Biochem. Soc. Trans.*, **1**, 982.

Bunn, C. R., and Matrone, G. (1966). *J. Nutr.*, **30**, 395.

Cotzias, G. C., Borg, D. C., and Selleck, B. (1961). *Amer. J. Physiol.*, **201**, 927.

Cotzias, G. C., Borg, D. C., and Selleck, B. (1962). *Amer. J. Physiol.*, **202**, 359.

Davies, N. T., Brenner, I., and Mills, C. F. (1973). *Biochem. Soc. Trans.*, **1**, 985.

Evans, G. W., and Cornatzer, W. E. (1970). *Fed. Proc.* **29**, 695.

Evans, G. W., Majors, P. F., and Cornatzer, W. E. (1970). *Biochem. Biophys. Res. Commun.*, **40**, 1142.

Fischer, G. M., and Thind, G. S. (1971). *Arch. Environ. Health*, **23**, 107.

Friberg, L., Piscator, M., and Nordberg, G. F. (1971). *Cadmium in the Environment: An Epidemiologic and Toxicologic Appraisal*, Chemical Rubber Co., Cleveland.

Frieden, E. (1973). *Nutrition Reviews*, **31**, 41.

Gabbiani, G. (1966). *Experientia (Basel)*, **22**, 260.

Gunn, S. A., Gould, T. C., and Anderson, W. A. D. (1968). *Proc. Soc. Exptl. Biol. Med.*, **128**, 591.

Jacobs, E. E., Jacob, M., Sandani, D. R., and Bradley, L. B. (1956). *J. Biol. Chem.*, **223**, 147.

Jakubowski, M., Piotrowski, J., and Trojanowska, B. (1970). *Toxicol. App. Pharmacol.*, **16**, 743.

Kägi, J. H. R. (1970). *Abst. 8th Internat. Cong. Biochem.*, p. 130.

Kägi, J. H. R., and Vallee, B. L. (1960). *J. Biol. Chem.*, **235**, 3460.

Kägi, J. H. R., and Vallee, B. L. (1961). *J. Biol. Chem.*, **236**, 2434.

Kennedy, A. (1968). *Brit. J. Exptl. Path.*, **49**, 360.

Lyle, W. H., Green, J. N., Gore, V., and Vidler, J. (1968). *Postgrad. Med. J. Suppl. (Oct.)* 18.

Malcolm, D. (1973). "Cadmium in the Environment," *Inter-Research Council Committee on Pollution Research, Seminar, London*, p. 16.

Margoshes, M., and Vallee, B. L. (1957). *J. Am. Chem. Soc.*, **79**, 4813.

Mills, C. F., Bremner, I., and Davies, N. T. (1973). "Cadmium in the Environment," *Inter-Research Council Committee on Pollution Research, Seminar, London*, p. 10.

Mills, C. F., and Dalgarno, A. C. (1972). *Nature (Lond.)*, **239**, 171.

Nordberg, G. F. (1971). *Environmental Physiology*, **1**, 171.

Nordberg, G. F., and Nishiyama, K. (1972). *Arch. Environ. Health*, **24**, 209.

Nordberg, G. F., Piscator, M., and Lind, B. (1971). *Acta Pharmacol. Toxicol.*, **29**, 456.

Nordberg, G. F., Nordberg, M., Piscator, M., and Vesterborg, O. (1972). *Biochem. J.*, **126**, 491.

Petering, H. G., Johnson, M. A., and Stemmer, K. L. (1971). *Arch. Environ. Health*, **23**, 93.

Piotrowski, J. K., Bolonowska, W., and Sapota, A. (1973). *Acta Biochim. Polonica*, **20**, 207.

Piscator, M. (1964). *Nord. Hyg. Tidsk.*, **45**, 76.

Piscator, M. (1966). *Proteinuria in Chronic Cadmium Poisoning*, K. L. Beckman, Tryckerier AB, Stockholm.

Porter, H. (1970). *Trace Element Metabolism in Animals* (ed. Mills, C. F.), E. and S. Livingstone, Edinburgh.

Porter, H., and Hills, J. R. (1974). In *Trace Element Metabolism in Animals—2, Proc. 2nd Internat. Cong.*, University Park Press, Baltimore.

Pulido, P. Kägi, J. H. R., and Vallee, B. L. (1966). *Biochemistry*, **5**, 1768.

Schroeder, H. A. and Vinton, W. H. (1962). *Amer. J. Physiol.*, **202**, 515.

Schroeder, H. A., Kroll, S. S., and Little, J. W. (1966). *Arch. Environ. Health*, **13**, 788.

Shaikh, Z. A., and Lucis, O. J. (1970a). *Fed. Proc.*, **29**, Abs. 298.

Shaikh, Z. A., and Lucis, O. J. (1970b). *Experientia (Basel)*, **29**, 301.

Shaikh, Z. A., and Lucis, O. J. (1970c). *Proc. Canad. Fed. Biol. Sciences*, **13**, 158 (Abs. 614).

Starcher, B. C. (1969). *J. Nutr.*, **97**, 321.

Underwood, E. J. (1956). *Trace Elements in Human and Animal Nutrition*, Academic Press, New York.

Webb, M. (1972a). *Biochem. Pharmacol.*, **21**, 2751.

Webb, M. (1972b). *Biochem. Pharmacol.*, **21**, 2767.

Webb, M. (1972c). *J. Reproduct. Fertil.*, **30**, 83.

Wisniewska, J. M., Trojanowska, B., Piotrowski, J., and Jakubowski, M. (1970). *Toxicol. App. Pharmacol.*, **16**, 754.

Yoshikawa, H. (1970). *Ind. Health*, **8**, 184.

10

The Significance of Multielement Analyses in Metal Pollution Studies

T. L. COOMBS

10.1. Introduction

International concern over the increasing hazards of industrial and domestic pollutants has focused particular attention on the toxic effects of heavy metals, exemplified by the effects of organic mercurials on fish and fish predators and on humans (Jernelov, 1972; Ui, 1971). Since then the effects of lead, cadmium, copper, and chromium have been or are currently being reexamined. When the hazard is manifest as an acute lethal episode, the end result is immediately apparent and investigation and prevention become prompt. When sublethal concentrations are present, however, the "signs and symptoms" become much more subtle, any toxic damage remains undetected for long periods, unless specifically sought after, and remedial action may become more difficult or even impossible. This sublethal aspect has hitherto received insufficient experimental attention, most probably because of the inherent difficulties in (a) predicting what compounds should be examined and (b) assessing their effects over a sufficiently long period of exposure.

In the marine environment it has been recognized that a greater potential

T. L. COOMBS • Institute of Marine Biochemistry, Aberdeen, Scotland.

hazard exists in estuarine and near-shore areas than in the open ocean, because of their proximity to sites of industrial and domestic activity, resulting in concentration of specific pollutants by runoff or by biological activity of the inhabiting organisms. It is for such reasons that the Institute of Marine Biochemistry has initiated studies on the biochemical role of trace metals in estuarine and coastal organisms (Coombs, 1972; Coombs et al., 1972) and on the effects of heavy metal pollutants on these systems. As an example of the work in progress some preliminary data on the effects of sublethal concentrations of cadmium on the plaice (*Pleuronectes platessa* L.) are presented. This work represents a collaborative effort of Dr. T. L. Coombs, Dr. Thelma Fletcher, and Mrs. Ann White and is considered to be particularly relevant in the context of this volume in that it illustrates an aspect in the study of metal toxins which merits much greater concern and experimental application, namely, the indirect effects produced on the other metals naturally present.

It may be hypothesized that a heavy metal toxin, in addition to producing a direct lethal effect by combining with essential biochemically functional groups, can also act by interfering with other metal ions present, either by suppression of their biological functioning or by suppression of their uptake, through competitive binding, i.e., development of a conditioned metal deficiency.

10.2. Investigation of Effects of Cadmium on the Plaice

10.2.1. Methodology

Following up our previous studies on the interaction of heavy metal ions with epithelial mucus from the plaice (Coombs et al., 1972), the experiments with cadmium were extended to examine its effects on other tissues. For this purpose plaice were freshly caught from an unpolluted area off the Aberdeenshire coast and transferred within a few hours of capture to a filtered sea water aquarium maintained at 12°C. The fish were kept under these conditions for at least 24 h before single fish, weighing between 200 and 300 g, were transferred to individual tanks, 30 × 50 × 20 cm, which contained 6 liters of aerated filtered sea water at 12°C, to which was added cadmium as $CdCl_2$ to give a final concentration of 2 ppm. The fish were exposed for periods of 4–28 days, and the cadmium-containing sea water was changed for a fresh 6-liter volume every 24 h. The fish were not fed before or during exposure. Controls, being fish maintained over the same period in similar tanks containing sea water without any added cadmium, were also examined. At the end of each exposure time each fish was exsanguinated and the blood separated into serum and blood cells, before killing by stunning and dissection, setting aside gills, liver, kidney, and spleen for metal analysis. Each tissue was weighed, homogenized in 2.5 volumes of 10 mM Tris buffer, pH 8.2, and a measured aliquot set aside for subcellular fractionation, before ashing the remainder in Pt at 450°C. The final ash was dissolved in 1 N HCl and the ash solutions analyzed for cadmium, copper, and zinc by atomic absorption spectrometry. The serum samples could be aspirated directly into the air–acetylene flame of the spectrometer. Since the weight of the spleen was somewhat low, the data on this tissue are not as detailed as on the other tissues. The tissue homogenates of liver and kidney were each centrifuged at 100,000 g for 1 h and the supernatants (cytosols) fractionated by gel-filtration chromatography on Sephadex G-75, using the 10 mM Tris buffer as the eluant. Each fraction of approximately 5 ml volume was analyzed for cadmium, copper, and zinc as well as absorbance at 280 and 250 nm.

10.3. Results

10.3.1. General Appearance

No lethal effects were produced in any of the fish, and apart from slight signs of starvation in the appearance of the skin and muscle in the fish exposed for 20 and 28 days, all appeared normal and healthy.

10.3.2. Tissue Concentrations of Cadmium, Copper, and Zinc

The concentrations in terms of $\mu g/g$ wet weight of tissue or $\mu g/ml$ of serum are shown in Figs. 10.1, 10.2, and 10.3. Significant amounts of cadmium are found in all of the tissues within 4 days of exposure. The concentration in the serum and blood cells remained fairly constant over the 28-day period, but in the gills, liver, and kidney the concentration decreased to a minimum on day 17 and then increased again to a level above the initial day 4 value. Trace amounts of cadmium are detected in the gills, liver, and kidney of the control fish, unexposed to the 2 ppm of cadmium.

For copper, there are two contrasting effects: in serum, blood cells, and gills the concentration of copper appears to be decreased compared to the concentration found in the controls, while for liver, kidney, and spleen the copper concentration is significantly increased.

For zinc, there are indications of a similar dichotomy between the concentrations in serum, blood cells, and gills and in liver, kidney, and spleen, but the differences are by no means as well marked as in the case of copper.

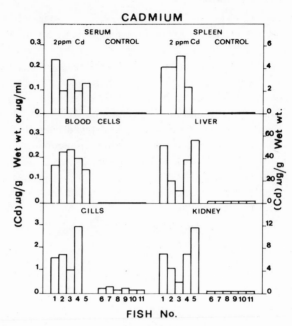

FIG. 10.1. Tissue concentrations of cadmium in plaice after exposure to 2 ppm Cd. Fish No. 1, 4 days; No. 2, 12 days; No. 3, 17 days; No. 4, 20 days; No. 5, 28 days. Fish Nos. 6–11 are controls, unexposed to Cd.

Similar changes in the metabolic interactions of copper and zinc with cadmium have been reported for liver and kidney in rats and mice (Evans and Cornatzer, 1970; Suzuki, 1972; Webb, 1972), in cows (Evans et al., 1970), and in rabbits (Piscator, 1964) injected with cadmium. These effects have been interpreted as being a consequence of the biosynthesis of a low-molecular-weight protein (10,000 daltons) named metallothionein, which contains a high proportion of cysteine residues and few aromatic amino acid residues. This protein binds cadmium, mercury, zinc, and copper and was first isolated from horse kidney (Kagi and Vallee, 1961). Addition of excess cadmium to metallothionein will displace any bound zinc and copper.

10.3.3. Gel-Filtration of Plaice Liver and Kidney Cytosols

Liver Cytosol. Fractionation of the liver cytosols produced chromatographic patterns typified by those of Fig. 10.4, which depict the fractionation of a control fish and a fish exposed for 12 days. For the cadmium-exposed fish, the figure shows four discrete metal-containing areas, labeled I–IV. Fraction I (40 ml eluate)

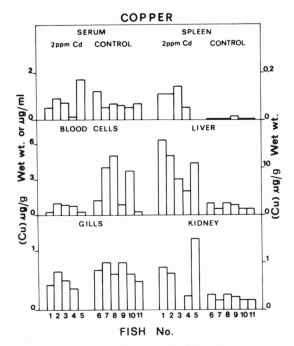

FIG. 10.2. Tissue concentrations of copper in plaice after exposure to 2 ppm Cd. Fish No. 1, 5 days; No. 2, 12 days; No. 3, 17 days; No. 4, 20 days; No. 5, 28 days. Fish Nos. 6–11 are controls, unexposed to Cd.

occurs at the void volume of the Sephadex column and represents proteins excluded by the gel and of molecular weight >70,000 daltons. These proteins bind 23% Cd, 79% Zn, and 44% Cu. Fraction II (84 ml eluate) corresponds to proteins of molecular weight 25,000–30,000 daltons and contains 49% Cd, 4% Zn, and 31% Cu. This fraction displayed superoxide dismutase activity. This enzyme is a copper–zinc protein known also as hepatocuprein or hemocuprein (McCord and Fridovitch, 1969). Fraction III (109 ml eluate), corresponds to proteins of molecular weight 9000–12,000 daltons and contains 18% Cd, no Zn, and 11% Cu. Finally Fraction IV (130 ml eluate) which contains no Cd, 8% Zn, and 12% Cu, probably represents either free metal ions or metal complexed to compounds of very small molecular weight. For the control fish, there is no detectable cadmium in any of the fractions and, while zinc is present in Fractions I (58%), II (10%), and IV (33%), copper is found only in Fractions I (83%) and II (17%).

Fraction III seems to correspond to metallothionein as isolated from mammalian liver cytosol (Bremner et al., 1973). For the present, however, the amount of material isolated from the plaice is insufficient to characterize this

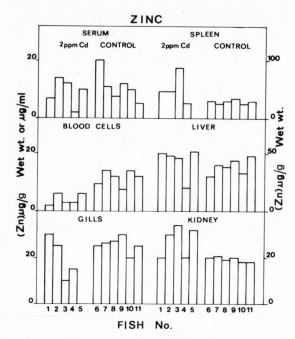

FIG. 10.3. Tissue concentrations of zinc in plaice after exposure to 2 ppm Cd. Fish No. 1, 4 days; No. 2, 12 days; No. 3, 17 days; No. 4, 20 days; No. 5, 28 days. Fish Nos. 6–11 are controls, unexposed to Cd.

material in terms of free –SH groups, absorption spectrum, and amino acid composition and establish that this is definitely metallothionein. It would appear that fish not stressed with cadmium do not contain in their liver any large amount of "metallothionein." When the fish are stressed, however, the cadmium is not exclusively bound to Fraction III but is distributed among the other metalloproteins of the liver.

Kidney Cytosol. Fractionation of the kidney cytosol produces patterns that differ from those obtained with the liver (Fig. 10.5). There are only two major metal-containing fractions and the position of one of them varies. For the 12-day cadmium-exposed fish, Fraction I (95 ml eluate) appears at the void volume of the Sephadex column and contains all of the cadmium, 70% Zn, and 31% Cu, while Fraction II (95 ml eluate) appears at the same position as the "metallothionein" of the liver cytosol chromatogram, but contains no Cd and yet contains 30% Zn and 69% Cu. For the control fish, the first fraction (35 ml eluate) is at the void volume and contains 82% Zn and 16% Cu but the second fraction (129 ml eluate) is not at the position for metallothionein but appears at the same position as Fraction IV of the liver cytosol chromatogram and contains

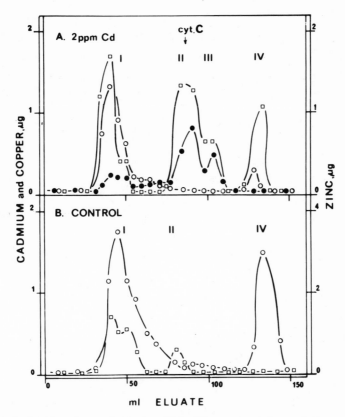

FIG. 10.4. Gel-filtration on Sephadex-G75 of liver cytosols from plaice, unexposed and exposed for 12 days to 2 ppm Cd. The livers were homogenized in 10 mM Tris buffer, pH 8.2, at 1°C and centrifuged at 100,000g for 1 h. The supernatant was then fractionated on the 1.5 × 80 cm Sephadex column using the same Tris buffer as the eluant and collecting 5-ml fractions at 4°C. ●—●, Cd; ○—○, Zn, □—□, Cu. The elution volume for cytochrome c used for column calibration is indicated.

12% Zn and 84% Cu. For the kidney therefore there has been a translocation of both zinc and copper in response to the influx of cadmium.

10.4. Discussion

The above investigation has shown that exposure of plaice to a sublethal concentration of cadmium, while to all outward appearances resulting in no deleterious effects, in reality has caused significant changes in the zinc and copper dis-

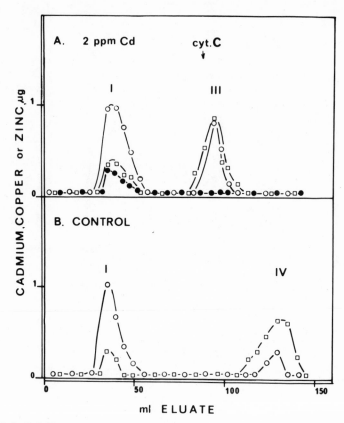

FIG. 10.5. Gel-filtration on Sephadex-G75 of kidney cytosols from plaice, unexposed and exposed for 12 days to 2 ppm Cd. The kidneys were homogenized in 10 mM Tris buffer, pH 8.2, at 1°C and centrifuged at 100,000g for 1 h. The supernatant was then fractionated on the 1.5 × 80 cm Sephadex column using the same Tris buffer as the eluant and collecting 5-ml fractions at 4°C. ●—●, Cd; ○—○, Zn; □—□, Cu. The elution volume for cytochrome c used for column calibration is indicated.

tributions in the tissues. These changes could potentially result in a conditioned metal deficiency in blood cells, gills, and serum, while mobilizing liver and kidney stores with the production of a low-molecular-weight protein suggestive of metallothionein. The biochemical consequences of these changes have not yet been studied and should be a prime concern in future experimentation. Analysis of this system for cadmium alone would not have revealed these changes and the results presented above have provided an example of the value of a multielement investigation as opposed to the more usual single-element analysis carried out in metal pollution studies.

References

Bremner, I., Davies, N. T., and Mills, C. F. (1973). "The effect of zinc deficiency and food restriction on hepatic zinc proteins in the rat," *Biochem. Soc. Trans.* **I**, 982–985.

Coombs, T. L. (1972). "The distribution of zinc in the oyster *Ostrea edulis* and its relation to enzymic activity and to other metals," *Marine Biol.* **12**, 170–178.

Coombs, T. L., Fletcher, T. C., and White, A. (1972). "Interaction of metal ions with mucus from the plaice (*Pleuronectes platessa* L.)," *Biochem. J.* **128**, 128–129P.

Evans, G. W. and Cornatzer, W. E. (1970). "Copper and zinc metalloproteins in the rat," *Fed. Proc.* **29**, 695.

Evans, G. W., Majors, P. F., and Cornatzer, W. E. (1970). "Mechanism for cadmium and zinc antagonism of copper metabolism," *Biochem. Biophys. Res. Comm.* **40**, 1142–1148.

Jernelov, A. (1972). Conversion of mercury compounds. In *Chemical Fallout, Current Research on Persistent Pesticides* (ed. Miller, M. N., and Berg, G. G.), Charles C Thomas, Springfield, Ill.

Kägi, J. H. R., and Vallee, B. L. (1961). "Metallothionein: a cadmium- and zinc-containing protein from enquine renal cortex," *J. Biol. Chem.* **236**, 2435–2442.

McCord, J. M. and Fridovich, I. (1969). "Superoxide dismutase, an enzymic function for erythrocuprein (hemocuprein)," *J. Biol. Chem.* **244**, 6049–6055.

Piscator, M. (1964). "Om kadmium normala manniskonjurar samt redogorelse för isolering av metallothionein ur lever fran kadmium exponerade kaniner," *Nord. Hyg. Tidskrift* **45**, 76–82.

Suzuki, Y. (1972). "Effects of cadmium-binding protein on metal distribution in supernatant of the liver homogenate of rat," *Ind. Health* **10**, 52–55.

Ui, J. (1971). "Mercury pollution of sea and freshwater and its cumulation into water biomass," *Rev. Int. Ocean. Med.* **22-23**, 79–128.

Webb, M. (1972). "Binding of cadmium ions by rat liver and kidney," *Biochem. Pharm.* **21**, 2751–2765.

11

Potentially Persistent Industrial Organic Chemicals Other than PCB

V. ZITKO

The widespread contamination of the environment by polychlorinated biphenyls (PCB) demonstrated that persistent chemicals should not be incorporated into products with uncontrollable ultimate fate and that extreme care must be taken to minimize the discharge or leakage of such compounds into the environment.

It is hoped that as a result of voluntary actions by industry, recommendations of international organizations, and regulatory actions, the use of PCB has been limited to essential applications. However, it is not known what compounds are used or planned to be used to replace PCB in the nonessential applications, and little is known about other potentially persistent industrial chemicals.

This paper summarizes some information, based mainly on industrial and patent literature, on compounds and preparations which are likely to be used as PCB substitutes, and on some other industrial chemicals.

The term "industrial chemicals" covers a wide variety of synthetic chemicals used as final products, additives, or intermediates, but excluding uses based on biological activity. Accordingly, polyethylene, dioctyl phthalate, and vinyl acetate are industrial chemicals, whereas pesticides used on the basis of their biological activity are not considered industrial chemicals in the present context.

V. ZITKO ● Fisheries Research Board of Canada, Biological Station, St. Andrews, New Brunswick EOG 2XO, Canada.

Persistence does not have a generally accepted definition. In this paper, compounds which remain unchanged under a variety of environmental conditions for a year or longer are classified as persistent.

11.1 Polychlorinated Terphenyls (PCTs)

PCTs were basically used for the same purposes as the higher-chlorine grades of PCB. Past and present production data are not available.

PCT's were first detected in the environment by Zitko et al. (1972) in Canada and were recently, in higher levels, reported in wildlife species from Europe (Mestres and Illes, 1973; Freudenthal and Greve, 1973) and in human fat from Japan (Doguchi, 1973; Doguchi et al., 1974; Doguchi and Fukano, in press). PCTs were also detected in food packaging material (Villeneuve et al., 1973).

Monsanto Organic Chemical Division introduced recently the Aroclor 6000 series (6040, 6050, 6062, 6070, and 6090), consisting of blends of Aroclor 5460 (a polychlorinated terphenyl preparation with 60% chlorine) and Aroclor 1221B (a monochlorinated biphenyl preparation), with recommended uses for delayed-tack, emulsion, pressure-sensitive, and hot-melt adhesives, sealants, caulking compounds, paints, and lacquers (Monsanto, 1972).

Because of their higher molecular weight, PCTs may be somewhat less mobile in the environment than PCBs, but from the toxicity and accumulation point of view, PCTs would present the same problems as PCBs.

According to unconfirmed reports, Monsanto has discontinued the production of PCTs.

11.2. Chlorinated Paraffins

Low-molecular-weight chlorinated and fluorinated aliphatics, such as chloroform, tetrachloro- and tetrafluoromethane, trichlorofluoromethane, dichloro difluoromethane, and tetrachloroethylene, used mainly as solvents, refrigerants and aerosol propellants, were recently detected in the atmosphere in levels between 0.1 and 5 ppb (parts per 10^9) in geographically widely separated area (Lovelock, 1972; Lovelock et al., 1973; Murray and Riley, 1973; Su and Goldberg, 1973; Gassmann, 1974; Lillian and Singh, 1974; Simmonds et al., 1974) Tetrachloromethane may be of natural origin, but the others are man-made and show surprisingly high persistence. For example, the global distribution of trichlorofluoromethane reasonably well coincides with a theoretical one, based on the total production of this compound (Lovelock et al., 1973), and dichlorofluoromethane may be even more persistent (Su and Goldberg, 1973). Little known about the effects of these compounds on the environment, and there is a need for further research in this area. It was reported that chlorofluoromethanes may decompose on ultraviolet irradiation in the upper atmosphere to yield chlorine, which, in turn, may decompose ozone (anonymous, 1974a).

High-molecular-weight chlorinated paraffins (C_{21}-C_{28}, 32-70% chlorine), were recently suggested as PCB substitutes in coatings, adhesives, and sealants based on chlorinated rubber, styrene–butadiene rubber, polyvinyl acetate, and polysulfide resins (Dover Chemical Corporation, 1972a). Chlorinated paraffins have been used since about 1930 as fire retardants, plasticizers, lubricants, antistatic agents, and additives in machine tool oils, paints, and tanning compositions.

Little is known about the environmental behavior, fate, and toxicity of chlorinated paraffins. Analytical techniques for chlorinated paraffins are not as well developed as those for PCB, and at the moment chlorinated paraffins can only be quantified by measuring the hydrochloric acid generated on their combustion (Zitko, 1973). No suitable conditions for their analysis by gas chromatography have been reported. The presence of the 40% and 50% chlorine grades can be confirmed by dechlorination with sodium bis(2-methoxyethoxy) aluminum hydride and gas chromatography of the resulting paraffins. Chlorinated paraffins with 70% chlorine yield under these conditions a highly fluorescent product (Zitko, 1974a).

Chlorinated paraffins were not irritant to human skin, and no mortality occurred in guinea pigs and rats after a single oral dose of 25 and 50 g/kg of a chlorinated paraffin with 70% chlorine, respectively (Dover Chemical Corporation, 1972b). According to Abasov (1970), minimum lethal dose, LD_{50}, and LD_{100} were 19, 21.85, and 24.0, and 24.5, 26.1, and 28.0 g/kg in mice and rats, respectively. The chloroparaffin did not accumulate in the animals.

Preliminary experiments indicate that, in comparison with PCB, chlorinated paraffins are much less, if at all, accumulated by fish when these are exposed to chlorinated paraffins adsorbed on silica, or fed contaminated food. On the other hand chlorinated paraffins are very likely toxic to fish when present in the food at 10 and 100 μg/g (Zitko, 1974b).

The annual production of chlorinated paraffins in the United States was 28 × 10^6 kg in 1969 (United States Tariff Commission, 1971) and now probably exceeds that of PCB.

Chlorinated paraffins have not yet been detected in the environment but deserve further research attention.

1.3. Chlorobiphenyl Derivatives

Alkylated (mostly isopropylated) chlorinated biphenyls and terphenyls, containing 1-3 chlorine atoms and 0.2-2.5 alkyl groups per molecule, were patented as dielectric liquids (Progil, 1971). Alkylated biphenyls and terphenyls were patented as solvents for pressure-sensitive recording paper (Matsukawa et al., 1972). There are no data on the persistence and toxicity of alkyl and alkylchloro biphenyls and terphenyls. It is likely that the highly substituted compounds may be quite persistent.

Chlorofluorobiphenyls have been patented for hydraulic fluids (Boschan et al., 1970). Their behavior may be similar to that of PCB.

Chlorobiphenyls and their esters were patented as fungicides: 3-chlorobiphenyl-2-ol and 5-chlorobiphenyl-2-ol for rubber (Tsurumaru and Tsubaki, 1972), nonachlorobiphenylol acetate and octachlorobiphenyldiol diacetate for textiles (Pechmeze, 1971, 1972).

There is no information on the environmental properties of chlorobiphenylols. The lower-chlorinated biphenylols are also of interest as PCB metabolites (Hutzinger et al., 1972; Yoshimura and Yamamoto, 1973). A number of these were prepared and their analytical properties were studied (Hutzinger et al., 1974; Zitko et al., 1974).

Nitrogen derivatives of PCB, prepared by reacting PCB with amines such as N,N-dimethylpropanediamine, diethylenetriamine, or with ammonia, were patented as microbiocides (Merianos et al., 1973). Again no further data on these compounds are available.

The preparation of bis(chloromethyl)octachlorobiphenyls, serving as intermediates for dyes, plastics, and plant protective agents, was patented (Woppert and Deiss, 1970).

11.4. Other Chlorinated Compounds

Halogenated selenophene and tellurophene, such as tetrachloroselenophene, were patented as additives for fire-resistant hydraulic fluids (McCord et al., 1973). In addition, these fluids contained tributyl and tricresyl phosphate. Additives are needed to maintain the fire resistance of otherwise flammable hydraulic fluids, but should be screened for possible environmental hazards before a wide-scale application.

Certain chlorinated cyclopentadiene-furan (or thiophene) adducts such as 1,2,3,4,6,7,8,9,10,10,11,11-dodecachloro-1,4,4a,5a,6,9,9a,9b-octahydro-1,4:6,9-dimethanodibenzofuran were patented as fire retardants for polyolefins and ABS copolymers (Boyer, 1971; Hooker Chemical Corporation, 1973 Krackeler, 1974). These compounds have some structural features of cyclodiene pesticides and some of chlorinated dibenzofurans, and their environmental and toxicological properties should be investigated. The same is true about related chlorinated norbornene derivatives, patented as fire retardants for polyolefins (Gloor, 1971; Cyba, 1973).

Mono-, di-, and trichloronaphthenic acids were suggested as extractants of heavy metals from aqueous solutions (Babaev, 1973), and chlorinated fatty acid esters (C_{8-24} acids, C_{1-8} alcohols) containing 40% chlorine were patented as plasticizers (Yagi et al., 1973). Esters of chlorinated stearic acid, such as methyl pentachlorostearate, may be used as fireproofing additives in acrylic fibers (Blackburn and Misenheimer, 1973).

A list of other industrial halogenated compounds is available (Zitko and Choi, 1971).

The industrial use of brominated compounds may be increasing. This is probably due to some advantages in their properties as compared to those of the corresponding chlorinated compounds, and to perspectively decreasing price of bromine caused by a decreasing demand for ethylene bromide as additive in leaded gasoline.

Hexabromobenzene (Hirami et al., 1973; Yamamoto et al., 1973), penta-bromotoluene (Morita and Shimizu, 1973), and polybrominated biphenyls (Celanese Corporation, 1973; Koyama, 1973; Wurmb and Pohlemann, 1973) are used primarily as fire retardants in plastics. Tetrabromo-3,4-dihydroxyhexane (Papa and Proops, 1973), tetrabromodiphenylamine (Kato et al., 1973), tetra-bromobisphenol A ethers (Kobayashi et al., 1973; Inada et al., 1974), and chlorinated norbornyl pentabromophenyl ethers (Yamazaki et al., 1973) were patented for similar purposes. Hepta- and octabromo-3-(trifluoromethyl)di-phenyl ether were suggested as stable heat-transfer liquids (Schlafke and Jenkner, 1974).

Production data for the above compounds are not available, and their toxicological and environmental properties have received relatively little attention. Brominated aromatic hydrocarbons will probably fairly closely resemble their chlorinated analogs, and their persistence may increase with increasing degree of bromination. Compounds with a low degree of bromination, such as bromobenzene, are readily metabolized (Sipes et al., 1974). Hexa- and octa-bromobiphenyl were similar in accumulation and toxicological properties to the corresponding PCB preparations (Cecil et al., 1972; Norris et al., 1973). On the other hand, octabromodiphenyl oxide accumulated in tissues to a much smaller extent than octabromobiphenyl (Norris et al., 1973). There may be some differences between bromo- and chloro-substituted aromatic hydrocarbons, caused by lower volatility and higher molecular weight of the former compounds, lower stability of the carbon–bromine bond in comparison to that of the carbon–chlorine bond, and the study of environmental aspects of brominated industrial chemicals should be encouraged.

1.5. Polyphenyl Ethers

Diphenyl ether is a well-known heat-transfer fluid. Ethylated diphenyl ether and polyphenyl ethers such as bis(phenoxyphenyl) ether and biphenylyl phenyl ether were recently patented as heat-transfer fluids (Jackson et al., 1972), and a number of diphenoxybiphenyls and phenoxyphenoxy biphenyls were prepared and characterized (Hammann and Schisla, 1972; Ouliac, 1972).

The low-molecular-weight members of this series are probably relatively easily biodegradable; the higher-molecular-weight compounds may not be very mobile in the environment. The impurities in polyphenyl ethers, such as *m*-dibromobenzene, *m*-bromodiphenyl ether, and *m*-bis(*m*-bromophenoxy)benzene (Utkin et al., 1972) may be of some interest.

A series of silylated polyphenyl ethers were recently described (Fink, 1973).

Chlorinated diphenyl ethers would probably be similar in their environmental and toxicological properties to PCB. A number of chlorinated diphenyl ethers and related compounds have recently been described (Babin et al., 1973).

11.6. Hindered Phenols

Hindered phenols contain bulky substituents, usually *tert*-butyl groups, in positions *ortho-* to the phenolic hydroxyl, and are used as antioxidants in a variety of products, ranging from plastics to food. Since the phenolic hydroxyl is sterically protected, these compounds may be quite persistent, and a number of hindered phenols have recently been identified in Rhine water (Guesten et al., 1973).

11.7. Organosilicone Compounds

The heat-transfer properties of polymethyl siloxanes, polymethylpheny siloxanes, and arylaroxysilanes have been described (Sobolevskii et al., 1972) and various other applications of organo-modified silicones have been suggeste (Union Carbide, 1972).

Little is known about the environmental behavior of these compounds. It i likely that most of them will be slowly hydrolyzed in the environment and b relatively harmless. However, some relatively exotic organosilicone compound are highly toxic (Voronkov, 1973).

11.8. Evaluation of Environmental Impact

The number of industrial chemicals is very large and is increasing steadil Any compound produced on an industrial scale reaches the environment. Tł degree of contamination depends on the amount produced, usage patterns, and transport and fate of the compound in the environment. The last two properties are determined largely by physical and chemical properties such as volatility, solubility, stability, etc. The dispersal of a compound in the environment is affected mainly by its physical properties, whereas chemical properties determine its persistence.

Persistence is only one factor determining the environmental impact of a chemical, but it was this property which focused attention on compounds such as hexachlorobenzene, PCB, and PCT. There is at the moment no exact method for the prediction of persistence of a compound. Available evidence suggests that both very small, highly substituted molecules and highly substituted aromatic compounds are more persistent than compounds with other structural features. The type and distribution of substituents affect persistence, but quantitative predictions cannot be made as yet.

The biological activity of chemicals and of their transformation and degradation products is an important factor determining their environmental impact. Quantitative structure–activity relationships are not available, except for some structurally closely related groups of compounds and limited ranges of biological activities. Problems encountered in establishing such relationships have recently been discussed (Rose, 1974).

Acute toxicity data are probably available for the majority of industrial chemicals. On the other hand, chronic effects of most of them are unknown. High chronic toxicity may be detected quite early in occupationally exposed workers, but this warning sign failed in the case of PCBs, possibly since data on their environmental persistence and mobility were not available at that time. Low chronic toxicity, or effects appearing only after a prolonged exposure, may remain undetected for many years, as was demonstrated recently in the case of vinyl chloride. In 1930, this compound was considered "less harmful than chloroform and carbon tetrachloride and similar in toxicity to ethyl chloride" (Patty et al., 1930). In 1966, the conclusion was that "although the experimental data are conflicting, the preponderance indicates a compound of relatively low toxicity" (Committee on Threshold Limit Values, 1966), and in 1972 "exposure to 300 ppm or above for a working lifetime together with a very low level of vinylidene chloride may result in slight changes in certain physiologic and clinical laboratory parameters" (Kramer and Mutchler, 1972). In 1974, angiosarcoma of the liver was detected in some workers exposed to high levels of vinyl chloride in the past, and also diagnosed in rats exposed to more than 250 ppm of vinyl chloride, 4 hours a day, 5 days a week, for 12 months (anonymous, 1974b).

These examples illustrate problems encountered in the evaluation of the environmental impact of chemicals. It is impossible to study every individual industrial chemical in detail and, at the same time, even a detailed study may not detect some long-term, chronic effects.

In contrast to pesticides, herbicides, and other compounds used on the basis of their biological activity, a comprehensive list of industrial chemicals is not available. Government-compiled lists (see, for example, United States Tariff Commission, 1971) are not complete and detailed enough, and the patent literature, which was the main source of information for many compounds discussed in this paper, does not provide production data and may not even accurately reflect the actual usage patterns of the patented compounds. A list of organic chemicals, including intermediates and by-products, produced in quantities larger than an arbitrarily selected amount should be compiled internationally and made available to scientists and agencies involved in environmental research. This list would help to determine the order of research priority.

11.9. Conclusions

Several classes of potentially persistent compounds which are, or are likely to be, used on a larger scale have been mentioned, and some problems of the evaluation of environmental impact of chemicals are discussed. Persistence is only one of many factors determining the impact of a chemical on the environment. There are no general rules for predicting the persistence of chemicals, although experimental data indicate that highly substituted small molecules and aromatic hydrocarbons are more persistent than other compounds.

The leakage of chemicals into the environment, both intentional and unintentional, is a fact of life. The important thing is to recognize the hazards and to eliminate the unnecessary risks.

References

Abasov, D. M. (1970). *Tr. Azerb. Nauch.-Issled. Inst. Gig. Tr. Profzabal.*, No. 5, 180.

Anonymous (1974a). *Industrial Research*, p. 17, August.

Anonymous (1974b). *Chem. Engng. News*, **52**, 16.

Babaev, V. A. (1973). *Khim. Zh.* **1**, 78.

Babin, E. P., Skavinskii, Y. P., Androkhov, N. A., Sedlova, L. N., Litoshenko, N. A., and Rudavskii, V. P. (1973). *Khim. Tekhnol.*, **43**.

Blackburn, W. A., and Misenheimer, J. R. (1973). *Ger.*, 1,569,147; *CA*, **80**, 146945.

Boschan, R. H., Nail, D. H., and Holder, J. P. (1970). *U.S.* 3,514,406; *CA*, **73**, 27321.

Boyer, N. (1971). *Ger. Offen.* 2,122,300; *CA*, **76**, 86574.

Cecil, H. C., Bitman, J., Fries, G. F., Smith, L. W., and Lilie, R. J. (1972). *ACS Division of Water, Air and Waste Chemistry*, **12**, 86.

Celanese Corp. Fiber Industries Ltd. (1973). *Brit.* 1,340,013; *CA*, **81**, 4640.

Committee on Threshold Limit Values (1966). *American Conference of Governmental Industrial Hygienists*, Cincinnati, Ohio.

Cyba, H. A. (1973). *U.S.* 3,723,383; *CA*, 79, 32501.

Doguchi, M. (1973). "Chlorinated hydrocarbons in the environment in the Kanto plain and Tokyo Bay, as reflected in fishes, birds and man," in *New Methods in Environmental Chemistry and Toxicology* (ed. Coulston, F., Korte, F., and Goto, M.), pp. 269–289, International Academic Printing Co., Totsuka, Tokyo.

Doguchi, M., Fukano, S., and Ushio, F. (1974). *Bull Environ. Contam. Toxicol.*, 11, 157.

Doguchi, M., and Fukano, S., *Bull. Environ. Contam. Toxicol.* (in press).

Dover Chemical Corporation (1972a). *Bulletins* 544,545.

Dover Chemical Corporation (1972b). *Bulletins* 529,530.

Fink, W. (1973). *Helv. Chim. Acta*, 56, 355.

Freudenthal, J., and Greve, P. A. (1973). *Bull. Environ. Contam. Toxicol.*, 10, 108.

Gassmann, M. (1974). *Naturwissenschaften*, 61, 127.

Gloor, W. E. (1971). *U.S.* 3,576,784; *CA*, 75, 37343.

Guesten, H., Koelle, W., Schweer, K. H., and Stieglitz, L. (1973). *Environ. Lett.*, 5, 209.

Hammann, W. C., and Schisla, R. M. (1972). *J. Chem. Engng. Data*, 17, 110, 112.

Hirami, M., Tomoaki, S., and Saitoh, H. (1973). *Japan.* 73 28,970; *CA*, 80, 134725.

Hooker Chemical Corporation (1973). *Brit.* 1,305,834; *CA*, 78, 160503.

Hutzinger, O., Nash, D. M., Safe, S., and DeFreitas, A. S. W., Norstrom, R. J., Wildish, D. J., and Zitko, V. (1972). *Science*, 178, 312.

Hutzinger, O., Safe, S., and Zitko, V. (1974). *J. Ass. Off. Anal. Chem.*, 57(5), 1061–1067.

Inada, H., Ogawa, A., and Kawasaki, Y. (1974). *Japan Kokai*, 74 20,155; *CA*, 81, 25363.

Jackson, L. L., Seifert, W. F., and Collins, D. E. (1972). *Ger. Offen.* 2,215,433; *CA*, 78, 32405.

Kato, T., Ohhira, T., and Masuda, Y. (1973). *Japan. Kokai* 73 95,445; *CA*, 80, 146901.

Kobayashi, S., Akatsu, T., and Kawashima, T. (1973). *Japan.* 73 18,099; *CA*, 81, 4587.

Koyama, M. (1973). *Japan. Kokai*, 73 44,346; *CA*, 80, 121832.

Krackeler, J. J. (1974). *Brit.* 1,343,272; *CA*, 81, 4470.

Kramer, C. G., and Mutchler, J. E. (1972). *Amer. Industrial Hygiene Assoc. J.*, 33, 19.

Lillian, D., and Hanwant Bir Singh (1974). *Analyt. Chem.*, 46, 1060.

Lovelock, J. E. (1972). *Atmospheric Environ.*, 6, 917.

Lovelock, J. E., Maggs, R. J., and Wade, R. J. (1973). *Nature (Lond.)*, 241, 194.

Matsukawa, H., Kiritani, M., Yoshida, M., and Ishige, S. (1970). *Ger. Offen.* 2,142,173; *CA*, 77, 36688.

McCord, R. S., Nail, D. H., and Sheratte, M. B. (1973). *U.S.* 3,730,898; *CA*, 79, 44208.

Merianos, J. J., Shay, E. G., Adams, P., and Petrocci, A. N. (1973). *U.S.* 3,733, 421; *CA*, 79, 42132; *U.S.* 3,755,636; *CA*, 79, 104918; *U.S.* 3,759,995; *CA*, 79, 126057.

Mestres, R., and Illes, S. (1973). *Trav. Soc. Pharm. Montpellier*, 33, 201.

Monsanto (1972). *Aroclor Plasticizers.*

Morita, Ko, and Shimizu, I. (1973). *Japan Kokai*, 73 90,338; *CA*, 81, 4499.

Murrary, A. J., and Riley, J. P. (1973). *Nature (Lond.)*, 242, 37.

Norris, J. M., Ehrmantraut, J. W., Gibbons, C. L., Kociba, R. J., Schwetz, B. A., Rose, J. Q., Humiston, C. G., Jewett, G. L., Crummett, W. B., Gehring, P. J., Tirsell, J. B., and Brosier, J. S. (1973). *Appl. Polymer Symposium*, No. 22, 195.

Ouliac, R. (1972). *Peintures-Pigments-Vernis*, 48, 604.

Papa, A. J., and Proops, W. R. (1973). *U.S.* 3,779,953; *CA*, 80, 134305.

Patty, F. E., Yant, W. P., and Waite, C. P. (1930). *U.S. Pub. Health Service, Reprint No. 1405.*

Pechmeze, J. P. E. (1971). *Ger. Offen.* 2,116,786; *CA*, 76, 73653.

Pechmeze, J. P. E. (1972). *Fr. Demande* 2,085,349; *CA*, 77, 136271.

Progil, S. A. (1971). *Fr.* 1,603,289; *CA*, 76, 105416.

Rose, F. L. (1974). *Proc. Roy. Soc. Lond. B*, 185, 159.

Schlafke, R., and Jenkner, H. (1974). *Ger. Offen.* 2,241,339; *CA*, **80**, 133011.
Simmonds, P. G., Kerrin, S. L., Lovelock, J. E., and Shair, F. H. (1974). *Atmospheric Environ.*, **8**, 209.
Sipes, I. G., Gigon, L., and Krishna, G. (1974). *Biochem. Pharmacol.*, **23**, 451.
Sobolevskii, M. V., Zhigalin, G. Y., Ruznyaeva, V. S., and Grinevich, K. P. (1972). *Khim. Promysl.*, **48**, 494.
Su, C. W., and Goldberg, E. D. (1973). *Nature (Lond.)*, **245**, 27.
Tsurumaru, H., and Tsubaki, K. (1972). *Japan.* 72 07,621; *CA*, **77**, 141198.
Union Carbide (1972). *Organo-Modified Silicones.*
United States Tariff Commission (1971). *Synthetic Organic Chemicals, U.S. Production and Sales, 1969*, Washington.
Utkin, V. A., Kobrina, V. N., Khmel'nitskii, A. G., and Egorova, T. G. (1972). *Khim. Teknol. Topl. Masel*, 51.
Villeneuve, D. C., Reynolds, L. M., Thomas, G. H., and Phillips, W. E. J. (1973). *J. Ass. Offic. Anal. Chem.*, **56**, 999.
Voronkov, M. G. (1973). *Chem. in Britain*, **9**, 411.
Woppert, H., and Deiss, H. (1970). *Ger. Offen.* 1,810,540; *CA*, **73**, 76831.
Wurmb, R., and Pohlemann, H. (1973). *Ger. Offen.* 2,226,931; *CA*, **80**, 121788.
Yagi, I., Katsumata, S., Okado, R., and Tsutsumi, Y. (1973). *Japan.* 73 33,975; *CA*, **81**, 4520.
Yamamoto, M., Hirami, M., Sasaki, T., Saito, H., and Iwabuchi, K. (1973). *Japan.* 73 07,846; *CA*, **80**, 121883.
Yamazaki, S., Takemura, A., Kojima, K., and Ishida, Y. (1973). *Japan.* 73 09,936; *CA*, **80**, 121815.
Yoshimura, H., and Yamamoto, H. (1973). *Chem. Pharm. Bull.*, **21**, 1168.
Zitko, V., and Choi, P. M. K. (1971). "PCB and other industrial halogenated hydrocarbons in the environment," *Fish. Res. Board Can. Tech. Rept. No. 272*, 55 pp.
Zitko, V., Hutzinger, O., Jamieson, W. D., and Choi, P. M. K. (1972). *Bull. Environ. Contam. Toxicol.*, **7**, 200.
Zitko, V. (1973). *J. Chromatogr.*, **81**, 152.
Zitko, V. (1974a). *J. Ass. Off. Anal. Chem.*, **57**(6), 1253–1259.
Zitko, V. (1974b). *Bull. Environ. Contam. Toxicol.*, **12**(4), 406–411.
Zitko, V., Hutzinger, O., and Choi, P. M. K. (1974). *Bull. Environ. Contam. Toxicol.*, **12**(6), 649–653.

12

The Influence of Polychlorinated Biphenyl Compounds on Hepatic Function in the Rat

D. J. ECOBICHON

The presence of polychlorinated biphenyls (PCBs) in a variety of wildlife species around the globe has indicated that these commonly used industrial chemicals are posing a serious problem of environmental pollution (Holmes et al., 1967; Jensen, 1966; Jensen et al., 1969; Koeman et al., 1969; Lincer and Peakall, 1970; Prestt et al., 1970; Risebrough et al., 1968; Zitko and Choi, 1971). Because of their low volatility, their chemical stability, and lipid solubility, PCBs have been detected in eco-systems, showing biological magnification as one examines residues in food chains. High concentrations in aquatic, avian, and terrestrial life have been detected in highly industrialized regions of the world. The now-famous "Yusho oil" disaster in Japan and a recent fish-meal problem in the United States point to the "epidemics" which may occur as a result of leakage of heat transfer media in food processing factories (Kuratsune et al., 1971; Miller, 1971; Murai and Kuroiwa, 1971; Nishizumi, 1970; Pichirollo, 1971). Against the latter occurrences it is difficult to guard, but it is possible to prevent the generalized pollution of the environment with these agents.

D. J. ECOBICHON • Department of Pharmacology, Faculty of Medicine, Dalhousie University, Halifax, Nova Scotia, Canada.

Polychlorinated biphenyls are marketed under a variety of trade names—Aroclors, Phenoclors, Clophens, Kanechlors, to name a few of the more commonly found preparations. Toxicologic assessment of these mixtures has been complicated by the heterogeneity of the PCB congeners, by marked differences in physical and chemical properties influencing the rates of absorption, distribution, metabolism, and excretion, and by the possible presence of such toxic impurities as chlorinated dibenzofurans and dibenzo-p-dioxins (Zitko and Choi, 1971; Vos et al., 1970). A statement by Tucker and Crabtree (1970) suggested that sublethal effects were directly correlated with the chlorine content, while lethal effects were inversely correlated. As techniques of definitive analysis have developed, studies have revealed that commercially available PCBs are extremely complex, as can be seen in Fig. 12.1, which demonstrates the congener composition of Aroclors (Monsanto Industrial Chemicals, St. Louis, Mo.; Sissons and Welti (1971); Webb and McCall, 1972). With the exception of Aroclor 1016 and 1232, it can be seen that one predominant congener, composed of a number of isomers, is found in each Aroclor preparation and, as the percentage of chlorine increases, the congener shifts from a mono- to a tri- to a tetra- to a pentachlorobiphenyl.

The ability of acute or chronic administration of PCBs to alter hepatic function in the form of ultrastructural changes and the induction of a variety of drug-detoxifying enzymes have been well documented (Allen and Abrahamson, 1973; Bennett et al., 1938; Benthe et al., 1972; Bickers, et al., 1972; Chen et al., 1973; Fujita et al., 1971; Kimbrough, 1972; Kimbrough et al., 1972; Koller and Zinkl, 1973; Litterst et al., 1972; Miller, 1944; Nishizumi, 1970; Norback and Allen, 1972; Villeneuve et al., 1971; Vos and Koeman, 1970). If it were possible to separate the complex mixtures, one could examine several facets of the toxicology of these chemicals and several questions could be posed and, perhaps, answered. Do the various congeners possess the same toxicologic properties, i.e., do dichlorobiphenyls have the same effect as hexachlorobiphenyls? Do all of the tetrachlorobiphenyl isomers produce the same toxicologic response following administration? Are the pathologic and toxicologic alterations observed due to the biphenyl nucleus itself, to the position(s) occupied by individual chlorine atoms, or to the number of chlorines present on the biphenyl nucleus? Since hepatic enzyme induction has been a well-characterized phenomenon, we decided to attempt to answer some of the above questions using the changes in enzyme activity as an index of structure–activity relationship. A study of the influence of a series of commercial Aroclors and a series of isomerically pure chlorobiphenyls of known degree and position of chlorination on hepatic function was conducted, examining enzymatic and ultrastructural changes in the tissue. The results presented here represent our findings to date. Many of the data have been published recently (Ecobichon and Comeau, 1974; Johnstone et al., 1974).

Preliminary experiments showed that a repeated intraperitoneal dose of com

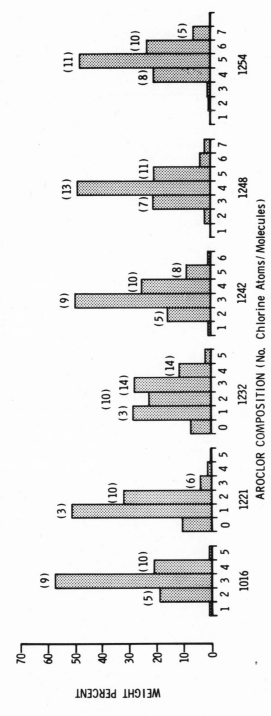

FIG. 12.1. The congener composition of commercially available Aroclors, based on the weight percentage of biphenyls bearing different numbers of chlorine atoms/molecule. The numbers in parentheses represent the number of isomers found for any one chlorobiphenyl. Data were obtained from reports by Webb and McCall (1972) and Sissons and Welti (1971), and from information supplied by the Monsanto Industrial Chemicals Company.

mercially available PCBs at a concentration of 50 mg/kg would cause measurable ultrastructural and enzymatic changes in rat liver. Since the object of these experiments was to elicit responses which, hopefully, could be related to the structures (of the pure chlorobiphenyls), we injected young male Wistar strain rats intraperitoneally with 50 mg/kg/day of the agent, dissolved in peanut oil, for three consecutive days, the animals being killed 96 h after the last injection. The livers were quickly removed, samples were taken and stained for light and electron microscopy, and the remaining hepatic tissue was prepared for enzymatic assays. The assays included representative functions of the microsomal monooxygenases, reductases, hydrolases (carboxylesterases), and conjugating enzymes. The agent-treated animals were compared with vehicle-treated control animals.

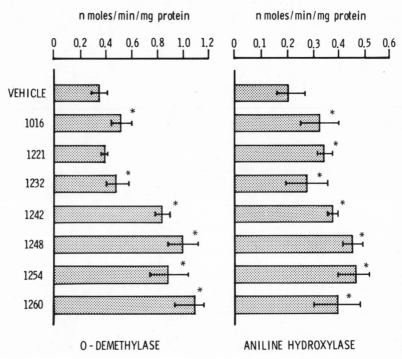

FIG. 12.2. The effects on hepatic p-nitroanisole O-demethylase and aniline hydroxylase of young male rats treated with a series of commercial Aroclor preparations. The animals were injected intraperitoneally for three consecutive days at a dose of 50 mg of agent/kg body weight and were killed 96 h after the last injection. Activities are expressed as nanomoles of product formed/min/mg of protein. The bars represent the mean enzymatic activities, the horizontal lines the standard deviations of the means of 18 control (vehicle-treated) animals and six animals per treated group. The asterisk signifies statistically significant differences from control values at $p < 0.05$.

As is shown in Fig. 12.2, significant increases in p-nitroanisole O-demethylase, a mixed-function oxidase, were observed following treatment with all Aroclors except Aroclor 1221. As the percentage weight of chlorine increased, more pronounced effects were observed, though there were no statistically significant ($p > 0.05$) differences between Aroclors 1248, 1254, and 1260. For aniline hydroxylase, another mixed-function oxidase, significant increases were observed for all agents tested, though more pronounced effects were observed with the more highly chlorinated Aroclor mixtures.

Figure 12.3 is a summary of the influence of the commercial Aroclors on hepatic carboxylesterase activity in young male rats. The enhancement of activity was not as great as that observed for the mixed-function oxidases, the maximum increase being only twofold higher than the control activity. Of the mixtures tested, significant increases were observed for all, with the exception of Aroclor 1232 and 1242. The greatest increases were observed following treatment with Aroclor 1254 and 1260.

The influence of the commercial Aroclor mixtures on two quite different hepatic "synthetic" conjugating enzymes, bromosulfophthalein (BSP)-glutathione "conjugase" and p-nitrophenol–glucuronic acid "conjugase," is

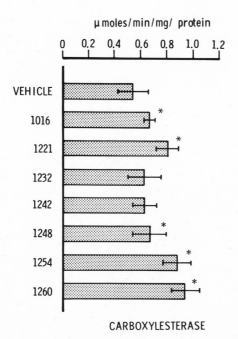

CARBOXYLESTERASE

FIG. 12.3. The effects on hepatic nonspecific carboxylesterase of young male rats treated with a series of commercial Aroclor preparations. For details, see caption to Fig. 12.1.

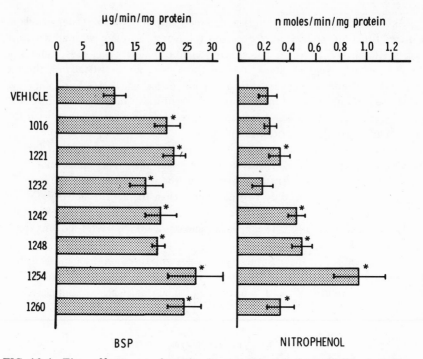

FIG. 12.4. The effects on hepatic bromosulfophthalein (BSP)–glutathione "conjugase" and *p*-nitrophenol–glucuronic acid "conjugase" of young male rats treated with a series of commercial Aroclor preparations. For details, see caption to Fig. 12.1.

shown in Fig. 12.4. Biphenyl (not shown) itself caused increases in BSP "conjugase" comparable to the increases observed for the various Aroclors. In contrast, the response of hepatic *p*-nitrophenol "conjugase" following treatment with Aroclors was markedly different. With the exception of Aroclor 1016 and 1232, significantly ($p < 0.05$) higher levels of enzyme activity were observed for the Aroclors tested. A highly significant increase was observed in rats treated with Aroclor 1254, the activity being fourfold higher than that of control animals and twofold higher than that observed in animals treated with Aroclor 1248 and 1260.

The results of these short-term acute studies with a series of Aroclor preparations of varying degree of chlorination would suggest that increased enzyme activity was, on the whole, related to the chlorine content. The data presented in Fig. 12.1, when compared to the experimental results in Figs. 12.2–12.4, suggest that a greater effect would be obtained with a pentachloro- than with a trichlorobiphenyl. Experiments similar to the above have indicated more marked induction of hepatic enzymes by Aroclor 1254 than by Aroclor 1016 or 1221 (Bickers et al., 1972; Villeneuve et al., 1971).

The availability of some isomerically pure chlorobiphenyls of known degree and position of chlorination prompted us to study the effects of these compounds on a number of functionally diverse, hepatic, drug-metabolizing enzymes of the rat. The biological activities of these agents, administered (ip) at a concentration of 50 mg/kg/day for three consecutive days followed by four days without treatment to maximize the effect, were compared to the inductive responses elicited by o,p'- and p,p'-DDT, Aroclor 1254 and 1260, and biphenyl. In addition to the microsomal mixed-function oxidases (N-demethylase, O-demethylase and aniline hydroxylase), microsomal nitroreductase, carboxylesterase, and cytoplasmic BSP "conjugase," the sleeping time induced by 40 mg/kg of pentobarbitone was measured (Johnstone et al., 1974).

To summarize the results of treatment with the isomerically pure chlorobiphenyls, biphenyl and 4-monochlorobiphenyl did not cause induction of hepatic drug-metabolizing enzymes. Microsomal mono-oxygenases were markedly induced by pure hexa- and octachlorobiphenyls and by di- and tetrachlorobiphenyls with chlorines substituted at the 3 and 4 positions of the rings. Nitroreductase and carboxylesterase activities were affected only by the highly chlorinated biphenyls, whereas all agents, including biphenyl, caused a marked induction of BSP "conjugase."

Recent experiments have extended the investigation to a series of pure isomers of di-, tri-, and tetrachlorobiphenyls in an attempt to confirm the importance of the position of the chlorine on the ring structure. The results indicate that not all isomers of di- or tri- or tetrachlorobiphenyls possess the same toxicologic properties. To date, results have demonstrated that a chlorine on the 4 position causes a more marked induction of hepatic enzyme activity than does a chlorine at any other position. A substitution at the 3 position is next in importance, followed by a substitution at the 2 position. It would appear that the varying response of the Aroclors is highly dependent upon (a) the degree of chlorination of the biphenyl nucleus (the higher the amount of chlorine, the greater the effect) and (b) the isomer composition of the predominating chlorobiphenyl in the Aroclor mixture.

Acknowledgment

The author wishes to thank the ASP Biological and Medical Press, Amsterdam for permission to reproduce Figs. 12.1 to 12.4, which are also to be published in *Chemico-Biological Interactions*, 9, 341–350 (1974).

References

Allen, J. R., and Abrahamson, L. J. (1973). *Arch. Environ. Cont. Toxicol.*, **1**, 265.
Bennett, G. A., Drinker, C. K., and Warren, M. F. (1938). *J. Ind. Hyg. Toxicol.*, **20**, 97.
Benthe, H. F., Schmoldt, A., and Schmidt, H. (1972). *Arch. Toxikol.*, **29**, 97.
Bickers, D. R., Harber, L. C., Kappas, A., and Alvares, A. P. (1972). *Res. Commun. Chem. Path. Pharmacol.*, **3**, 505.
Chen, P. R., Mehendale, H. M., and Fishbein, L. (1973). *Arch. Environ. Contam. Toxicol.*, **1**, 36.
Ecobichon, D. J., and Comeau, A. M. (1974). *Chem.-Biol. Interactions*, **9**, 341.
Fujita, S., Tsuji, H., Kato, K., Saeki, S., and Tsukamoto, H. (1971). *Fukuoka Acta Med.*, **62**, 30.
Holmes, D. C., Simmons, J. H., and Tatton, J. O'G. (1967). *Nature (Lond.)*, **216**, 227.
Jensen, S. (1966). *New Scientist*, **32**, 612.
Jensen, S., Johnels, A. G., Olsson, M., and Otterlund, G. (1969). *Nature (Lond.)*, **224**, 247.
Johnstone, G. J., Ecobichon, D. J., and Hutzinger, O. (1974). *Toxicol. Appl. Pharmacol.*, **28**, 66.
Kimbrough, R. D. (1972). *Arch. Environ. Health*, **25**, 125.
Kimbrough, R. D., Linder, R. E., and Gaines, T. B. (1972). *Arch. Environ. Health*, **25**, 354.
Koeman, J. N., Ten Noever de Brauw, M. C., and de Vos, R. N. (1969). *Nature (Lond.)*, **221**, 1126.
Koller, L. D., and Zinkl, J. G. (1973). *Amer. J. Pathol.*, **70**, 363.
Kuratsune, M., Yoshimura, T., Matsuzaki, J., and Yamaguchi, A. (1971). *Natl. Inst. Environ. Health Meeting, Rougemont, N.C.*, Dec. 20–22.
Lincer, J. L., and Peakall, D. B. (1970). *Nature (Lond.)*, **228**, 783.
Litterst, C. L., Farber, T. M., Baker, A. M., and van Loon, E. J. (1972). *Toxicol. Appl. Pharmacol.*, **23**, 112.
Miller, J. W. (1944). *U.S. Public Health Report*, **59**, 1085.
Miller, R. W. (1971). *Teratol.*, **4**, 211.
Murai, Y., and Kuroiwa, Y. (1971). *Neurology*, **21**, 1173.
Nishizumi, M. (1970). *Arch. Environ. Health*, **21**, 620.
Norback, D. J., and Allen, J. R. (1972). *Environ. Health Perspect.*, **1**, 137.
Pichirollo, J. (1971). *Science*, **173**, 899.
Prestt, I., Jefferies, D. J., and Moore, N. W. (1970). *Environ. Pollut.*, **1**, 3.
Risebrough, R. W., Rieche, P., Peakall, D. B., Herman, S. G., and Kirven, M. N. (1968). *Nature (Lond.)*, **220**, 1098.
Sissons, D., and Welti, D. (1971). *J. Chromatog.*, **60**, 15.
Tucker, R. K., and Crabtree, D. G. (1970). *Handbook of Toxicity of Pesticides to Wildlife*, Publ. 84.
Villeneuve, D. C., Grant, D. L., Phillips, W. E. J., Clark, M. L., and Clegg, D. J. (1971). *Bull. Environ. Contam. Toxicol.*, **6**, 120.
Vos, J. G., and Koeman, J. H. (1970). *Toxicol. Appl. Pharmacol.*, **17**, 656.
Vos, J. G., Koeman, J. H., van der Maas, H. L., Ten Noever de Brauw, M. C., and de Vos, R. H. (1970). *Food Cosmet. Toxicol.*, **8**, 625.
Webb, R. G., and McCall, A. C. (1972). *J. Assoc. Offic. Anal. Chem.*, **55**, 746.
Zitko, V., and Choi, P. M. K. (1971). *Fisheries Research Board of Canada, Technical Report 272.*

13

The Accumulation and Excretion of Heavy Metals in Organisms*

JORMA K. MIETTINEN

13.1. Introduction

By the term "heavy metals" we usually understand, at least in the biological context, iron and metals denser than it. Some of these metals, e.g., iron, manganese, copper, cobalt, and zinc, are essential to many organisms, while others are either nonessential, harmful, or outright toxic. However, the concept of "essentiality" is under constant review, and "harmfulness" and "toxicity" vary widely with organism and concentration. All heavy metals are potentially harmful to most organisms at some level of exposure and absorption.

Three heavy metals which are toxic to most organisms at the lowest concentrations and which are probably never beneficial to living things are cadmium, mercury, and lead. Due to human activity, their presence in the environment has increased in some areas to levels which threaten the health of aquatic and terrestrial organisms, man included. Especially dangerous situations may arise

*Reprinted from Krenkel (ed.), *Progress in Water Technology*, Vol. 7, Pergamon Press, Oxford, 1974.

JORMA K. MIETTINEN • Department of Radiochemistry, University of Helsinki, Helsinki, Finland.

due to heavy metal compounds, such as methylmercury, which are efficiently enriched from one trophic level to another along the food chains.

Information regarding the accumulation and excretion of these three heavy metals and those of their compounds able to persist in the environment has therefore become highly desirable.

This review is concerned mainly with mechanisms and rates of absorption and excretion, with particular reference to biological half-times and accumulation. The primary emphasis is on accumulation in man, although other organisms, especially fish and shellfish which are important constituents of food chains leading to man, are also briefly treated. Only the most recent results and viewpoints are discussed, without full coverage of the earlier literature. In this respect, reference is made to the recent report of an international Task Group on Metal Accumulation (1973), which reviews the literature extensively.

13.2. Relevant Compounds, Corresponding Critical Organs in Man, and Scheme of Absorption (by Ingestion) and of Elimination

The compounds concerned and their critical organs in man are presented in Table 13.1. By critical organ we understand that organ in which the first undesirable functional changes occur under increasing intake of the toxicant. This is not necessarily the same organ in which the highest accumulation takes place. Sensitivity varies widely between individuals, and the critical concentrations usually form a Gaussian distribution within a population (Fig. 13.1). The varia-

Table 13.1. Some Toxic Heavy Metals and Compounds Thereof Occurring in Aquatic Food Chains and the Corresponding Critical Organs in Man

Compound	Critical organ
Cadmium (Cd^{2+})	Kidney
	Liver
Mercury (Hg^{2+})	Kidney
Methylmercury ($CH_4 Hg^{2+}$)	CNS[a]
Lead (Pb^{2+})	Hematopoetic system
	CNS and PNS[b]
	Kidney

[a]CNS, central nervous system.
[b]PNS, peripheral nervous system.

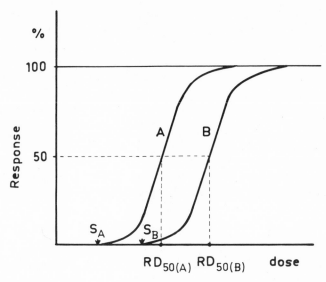

FIG.13.1. Dose–response curves obtained for two toxic substances, A and B, within a population. The most sensitive individuals (S) respond to a much lower dose than do 50% of the population (RD_{50}). The curves represent integrals of Gaussian distribution functions.

bility may be so great as to make one organ critical for one individual while a different organ can be so for another individual. This variability depends upon individual differences in retention and elimination rate, possibly even in the capacity to detoxify the toxic metal. It is known, for example, that mammals and even fish contain an adaptive protein, metallothionein, which can bind large amounts of mercury, cadmium, and zinc.

Absorption via ingestion is the only route by which heavy metals enter man from the aquatic milieu. In addition to this, however, man obtains heavy metals and their compounds from atmospheric pollution via inhalation. This source has to be reckoned with when the effects of these metals upon man's health are studied, since some occupational, industrial, and even urban environments may contribute significant amounts compared with the intake from food. Metals are to some extent absorbed directly from the lungs, but a portion of these in particulate form is transferred by mucociliary clearance into the gastrointestinal tract and may be absorbed there. In this paper, however, only intake via ingestion is considered.

In Fig. 13.2 a model for the absorption and elimination of metals is presented. The major source of mercury, cadmium, and lead is food, and, especially

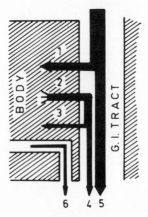

FIG. 13.2. A model for the absorption and elimination of heavy metals via the gastrointestinal tract: 1, absorption; 2, gross excretion; 3, reabsorption; 4, net excretion; 5, unabsorbed; 6, excretion via urine; 1 + 5, intake; 4 + 5 + 6, elimination.

for mercury and cadmium intake by man, aquatic food chains play an important role. In seafood, cadmium, lead, and ionic mercury exist primarily as bivalent cations, more or less loosely bound to proteins. Their availability to man, equal, whether from proteinate or from ionic solution, depends upon nutritional factors. A deficiency of dietary calcium increases the absorption of lead and cadmium (Six and Goyer, 1970; Kobayaski et al., 1971), while a deficiency of dietary iron increases the absorption of lead (Six and Goyer, 1972). In children, and in pregnant and lactating women, the absorption rates of lead and cadmium may be doubled due to their great demand for calcium. A low intake of protein and Vitamin D also increases cadmium absorption (Friberg et al., 1972). A low-protein diet may increase lead absorption as well (Milev et al., 1970).

Mercury is often present in seafood in the form of its organometallic compound, methylmercury. In Scandinavia, about 95% of the total mercury in fish is usually in this form (Westöö, 1969). Elsewhere, lower percentages have been reported, e.g., <50% in certain marine fish (blue marlin) of the Hawaiian area (Rivers et al., 1972). Selenium in the diet may influence the absorption of methylmercury (Ganther et al., 1972), and nutritional status may influence its retention, but these factors have not as yet been sufficiently well investigated.

In *marine animals* the direct uptake of metals from water via the gills (fish) or the sieve tubes (mollusks) is possible, although this factor probably does not play a major role except in heavily polluted areas. Methylmercury and the metal ions are all readily absorbed by plankton and bacteria, thus being mostly particle-bound in the sea water and able to be taken up only through food chains.

13.3. Absorption and Elimination of Cadmium in Man

One method of studying the absorption and retention of cadmium in man is the "balance study," i.e., measurement of intake and excretion in a number of subjects over a long period of time. Alternatively, an attempt may be made to estimate the approximate cadmium intake of individuals for whom kidney and liver analyses have been performed *post mortem*. Both of these methods are extremely tedious and require a large number of subjects, since the intake of cadmium varies daily, weekly, seasonally, and perhaps even over longer periods for most individuals. The bulk of the human cadmium burden is usually obtained by utilizing certain foods, e.g., kidney, liver, some cereals, or seafood, which the majority consume only occasionally. As the retained amount is very small compared with the amounts taken in and excreted, its reliable quantitative determination would require high accuracy of the analytical method. This is why cadmium balance studies have not, thus far, resulted in a reliable figure regarding the percentage of retention.

Use of the radioisotope ^{115m}Cd and the wholebody counting technique, however, provides for the precise, direct determination of the retained fraction. Unfortunately, the physical half-life of ^{115m}Cd (43 days), although highly useful for the determination of retention, is too short to permit determination of the biological half-time of the slowly excreted portion of the element, which appears to be quite long, of the order of years.

A study on cadmium metabolism in man has been recently reported (Rahola et al., 1972a, b) in which a single oral dose of labeled, mostly protein-bound cadmium, was administered to each of five voluntary male subjects ranging in age from 19 to 50 years. The labeled dose was carefully prepared to resemble normal food. The radioisotope and a solution of stable carrier were mixed with homogenized calf kidney cortex and kept under refrigeration overnight. Analysis demonstrated that approximately 80% of the cadmium became protein-bound. Portions of the homogenate containing 100 μg Cd and 4.8–6.1 μCi ^{115m}Cd were mixed with dressing and served to the volunteers as a sandwich.

Whole-body counting, as well as the analysis of feces and urine samples which were collected quantitatively during the first days following the administration of the dose, revealed that approximately 75% of the ingested ^{115m}Cd activity was eliminated within 3–5 days and 94% within 10–15 days. This elimination occurred primarily via the feces, with only a minor portion being excreted in urine (Fig. 13.3). The elimination equation was biexponential (Fig. 13.4), the biological half-time of the fast component being about 2.5 days. The mean percentage of the slow component in the five individuals was 5.9 ± 0.5% of the dose. The biological half-time of the slow component could not be determined due to the low percentage of 0.935 MeV gamma rays emitted by ^{115m}Cd

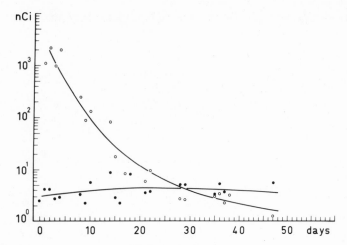

FIG. 13.3. Daily excretion of ^{115m}Cd in feces (○) and urine (●) (average of five volunteers).

in its decay and its short physical half-life (43 days). Some idea regarding this component is obtainable from autopsy data.

Such data regarding cadmium concentration in the human kidney at 10-year age intervals were published by Schroeder et al. (1961). Their results reveal an almost linear increase until approximately 40 years of age and a similar decrease after 50 years. Data collected from differing populations were compared by Friberg et al. (1972). According to this study, the maximum concentration of cadmium is approached in most cases at the age of 30–40 years, while the half-saturation value based upon the maximum appears to occur at about 18 years (12–24 years). The accumulation curve once again appears to be nearly linear.

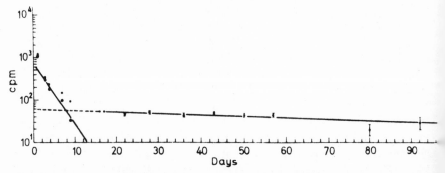

FIG. 13.4. Whole-body retention by an individual male subject of ^{115m}Cd resulting from a single oral dose of cadmium.

A biological half-time of 18 years for cadmium would correspond to an average daily retention of about 1.6 μg, thus indicating an average daily intake of 26 μg (assuming 6% retention). These figures are feasible for the first 18 years of age if the adult intake is 50 μgCd/day (Friberg et al., (1972). The linearity of the accumulation curve may be due to increased Cd intake with advancing age (as a result of, for example, increased food consumption, greater use of kidney and liver, and the onset of smoking at 14–18 years). In light of these evaluations, a biological half-time of approximately 15–20 years appears likely for the slow component of cadmium excretion.

Cadmium circulates in blood primarily bound to red cells. It is evidently bound partly to hemoglobin and partly to metallothionein (Friberg et al., 1972).

Regarding the transport of cadmium, the plasma fraction is probably more important than that of the red cells.

13.4. Absorption and Elimination of Cadmium in Fish and Mollusks

The retention and elimination of cadmium in rainbow trout was studied utilizing food labeled with $^{109}Cd^{2+}$ and whole-body counting the live fish. The results (Fig. 13.5) demonstrated that the bulk of the ^{109}Cd activity was rapidly eliminated, the excretion following a power, rather than an exponential function. After 42 days, about 1% of the administered dose was retained in the whole body, the elimination rate then being quite slow (Jaakkola et al., 1972). In nature, the following concentration factors have been measured (Preston, 1973): fish 10^2, crustaceans 10^3, mollusks 10^3-10^4 (10^5), plankton 10^4, and seaweed 10^2-10^3.

The main vehicles of cadmium intake by man from marine biota are mollus-

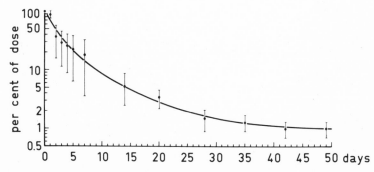

FIG. 13.5. Elimination of cadmium from rainbow trout (*Salmo gairdnerii*) determined by whole-body counting. Points indicate average retention by six fish; bars indicate one standard deviation.

can shellfish and the brown flesh of the crab, which may contain high levels of cadmium in polluted areas. Pelagic fish are low in cadmium, as are coastal fish, even in polluted areas (Jaakkola et al., 1973). This suggests that there is no important food chain effect, since high concentrations would then be found in predatory and aged fish. It should be mentioned here that one important terrestrial source of cadmium is kidney of aged horse, elk, and reindeer. Kidney of aged horse may contain 50–200 ppm Cd, and one meal consisting of such kidney would correspond to a whole year's normal intake.

13.5. Metabolism of Inorganic Mercury and Methylmercury in Man and Its Implications

Two studies have been published on the absorption and elimination of methylmercury in man. Åberg et al. (1969) administered ionic methylmercury to three male volunteers and obtained an absorption of 95% and a half-time of 70–74 days. Miettinen et al. (1971) gave protein-bound methylmercury to fifteen volunteers and obtained nearly the same retention (94%) and half-time (76 ± 3 days) (Table 13.2). We also studied inorganic mercury in the same way

Table 13.2. Biological Half-time of ^{203}Hg Activity in the Whole Body after Oral Administration of Protein-Bound CH$_3$^{203}Hg (Error Marked as One Standard Deviation of the Mean)

Volunteer	$T_{1/2}$ biol (days)	Volunteer	$T_{1/2}$ biol (days)
♀		♂	
AE	52	RE	72
EH	69	AH	88
LJ	73	PK	87
AN	88	JK	74
KR	87	MM	78
LU	56	JM	70
		VM	78
		RP	93
		HT	74
Mean	71 ± 6	Mean	79 ± 3
Mean of whole group 76 ± 3			

(Rahola et al., 1973), administering protein-bound and ionic inorganic mercury to 10 volunteers and obtaining a retention of 15% and half-time of 42 ± 3 days (Fig. 13.6). No difference between the two forms was observed. All of these studies were performed utilizing ^{203}Hg-labeled doses and the whole-body counting technique. In animals, both inorganic mercury and methylmercury follow a biexponential elimination equation, although the fast component is not always easily measurable, being too short. It may be assumed that the fast component primarily reflects the blood and plasma level, while the slow component reflects the intracellular level in flesh, liver, and other tissues.

The ratio of the amount of mercury in the red blood cells to that in the plasma is 10 for methylmercury and 0.4 for inorganic mercury; thus, it is a simple matter to calculate the content of each in cases when both compounds are present simultaneously. However, the half-times of both compounds in the blood are considerably shorter than in the whole body. Following the administration of a single dose, the half-time of methylmercury in the red blood cells was 50 ± 7 days, while that of inorganic mercury was 16 days. If the elapsed time since the beginning of mixed intoxication is known, then the content of mercury in the body may be calculated from the blood levels, at least in cases of intoxication due to a single dose. Chronic cases require other calculations, which may be difficult if both inorganic mercury and methylmercury are present in the diet.

It is quite reasonable to assume that different mercury compounds may be present in different populations. Figure 13.7 presents data compiled by Suzuki (personal communication). These data can be interpreted as meaning that Swedish fish consumers contain practically pure methylmercury (RBC/plasma

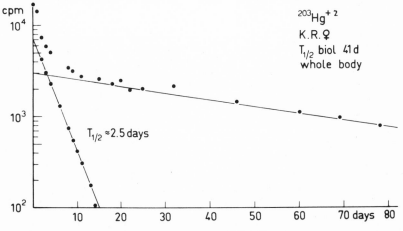

FIG. 13.6. Typical retention curve of ^{203}Hg^{2+} in the whole body.

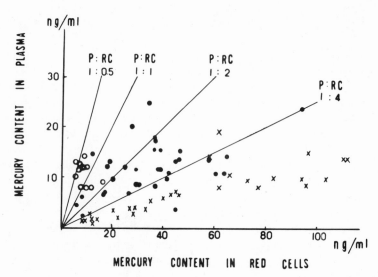

FIG. 13.7. Mercury content in plasma versus red blood cells of some populations, according to Suzuki (personal communication). ○ Japanese-Americans in Honolulu. ● Japanese in Tokyo and surroundings. × Swedes consuming fish up to three times per week.

ratio = 10), while the Japanese-Americans in Honolulu would contain nearly pure inorganic mercury (RBC/plasma ratio = 0.5) and the Japanese in Tokyo ¼ methylmercury and ¾ inorganic mercury. Both rice and the Pacific fish, the prime sources of dietary mercury in the Pacific islands, seem to contain an important proportion of their mercury in the inorganic form (at least the blue marlin), thus explaining the results of Fig. 13.7. In the blood, most mercury is eliminated by the plasma fraction.

13.6. Biological Half-time of Mercury Compounds in Aquatic Animals

Several studies (Miettinen et al., 1969, 1972; Järvenpää et al., 1970; Tillander et al., 1972; Ruohtula and Miettinen, 1975) have been performed in which labeled mercury compounds (Hg^{2+} or methyl-, ethyl-, propyl-, or phenyl-Hg) have been introduced into aquatic animals by means of food, intramuscular injection, or direct uptake from the surrounding water, and the absorption, distribution, and rate of elimination have been studied by whole-body counting of the individual labeled animal. The effects of the administration route, the concentration of the compound in the animal, and the ambient water temperature upon the rate of elimination have also been studied.

Briefly summarized, the excretion rate varies greatly among the different species, but usually follows a biexponential equation. The biological half-time at an ambient water temperature of the fast component usually varies from 1 to 10 days, while the slow one ranges from 200 to 1200 days. The excretion rate at 15°C is twice as fast as that at 4°C. Fresh, brackish, and salt water species were found to have broadly similar rates of excretion. When the concentration of methylmercury in fish increases, the biological half-time of mercury decreases: in rainbow trout, dosed with $Me^{203}Hg$, a concentration of 0.4 mg Hg/kg is eliminated with a half-time of 340 days, while a concentration of 4 mg Hg/kg is eliminated with a half-time of 170 days. Ionic and protein-bound methylmercury have similar rates of elimination when orally administered, but methylmercury absorbed by rainbow trout directly from aquarium water via the gills is eliminated faster (half-time: 268 days) than methylmercury administered orally as, for instance, a proteinate (half-time: 326 days). The half-times of inorganic Hg and phenyl- and methyl-Hg in mussel (*Pseudanodonta complanata*) were 23, 43, and (depending on age) 100–400 days, respectively, while the half-times of methyl-, ethyl-, and propyl-Hg in rainbow trout were 346, 119, and 233 days, respectively. Thus, of all these compounds, methylmercury has the slowest rate of elimination.

Both injected and orally administered methylmercury have approximately the same rate of elimination in fish, while inorganic mercury, when injected intramuscularly, is eliminated several times more slowly than when dosed in food. Methylmercury administered orally to the seal has a very long biological half-time (about 500 days). The biological half-times of the slow component of ^{203}Hg elimination for ionic and protein-bound methylmercury in three species of fish are displayed in Table 13.3.

13.7. Absorption and Elimination of Lead in Man

The gastrointestinal absorption of lead in man is quite variable, between 1 and 16% (Kehoe, 1961; Hursh and Suomela, 1967), and is age-dependent, being highest in the young. In blood, lead is bound to the red cells. The plasma-to-red-cell ratio of lead is the smallest for any metal (0.01), yet lead passes into the brain more easily than cadmium, although it does not accumulate there (Schroeder and Tripton, 1968). More lead concentrates in cortical gray matter and basal ganglia than in cortical white matter in cases of lead poisoning (Klein et al., 1970). Organolead compounds penetrate the brain quite readily, especially the monovalent triethyl lead, which the organism readily forms from tetra-

Table 13.3. Biological Half-time of the Slow Component of Excretion for Ionic and Protein-Bound Methylmercury in Three Species of Fish: Flounder, Pike, and Eel. Gulf of Finland, Tvärminne Zoological Station (Salinity 0.6%)

Fish	Route of administration and form of methylmercury	$T_{1/2}$ biol (days)	Number of fish
Flounder	*per os*, proteinate	780 ± 120	9
(*Pleuronectes flesus*)	*per os*, ionic	700 ± 50	7
	intramuscular, ionic	(1200 ± 400)	10
Pike	*per os*, proteinate	750 ± 50	5
(*Esox lucius*)	*per os*, ionic	640 ± 120	2
	intramuscular, ionic	780 ± 80	3
Eel	*per os*, proteinate	910 ± 40	4
(*Anguilla vulgaris*)	*per os*, ionic	1030 ± 70	4
	intramuscular, ionic	1030 ± 80	2

ethyl lead. In this respect, they resemble methylmercury. The cells evidently are not adequately protected against monovalent metal compounds which mimic alkalies. The gastrointestinal excretion of lead is low, of the order of one or a few percent (Hursh and Suomela, 1967). In the kidney, a tubular reabsorption mechanism exists for lead in acutely exposed subjects with high blood levels (>100 μg Pb per 100 ml) and probably also in cases of normal lead burdens (Vostal, 1963, 1972). Details of the tubular mechanism are still unknown since the low level of lead in plasma has thus far made analysis difficult. Modern methods, especially the graphite oven technique for atomic absorption spectrophotometry, have substantially increased the possibility of analyzing plasma lead in normal persons.

Lead excretion via milk correlates with blood levels and may reach high values (0.3 ppm) in cows exposed to lead (Hammond and Aronson, 1964).

The primary difficulty in studies of lead absorption and retention is its strong affinity to bone. The half-time of lead in human bone is not known, but the ICRP uses 10 years as the first approximation (ICRP 2, 1959). There exist two or three components with different mobilities, and excretion follows more a power function than an exponential one. The liver is another site for the storage of lead. This partition of lead between the liver and bone as well as its normally very low plasma level render it difficult to evaluate the relationships between lead concentration in blood, the critical organs, and urine under normal exposure, but much information exists regarding current exposure (Hernberg, 1972). Lead in blood and urine reflect current exposure well. The blood level is considered to be more reliable, since metabolic factors may influence renal handling of lead.

Lead metabolism in the mussel was recently studied by Kauranen and Järvenpää (1972) utilizing ^{210}Pb. The biological half-time for the soft parts of *Mytilus edulis* was 300 days, that for the shell nonmeasurable (long). In two other marine organisms, *Mesidotae entomon* and *Harmatoe* sp., the values were 170 and 50 days, respectively. A short component of a few days exists in all these species.

13.8. Conclusion

Mechanisms detailing the absorption and excretion of heavy metals in animals and man are still only rather vaguely known. In the case of methylmercury, however, a reliable mathematical model exists. Although common features exist among the various metals which permit the drawing of general schemes such as that illustrated in Fig. 13.2, the differences among the metals are more marked. In particular, the mechanisms involved in renal excretion are not completely known. The use of radioactive or stable isotopes and new analytical methods make experimental studies easier. Better epidemiological data are necessary in order to be able to evaluate the significance of the parameters of general environmental exposure, which is chronic and at low level.

References

Åberg, B., Ekman, L., Falk, R., Greitz, U., Persson, G., and Snihs, J. O. (1969). "Metabolism of methylmercury (^{203}Hg) compounds in man: excretion and distribution," *Arch. Environ. Health*. 19, 478–484.

Friberg, L., Piscator, M., and Nordberg, G. (1972). *Cadmium in the Environment*, Chemical Rubber Co., Cleveland, Ohio.

Ganther, H. E., Goudie, C., Sunde, M. L., Kopecky, M. J., Wagner, P., Oh, S.-H., and Hoekstra, W. G. (1972). "Selenium: relation to decreased toxicity of methylmercury added to diets containing tuna," *Science* 175, 1122–1124.

Hammond, P. B., and Aronson, A. L. (1964). "Lead poisoning in cattle and horses in the vicinity of a smelter," *Ann. N.Y. Acad. Sci.* 111, 569–611.

Hernberg, S. (1972). "The value of lead analyses in blood and urine as indices of body burden, accumulation in critical organs and exposure," *Proceedings of the XVIIth International Congress on Occupational Health*.

Hursh, J. B., and Suomela, J. (1967). "Absorption of ^{212}Pb from the gastrointestinal tract of man," *Acta Radiol.* 7, 108–120.

ICRP, 2, (1959). *Recommendations of the International Commission on Radiological Pro-*

tection, Report of Committee II on Permissible Dose for Internal Radiation, ICRP Publication 2, Pergamon Press, London.

Jaakkola, T., Takahashi, H., Soininen, R., Rissanen, K., and Miettinen, J. K. (1972). "Cadmium content of sea water, bottom sediment and fish, and its elimination rate in fish," *Radiotracer Studies of Chemical Residues in Food and Agriculture*, 69–75, IAEA-PI-469/7, IAEA, Vienna.

Jaakkola, T., Takahashi, H., and Miettinen, J. K. (1973). "Cadmium content in sea water, bottom sediment, fish, lichen and elk in Finland," *Environmental Quality and Safety, Global Aspects of Chemistry, Toxicology and Technology as Applied to the Environment*, Vol. II, pp. 230–237 (ed. Coulston, F., and Korte, F.), Academic Press, New York.

Järvenpää, T., Tillander, M., and Miettinen, J. K. (1970). "Methylmercury: half-time of elimination in flounder, pike and eel," *Suomen Kemistilehti* B43, 439–442.

Kauranen, P., and Järvenpää, T. (1972). "Biological half-times of ^{210}Po and ^{210}Pb in some marine organisms," *Department of Radiochemistry, University of Helsinki, Annual Report, May 1972*.

Kehoe, R. (1961). "The metabolism of lead in man in health and disease," *J. Roy. Inst. Publ. Health*. 24, 81–97, 101–120a, 129–143, 177–203.

Klein, M., Namer, R., Harpur, E., and Robin, R. (1970). "Earthenware containers as a source of fatal lead poisoning," *New Engl. J. Med.* 283, 669.

Kobayashi, J., Nakahura, H., and Hasegawa, T. (1971). "Accumulation of cadmium in organs of mice fed on cadmium polluted rice," *Jap. J. Hyg.* 26, 401–407 (in Japanese, with English summary).

Miettinen, J. K., Heyraud, M., and Keckes, S. (1972). "Mercury as hydrospheric pollutant. II, Biological half-time of methylmercury in four Mediterranean species: a fish, a crab and two molluscs," *Marine Pollution and Sea Life* (ed. Ruivo, M.), pp. 295–298, FAO Fishing News, London.

Miettinen, J. K., Tillander, M., Rissanen, K., Miettinen, V., and Ohmomo, Y. (1969). "Distribution and excretion rate of phenyl- and methylmercury nitrate in fish, mussels, molluscs and crayfish," *9th Japan Conference on Radioisotopes, Tokyo, May 1969*, paper B/(11)-17, pp. 474–478.

Miettinen, J. K., Rahola, T., Hattula, T., Rissanen, K., and Tillander, M. (1971). "Elimination of ^{203}Hg-methylmercury in man," *Ann. Clin. Res.* 3, 116–122.

Milev, N., Sattler, E.-L., and Menden, E. (1970). "Aufnahme und Einlagerung von Blei im Körper unter verschiedenen Ernährungsbedingungen," *Med. Ernähr.* 11, 29–32.

Preston, A. (1973). Cadmium in the marine environment of the United Kingdom," *Mar. Pollut. Bull.* 4, 105–107.

Rahola, T., Aaran, R.-K., and Miettinen, J. K. (1972a). "Half-time studies of mercury and cadmium by whole-body counting," *IAEA Symposium on the Assessment of Radioactive Organ and Body Burdens, Stockholm, Sweden, November 22-26, 1971*, pp. 553–562, IAEA-SM-150/13.

Rahola, T., Aaran, R.-K., and Miettinen, J. K. (1972b). "Retention and elimination of cadmium-115m in man," *Second European Congress on Radiation Protection, Budapest, Hungary, May 3-5, 1972*, pp. 213–218.

Rahola, T., Hattula, T., Korolainen, A., and Miettinen, J. K. (1973). "Elimination of free and protein-bound ionic mercury (^{203}Hg^{2+}) in man," *Ann. Clin. Res.* 5, 214–229.

Rivers, J. B., Pearson, J. E., and Schultz, C. D. (1972). "Total and organic mercury in marine fish," *Bull. Environ. Contam. Toxicol.* 8, 257–266.

Ruohtula, M., and Miettinen, J. K. (1975). "Retention and excretion of ^{203}Hg-labelled methylmercury in rainbow trout," *Oikos*, 24 (in press).

Schroeder, H. A., and Tipton, L. (1968). "The human body burden of lead," *Arch. Environ. Health.* **17,** 965–978.

Schroeder, H. A., Balassa, J. J., Brattleboro, V., and Hogencamp, J. C. (1961). "Abnormal trace metals in man: cadmium," *J. Chron. Dis.* **14**(2), 236–258.

Six, K. M., and Goyer, R. A. (1970). "Experimental enhancement of lead toxicity by low dietary calcium," *J. Lab. Clin. Med.* **76,** 933–943.

Six, K. M., and Goyer, R. A. (1972). "The influence of iron deficiency on tissue content and toxicity of injested lead in the rat," *J. Lab. Clin. Med.* **79,** 128–138.

Task Group on Metal Accumulation (1973). "Accumulation of toxic metals with special reference to their absorption, excretion and biological half-times," *Environ. Physiol. Biochem.* **3,** 65–107.

Tillander, M., Miettinen, J. K., and Koivisto, I. (1972). "Excretion rate of methylmercury in the seal, *Pusa hispida*," *Marine Pollution and Sea Life* (ed. Ruivo, M.), pp. 303–306, FAO Fishing News, London.

Vostal, J. (1963). "Mechanisms of lead excretion," *Biochem. Pharmacol.* **2,** 207.

Vostal, J. (1972). "General mechanisms of the renal and biliary excretion of toxic metals," *Proceedings of the XVIIth International Congress on Occupational Health.*

Westöö, G. (1969). "Methylmercury compounds in animal foods," *Chemical Fallout Current Research on Persistent Pesticides* (ed. Miller, M. W., and Berg, G. G.), pp. 75–93, Charles C. Thomas, Springfield, Ill.

Part III
WORKING GROUP
REPORTS

A

Entry, Distribution, and Fate of Heavy Metals and Organohalogens in the Physical Environment

Chairman: E. D. Goldberg

Members: K. I. Beynon, A. J. de Groot, J. C. Duinker, H.-J. Elster, R. L. Halstead, P. Heurteaux, A. Kloke, J. W. M. La Riviere, D. R. Miller, I. Price, A. N. Yule

Rapporteur: T. Duce

A.1. Atmosphere

A.1.1. Metals

A.1.1.1. Sources and Entry

Unlike the heavier organohalogen compounds such as DDT and PCBs, atmospheric trace metals have significant natural as well as anthropogenic sources. Thus one of the major problems in understanding trace metals and their transport in the atmosphere is distinguishing between the natural and anthropogenic components. While this is often relatively easy to do in or near urban areas, it becomes increasingly difficult on a regional and global scale.

In general, both natural and anthropogenic source strengths for trace metals in the atmosphere are poorly known. While reasonably accurate estimates have been made for man's atmospheric injection of some metals, such as lead and perhaps mercury, little information is yet available for the majority of trace metals, such as Ni, Cu, Mn, Mo, As, Sb, Zn, Cd, Cr, and Fe. Studies to determine the various anthropogenic processes (manufacturing industries, fuel combustion, garbage incineration, mining, etc.) which are sources for these metals as well as the respective source strengths must be encouraged.

There are major natural sources for trace metals in the atmosphere, including erosion or crustal weathering, volcanism, forest fires, and the ocean. Again, our knowledge of the source strengths is minimal. Estimates have been made of the total annual atmospheric particulate production by several of these natural sources, and the estimates vary by over an order of magnitude. In addition, the relative trace element composition of particles from erosion processes and from the ocean may differ from the average composition in their respective source area due to selective chemical processes occurring during particle formation. Our understanding of these natural processes and the composition of the particles produced needs additional study. The particle size and number distribution of atmospheric material produced from both natural and anthropogenic sources is also largely unknown.

The vapor phase apparently plays a major role in the atmospheric chemistry of mercury and there is some evidence that it may be important in the atmospheric cycle of some other trace metals, e.g., Se, Sb, Zn, Cd, As, and Pb (Zoller et al., 1974; Duce et al., 1974). All of these elements form relatively volatile inorganic or organic compounds, and all are found on particles in remote atmospheric areas at concentrations higher than would normally be expected from natural sources such as crustal weathering or the ocean. Considerable work is needed to confirm the observation that a vapor phase does exist at some point for these trace metals and, if so, what its chemical form and source is and whether it may be responsible for the relatively high concentrations observed for these metals in the atmosphere in nonurban areas. Potential sources for a vapor phase include anthropogenic high-temperature processes, volcanism, biological mobilization (e.g., methylated species), and general degassing of the earth's crust. There is a considerable body of evidence suggesting that the high atmospheric lead concentrations observed in remote areas in the northern hemisphere may be the result of the burning of lead alkyls in motor vehicles (Murozumi et al., 1969).

A.1.1.2. Distribution

While there is a growing body of information on the surface level concentration of many particulate trace metals in urban and near-urban air, there have been very few measurements of trace metal concentrations on the regional to global scales. Even in urban areas, information on the vertical profiles of metals in the troposphere and stratosphere is largely lacking. Very few particle size distribution studies of trace metals, except in a few urban areas, have been made. Until much more information is available on the horizontal and vertical concentration gradients and size distribution of the various trace metals, it will be very difficult to predict their transport rates within and removal rates from the atmosphere. Atmospheric measurements in remote areas in both the northern and southern hemispheres will be particularly important in ascertaining potential global transport of anthropogenic source trace metals.

If, as mentioned previously, a vapor phase exists for some trace metals in the atmosphere, measurement of both the particulate and vapor concentrations in urban and remote areas will be necessary to understand and predict the transport of these elements.

A.1.1.3. Fate

The ultimate fate of trace metals in the atmosphere is removal by precipitation or dry fallout. Techniques for measuring the removal rate of atmospheric particles by both mechanisms are available. However, since the total removal rate and the relative removal by the two processes depend upon the particle size distribution as well as the rainfall rate and amount at any particular geographic location, it is very difficult to extrapolate results from one area to another. Thus, measurements of the flux of trace metals from the atmosphere to the land and sea surface on a variety of scales—urban, regional, and global—and in a variety of climatic zones will be necessary.

Our knowledge of the residence time of atmospheric particulate matter is based largely on the use of artificial and natural radioactive nuclides in the atmosphere. Recent studies suggest that the mean atmospheric particle residence time is 4–10 days (Poet et al., 1972). However, very little information is available on the variation of particle residence time with particle size, except that particles with radii in the 0.1-1.0 μm range have residence times longer than larger particles. Thus, the particle size distribution of the various trace metals will influence their atmospheric residence time. However, there are presently insufficient data available to make any quantitative predictions of atmospheric residence times for the various trace metals.

A.1.1.4. Recommendations

1. The concentration and size distribution of atmospheric trace metals near the earth's surface and at various levels up to the stratosphere on urban, regional, and global scales should be measured.
2. Fluxes of trace metals to the atmosphere from both anthropogenic and natural sources and from the atmosphere back to the earth's surface in various geographic areas and climatic zones should be determined.
3. The possible existence and potential importance of a vapor phase in the atmospheric cycle of several of the trace metals should be ascertained.

A.1.2. Low-Molecular-Weight Halogenated Hydrocarbons

The atmosphere and surface ocean waters now contain a burden of low-molecular-weight halogenated hydrocarbons (LMHC) produced industrially. These include:

Substance	Use	Atmospheric concentration (ml/ml of air)
CCl_3F (freon-11)	Aerosol propellant	5×10^{-10}
CCl_2F_2 (freon-12)	Aerosol propellant	5×10^{-9}
CH_3CCl_3	Dry cleaning fluid	5×10^{-9}
$Cl_2C{=}CCl_2$	Dry cleaning fluid	2×10^{-9}
$Cl_2C{=}CHCl$	Dry cleaning fluid	5×10^{-9}

In addition CCl_4 and $CHCl_3$ are found at similar levels, but a natural production now seems probable for them.

To understand present exposure levels and to predict future ones, mass balance models and flow sheets can be constructed. Inasmuch as steady-state conditions most probably have not been attained for these substances in the environment, the models should reflect their increasing usages. The necessary data for model formulation, not yet completely available, are considered below.

A.1.2.1. Sources and Entry

Production figures for the United States are available for all of the five listed compounds. World data are usually obtained by extrapolation, a factor of three being commonly used.

The production is taken to be equivalent to the rate of atmosphere injection, since there is little storage of these materials in closed systems. Further, their atmospheric entry is disperse, probably closely related to population densities in countries with high per capita gross national products.

A.1.2.2. Distribution

Most of the analyses so far are at ground level and in the northern hemisphere. Wilkniss et al. (1973) measured CCl_3F and CCl_4 in marine atmospheres over North and South Pacific waters and the Ross Sea. A slight decrease was observed going from northern latitudes to the Antarctic for chlorofluorocarbon, while CCl_4 showed a nearly uniform global distribution. This latter point argues for a CCl_4 production from natural sources. A much more distinct difference between northern and southern Atlantic Ocean atmospheres for CCl_3F concentrations was observed by Lovelock et al. (1973). Here the northern airs contained nearly 50% or more of the LMHC than their southern counterparts. Clearly, more extensive analyses are required to establish the validity of these data.

Of greater importance are the residence times derived from such data on the basis of a steady statistification. Su and Goldberg (1973) obtain 30 years for CCl_2F_2, while Lovelock et al. (1973) report a value of ">10?" years. The latter authors, using a model with an exponentially growing rate of release with a doubling time of two years in the northern hemisphere between $35°$ and $55°N$, were able to match these observed distributions.

A.1.2.3. Fate

The fates of these LMHC, following their atmospheric residence, are poorly known. However, probably most of the fluorochlorocarbons released to the atmosphere may still be there, if residence times of decades are valid. Besides dissolution in the world's ocean, decomposition in the troposphere or stratosphere, by photochemistry or by oxidation, is possible. Altitude profiles of these hydrocarbons are urgently needed to assess the possibility of their destruction in the atmosphere.

On the basis of the data by Lovelock et al. (1973), Liss and Slater (1974) calculated a flux of 2% of the world's production from the atmosphere to the surface ocean waters. Using the same two-layer model for CCl_4, they find an escape of 5×10^{10} g/y from the ocean to the atmosphere and a flux of 1.4×10^{10} g/y from the atmosphere to the ocean. The obvious conclusion is that the oceans are a source of CCl_4.

A.1.2.4. Summary and Recommendations

There seems to be an increasing burden of low-molecular-weight halogenated hydrocarbons of industrial origin in the atmosphere. Their levels may be attaining values of 10^{-8} ml/ml of air. There are little or no data on such pesticide components as dichloropropane, which also may have significant levels.

These compounds at higher concentrations interfere with fermentation processes through reactions with B_{12} and have anesthetic properties. The possibility that they can attain unacceptable levels should be evaluated.

A.1.3. High-Molecular-Weight Halogenated Hydrocarbons

The compounds considered in this section include organochlorine pesticides (e.g., BHC, aldrin, dieldrin, DDT, and 2,4-D), together with compounds such as the PCBs, chlorinated terphenyls, and chlorinated naphthalenes; in addition, impurities in products (e.g., dioxins) and intermediates (e.g., hexachlorobutadiene) should be considered under this heading. Such impurities and intermediates have not yet, however, been detected in the atmosphere.

Pesticides have been reported to be present in the air and rainwater on the American and European continents and in the air over the Pacific and Atlantic Oceans. Fewer determinations have been made of PCBs, but they have been detected in the air over the Sargasso Sea and Scandinavia.

The amounts detected are small, as would be expected following the effect of dilution by large volumes of air. However, the presence of these small amounts has been sufficient to generate a range of interesting theories. The air has been implicated as a route for the global dispersion of organochlorine compounds, it has been implicated as an important sink for these compounds, and, alternatively, it has been suggested as an effective matrix for their photochemical or chemical destruction. Such concepts are important but the evidence to justify some of them is scant.

A.1.3.1. Sources and Entry

Organochlorine pesticides enter the atmosphere mainly during spraying and by evaporation from plants, soils, and waters. Losses by evaporation have not been adequately quantified under practical conditions. Such information is desirable, although it will be difficult to design realistic experiments. Evaporative losses of pesticides during manufacture, formulation, or from industrial effluents are probably small, but it would be better to base this conclusion on numerical data than on conjecture. Such data are of greatest interest for those compounds which have industrial as well as agricultural uses.

The main routes for the entry of pesticides into the atmosphere are known in principle, but there is a distinct need to study the routes of compounds such as the PCBs. Incineration of products containing them may well be an important route of entry. Attention should also be given to the extent to which such materials can evaporate during manufacture and usage and the extent to which they can evaporate following their disposal, such as in sewage sludge and landfill. Within this subclass of compounds there is particular scope for the handling or disposal procedures to be modified when the important route of entry has been established.

A.1.3.2. Distribution

Once in the atmosphere the organochlorine compound may be dispersed widely and this dispersal may be vertical as well as horizontal. The compounds may be absorbed onto particles (or aerosols) or may be entirely in the vapor phase. For compounds such as DDT most is probably in the vapor phase, although opposite views have been expressed (Aitkins and Eggleton, 1971; Stanley et al., 1971; Bidleman and Olney, 1974). Information on the other compounds is limited, and there is a clear need to establish the physical state of these compounds in the atmosphere.

Up to the present, most of the determinations of atmospheric concentrations of pesticides have been made in Europe or in the United States, in regions that are not entirely remote from areas of usage. It is impossible to quote average or typical values, but the units for expressing data are usually ng/m^3. The few determinations made in areas more remote from the use indicate lower concentrations. It is important that we obtain information on the atmospheric concentrations of these compounds, as a function of time, from a sufficient number of locations to enable the total atmospheric burden to be calculated. In addition, some attention should be paid to their vertical, as well as their horizontal distribution. If it can be shown that organochlorine compounds reach the stratosphere, then one can be confident that a range of reactive species, including ozone, can cause massive degradation, especially in the presence of the radiation at that altitude.

A.1.3.3. Fate

There is no doubt that organochlorine compounds can be removed from the atmosphere by physical processes such as washout by rain or by deposition of contaminated particles. Adsorption into soil, foliage, or water has also been considered to be a predominant and rapid mechanism for the removal of some compounds from air (Aitkins and Eggleton, 1971).

Laboratory studies have shown that some pesticides can be decomposed in air in the presence of sunlight. However, it is difficult to extrapolate from these experiments to outdoor conditions. Information is needed on the rate of any photochemical reactions under practical conditions, including the possible effect of particulates, although it is recognized that this will be difficult to achieve.

A.1.3.4. Summary and Recommendations

The atmosphere may not at first sight appear to be an important part of the physical environment in relation to the higher-molecular-weight organochlorine compounds, although it probably provides an important route for their global distribution. However, relevant studies could provide the answers to two critical questions: (1) Is the current atmospheric content of organochlorine compounds a significant part of the total global burden? (2) Is there an effective process in the atmosphere for the degradation of these compounds?

The most important points for attention may be summarized in the following recommendations:

1. The route of entry of PCBs, etc., into the atmosphere should be established.
2. The evaporative losses of organochlorine compounds should be quantified, particularly those during field usage but also those during manufacture and handling.
3. Global information should be collected on the atmospheric concentration of organochlorine compounds, and on their vertical and horizontal distribution as a function of time, so that atmospheric residence times can be assessed and an adequate input be made into models which calculate global burdens.
4. The physical state of the organochlorine compounds in the atmosphere should be investigated and an attempt made to establish whether they are bound to particles or aerosols or are in the vapor state.
5. Quantitative data on the processes for the removal of organochlorine compounds from the atmosphere should be obtained. More attention should be paid to photochemical and chemical degradation processes of organochlorine compounds in air, under conditions that can be related to their atmospheric state.

A.2. Soil

The soil, an essential multipurpose resource for man, is a reactive heterogeneous medium containing numerous different microenvironments in which many physical, chemical, and biological processes occur that affect the availability and toxicity of accumulated pollutants in space and time, depending on factors like soil type, climate, and vegetation. Thus cause–effect relationships are often complex, and deleterious effects may go unrecognized until a change in use takes place.

Although there is constant exchange of matter between soil and water as well as the atmosphere, soil, being a solid phase, may act as a final sink in which many persistent pollutants accumulate in an irreversible manner. In contrast to air and water, soil is only to a small extent amenable to natural or man-made processes for restoring its quality once pollution has occurred, and because of this, prevention of pollution by protection is the only rational approach to preservation of soil quality. Although natural background concentrations for heavy metals show a great variation, agreement on permissible levels is essential for effective management and development of realistic control measures.

The heavy metal contamination of soils is generally localized, whereas inputs of chlorinated hydrocarbons are more ubiquitous because of atmospheric and water transport, and because of widespread application and use in agriculture, forestry, and recreation.

In view of the increasing need for safe disposal of toxic chemicals and nuclear wastes, subsurface deposition by deep-well injection or disposal in salt layers and old mine pits is receiving more and more attention. The danger to soil quality by contamination from such sources is unknown due to lack of information on hydrological transport mechanisms and other forces to which the material may be subjected. Recent concern about marine pollution is now leading to national and international restrictions on the release of harmful chemicals into the sea and into surface waters. As a result, an increasing pressure is to be expected on the soil as a recipient of harmful and persistent waste residues.

A.2.1. Sources and Entry into Soils

Organic halogen compounds (OHCs) are mostly introduced into soils by man either directly, i.e., in fertilizers, pesticides, or other cultural practices, or indirectly, via industrial effluents, waste disposal, and atmospheric fallout. Higher-molecular-weight OHCs tend to persist and can accumulate in soils, being resistant to degradation and loss, and may have direct toxic effects on plants and animals dependent on the soil or indirect effects by reducing fertility or plant quality. These effects are of great concern to man, since they may affect the production of food and fiber. On the other hand, the soil system is a major part of the dynamic recycling process for organic compounds, and has a great capacity for binding or degrading introduced exotic organic chemicals, thereby limiting their availability for uptake into biological systems. These processes involve physical-chemical adsorption, conjunction, and direct degradation (e.g., hydrolysis, reduction), and enzymatic decomposition by soil microorganisms. OHCs can be lost from soil, either directly as synthetic chemicals or via their breakdown products, by runoff, volatilization, dust erosion, cropping, etc.

Sources of heavy metals in soils (Lisk, 1972) are as follows:

1. Metals contained natively in rocks and minerals from which the soil was formed.
2. Metals added as impurities in fertilizers and lime, as constituents of pesticides and manure, or as contaminants of sewage sludge.
3. Metals in debris from industrial and mining wastage, fossil fuel combustion products, wind-eroded soil particles, atomic testing, pollen, sea spray, and meteoric and volcanic material which settles or rains out.
4. Metals in soil particles displaced through water erosion, or metals dissolved or suspended in the water itself.

A.2.1.1. Entry from Air

Although the normal atmosphere (air) is contaminated with dust particles, the contamination of soils with heavy metals by this mechanism is relatively unimportant. For example, the normal concentration of mercury in air is about 0.01 $\mu g/m^3$, while that in volcanic emissions is about 20 $\mu g/m^3$ and that in special industrial plants as high as 20,000 $\mu g/m^3$. In many instances, the major part of the heavy metal emission in industrial and urban areas remains in a zone of 3 km around the center of emission (Kloke, 1972a,b). The 3–7 km zone around these cities is an area of lesser enrichment. In addition to the above distribution pattern for emissions, there is an enrichment zone, particularly for Pb, Cd, and other pollutants, of up to 50 m in width on either side of all highways (Kloke, 1972b,c; Lagerwerff and Specht, 1970; MacLean et al., 1969). Our present knowledge would indicate that these are the two main aerial mechanisms for heavy metal enrichment of soils.

The OHCs occur as vapors arising from industrial effluents, application practices, and residues, and in particulate forms such as dusts and aerosols, or associated with soil and smoke particles. PCBs and some of the more persistent organochlorine insecticides (DDT, dieldrin) are thought to be widely distributed due to aerial transport in dusts and by fallout and rainout.

A.2.1.2. Entry from Wastes

The trend to consider land, especially agricultural land, as a suitable medium for the disposal of urban wastes is supported by society in an attempt to reduce the pressure on other areas of the environment as "ultimate sinks for most wastes" (Webber, 1973). Land disposal of wastes must be made without damage to the ecological balance of the land or the total environment—land, water, air. It is important to distinguish between *disposal* and *utilization* (an approach favored by agriculture). If land is to be a repository of wastes—industrial, urban (including sewage sludge and garbage), agricultural—then precautions are required to avoid its pollution by contaminants in the waste, while utilizing the noncontaminants (nutrients, organic matter, etc.) to maintain and enhance the soil productivity. In order to develop the knowledge necessary to obtain the maximum benefit from these wastes and to minimize their harmful effects on the terrestrial ecosystem, it is necessary to have information on the physical, chemical, and microbiological properties of the wastes as well as on the various soil properties and their relationship to waste disposal or utilization.

Specific problems relating to land disposal of wastes include occurrence of pathogens, smell during application, risks to ground water, eutrophication due to leaching of nutrients, and contamination of the soil due to pesticides, heavy metals, and PCBs. The levels of heavy metals in an "urban" and "industrial" sludge from two municipalities in Sweden (Emmelin, 1973) are given below to illustrate the range in concentration of heavy metals found in sewage sludges. This variability demonstrates the need for control of application of this material to soil if quality and productivity are to be maintained.

Element	Urban sludge (per kg dry matter)	Industrial sludge (per kg dry matter)
Zinc	1-3 g	> 10 g
Copper	0.5-1.5 g	> 3 g
Manganese	0.2-0.5 g	> 2 g
Lead	0.1-0.3 g	> 1 g
Chromium	50-200 mg	> 1 g
Nickel	25-100 mg	> 500 mg
Cobalt	8-20 mg	> 50 mg
Cadmium	5-15 mg	> 25 mg
Mercury	4-8 mg	> 25 mg

OHCs may enter the soil as contaminants in industrial and urban wastes, and via contaminated food and animal wastes.

A.2.1.3. Entry from Direct Application

In the past organochlorine insecticides (DDT) have been applied directly to soils to control pest insects. Chlorinated herbicides (2,4-D) are still used in large amounts in agriculture and in brush-clearing operations. The application of heavy metals in fertilizers, lime, pesticides, and manures is considered generally of little significance in relation to existing background levels in the soil. Nevertheless, the inputs from these sources could be important locally if additions from other sources become significant.

A.2.1.4. Entry from Water

Irrigation water may be a source of heavy metals and OHCs in situations where water (industrial and sewage effluents, etc.) is held in impoundment for this purpose or enters into river systems subsequently used for irrigation. Sewage effluents may be diffused over soil surfaces for purposes of purification.

A.2.2. Distribution and Fate

Persistent chlorinated insecticides and industrial OHCs are not, as a rule, leached to a large extent from most soils with a significant clay and organic matter content. Less persistent industrial OHCs and chlorinated herbicides, however, have been found to leach through soil and contaminate ground water and waterways, either directly or as decomposition products. Soil-dwelling animals (e.g., earthworms) and plants have been found to absorb and accumulate OHCs from contaminated soils. These compounds may be removed by cropping and degradation, or be introduced into food chains and recycled back to soil and water sinks.

Water and dust erosion of contaminated soils have been found to redistribute persistent OHCs into previously "clean" areas on a local and global scale (Cohen and Pinkerton, 1966).

Persistent chlorinated organic compounds (DDT, PCB) have contaminated plants and animals and caused ecological effects long after their industrial or agricultural use has ceased. For example, in spruce budworm control operations in eastern Canada between 1952 and 1968, approximately 6000 tons of DDT was applied to 10,000,000 acres of forest land. In 1974, residues ($<$1 ppm) were found bound up in the surface organic layers of forest soil, in river and lake sediments (0.1 ppm), and water (0.1 ppb), and may still contribute to ecological magnification and population effects in higher animals. Plant residues have mostly dissipated, however, except as temporary receptacles of recycled residues (condensed vapors, dust, rainout, etc.). The "half-life" of DDT in forest soils has been estimated at approximately 10 years under these environmental conditions (Yule, 1973), but persistence of OHCs varies markedly in different soils (Edwards, 1966).

Persistent residues of several chlorinated insecticides and PCBs have not been found to inhibit growth or activity of soil microorganisms, but have altered numbers and caused qualitative changes in soil animal populations. Soil fertility and productivity have not been affected by the presence of these persistent residues, but contaminated crop plants grown on these soils have sometimes been considered unfit for human and domestic animal consumption. Acute effects on soil microorganisms and plants have been produced by chlorinated herbicides, requiring adjustment of crop rotations and land use.

The occurrence of persistent OHC residues in surface soil has resulted in spreading environmental contamination, and in continued introduction from this reservoir into biological food webs, resulting in ecological magnification and some deleterious effects on higher animals (e.g., fish and flesh-eating birds).

Our knowledge of the chemistry of toxic metals in soils is very incomplete and largely speculative (Lisk, 1972). In brief, metals in soils are found in minerals as part of their structure and as interstitial impurities, as inorganic precipitates, as inorganic ions, as components of organic compounds and microorganisms, as soluble and insoluble organic complexes or chelates, and as adsorbed ions on charged surfaces of clays, precipitates, and organic matter.

In general, the physical and chemical characteristics of the soil (texture, organic matter content, pH, etc.) influence the distribution and fate of the heavy metals in the system, and consequently control the transportation of these elements via leaching, plant uptake, and erosion (Halstead et al., 1969; Lagerwerff, 1967; MacLean, 1974a,b; MacLean et al., 1969). A major concern is that of the effect of heavy metal and other pollutants on "soil quality," as measured by physical and chemical changes, productivity, and crop quality. In addition, the secondary effects of these pollutants on microorganisms and other soil fauna should not be discounted. The need for acceptable "guideline levels" for heavy metals in soils is necessary for the development of suitable waste management practices that will be of benefit rather than harm to soils. The International Society of Soil Science, as well as individual countries, are involved in development of soil quality criteria with respect to heavy metals and other pollutants.

It is now appreciated that soil may account for between 0.5 and 20% of the dry matter intake of some herbivorous animals (e.g., sheep). Soil intake is influenced by the adequacy of herbage supplies, the physical characteristics of the soil, and the degree of foliar contamination by "splash up" during rainfall. Accurate definition of the chemical form of heavy metals contaminants of such soil is essential before the significance of this route of entry into animals can be assessed.

A.2.3. Recommendations

1. A quantitative inventory of sources and flow of pollutants to the soil is required.
2. Base-line inventories for establishment of soil quantity criteria are required, and increased coordination of countries in establishment of these criteria should be encouraged.
3. Research capability for improved waste management including recycling, particularly heavy metals, should be developed.
4. Criteria for the environmental acceptability of a potential pollutant should be set up.
5. Research programs should be developed oriented to an increased understanding of the transport mechanisms from soils leading to redistribution of pollutants in the ecosystem.

A.3. Water

A.3.1 Sources and Entry of Pollutants

Global knowledge concerning the total weight or volume of the organohalogen compounds and heavy metals produced is inadequate not only for individual chemicals and metals, but for the total production of these groups as a whole, including by-products and impurities in the final product. Even less well known is the transitional and ultimate environmental fate of individual chemicals once they leave the production center. On the other hand, some of the mechanisms of distribution and transport in the environment are beginning to be understood.

Pollutants entering the aquatic ecosystem do so by direct discharge to the water via industrial and urban effluents and surface runoff, and indirectly via aerial fallout. Only direct entry is considered here. The discharges of mercury as a by-product of the production of acetaldehyde and vinyl chloride, the direct discharge of a wide variety of heavy metals as by-products of the production of titanium dioxide, and the production and use of caustic soda manufactured by the mercury cell processes are but three examples of direct input. Chlorinated hydrocarbon insecticides and herbicides have been and continue to be applied directly to aquatic environments for the control of noxious insects and weeds, and to eradicate coarse fish prior to introduction of "desirable" game fish. Organohalogen compounds are discharged as wastes from the production of plastics, lubricants, and refrigerants and the poduction and formulation of chlorinated insecticides. Surface runoff from agricultural areas treated with chemical fertilizers and organic and inorganic pesticides may result in contamination of water by heavy metals from the former and chlorinated hydrocarbons and heavy metals from the latter. Additional heavy metal contamination of water is possible as a consequence of the use of cleaning agents (phosphate detergents) contaminated with metals. Deposition in landfill sites of municipal and industrial wastes may also lead to contamination of surface runoff and groundwater.

Many of the chlorinated hydrocarbons are strongly adsorbed to suspended matter, both in fresh water and sea water. Those molecules that have a significant water solubility can be detected both in suspended matter and in the water phase. The relative contribution of atmospheric fallout to organohalogen levels in estuarine regions will probably be smaller than for the open ocean on the basis of the amounts already present.

The fate and distribution of the pollutants varies according to the pH, water hardness, salinity, organic matter content, nutrient content, etc. of the receiving water. Chemical and physical transformations of both chlorinated hydrocarbons and heavy metals are possible, and residence time in the physical sphere varies according to a wide variety of physical, chemical, and biological parameters.

Pollutants may be removed from water by irrigation, with some of the pollutants entering the soil, plants, and atmosphere. Subsequent runoff may contain some of the original chemicals which may re-enter the system after a considerable delay and at some distance from the point of origin. Compounds picked up are those which were added intentionally to the soils (pesticides and fertilizers) or present in the natural state (heavy metals). It should be noted that sedimentary soils may contain high but natural levels of heavy metals.

A.3.2. Distribution and Fate in Water

In discussing the partition of pollutants between the aqueous and the solid phase, we must emphasize that as far as the latter is concerned, the extent to which adsorption processes of pollutants occur is highly dependent on the grain size composition. Since there is a preferred association of, for example, the heavy metals with the finest grains, relationships can be found between metal contents and grain size composition (de Groot, 1973). These relationships have to be taken into account when comparing pollution from one place to another. Much confusion originates from neglecting this.

The movement of heavy metals and organohalogen compounds in a river must be divided into transport in dissolved forms and transport by adherence of these substances to suspended material. The very diverse composition of this suspended matter and the binding properties of the relevant compounds make it particularly difficult to estimate the discharge.

Differences in composition of bed-load material and of suspended matter in the more superficial water layers of the system, both of which are dependent on the current velocity of the river, make it difficult to derive general conclusions from analytical data. Much more work must be done on the development of sampling procedures in this respect.

Nevertheless, calculations of this kind have been made on the discharge of metals for some rivers by combining water discharge, concentration of suspended matter in the river water, and the contents of heavy metals in the suspended matter. For a number of metals there seems to be a pronounced occurrence in the suspended material (de Groot, 1973). For the Rhine, the ratio of metal in water to metal in suspended matter was 1/2.6 for Pb and 1/1.8 for Cu. For an element like Ni, on the other hand, the ratio was reversed (1/0.3). Similar trends have been found for the lower regions of the Amazon and Yukon rivers, where the preferential occurrence of the metals in the suspended matter was even more extreme (Gibbs, 1973).

A global picture in this respect is lacking, however, and much more understanding is needed concerning the role of suspended matter, depending on local chemical and environmental conditions. In particular, the form in which metals and organohalogen compounds appear in the two phases and the factors governing the partition need a better understanding.

A.3.2.1. Particulate Transport

There are many factors which influence the metal content of suspended material. In the first place, the type of suspended matter depends on the velocity of the river currents. Under normal flow conditions of the river, the main component of the suspended matter is the so-called "original mud" (de Groot, 1973). For the Rhine this material originates mainly directly from the drainage area. Under conditions of high water discharge, the erosion of the river bed gives rise to the formation of a suspension with different sedimentary characteristics, referred to as "erosion mud." In consequence of processes of pedogenesis on the river bottom, this material forms aggregates of sufficient size which readily settle again when the high flow velocities are reduced at the place where the river enters areas of flood plains. The latter may be upstream with respect to the fresh-water tidal region.

The mud deposited under normal flow conditions in estuarine and coastal regions has been regarded for many years as representative of the material present in suspension. However, it has been pointed out recently that suspended matter contains components that do not settle out within the coastal sedimentation areas. Moreover, the metal levels in suspended matter are larger than the levels of the deposits, even after correction for the differences in grain size distribution (see Chapter 8). It is even possible that at least a part of these components never settle out at all.

The characteristics of the different forms of this suspended matter, apart from the granulometric composition after destruction of the organic matter, is of the highest importance. Besides differences in sedimentation characteristics, there exist appreciable differences in heavy metals content. For the Rhine it has been found that the metals supplied to the stream by industrial wastes adhere to the solids in decreasing amounts in the following order: suspended matter, original mud (the main component settling in shallow areas), and erosion mud. The distribution of the solid substances in the environment diminishes in the same order (i.e., the erosion mud is deposited very locally on the river flood plains; a part of the suspended matter, on the other hand, moves further away). Therefore, those constituents which have been contaminated in the most severe way have the most widespread distribution in the aquatic environment.

A more detailed insight into the relations between contamination characteristics and physical properties of the solid constituents or the aquatic environment is urgently needed, especially in view of the processes of bioaccumulation.

A.3.2.2. Chemical Transformations

Chemical transformations of pollutants can occur in water or sediment, and thus influence the distribution and transport of pollutants within the ecosystem and their effects on organisms. We must consider the possibility that oxidation or reduction processes may change their solubility and toxic effects. Heavy metals can be kept in the colloidal state or in solution by complex formation with organic compounds, under conditions in which they are normally insoluble or soluble in only trace amounts.

Detoxification can occur, or planktonic organisms can be influenced detrimentally, by heavy metals. This latter aspect is particularly important if organic complexes are involved which are broken down photochemically in the upper layers or, more generally, by microorganisms. Microorganisms can transform mercury into the more toxic methylmercury, for instance, while in the case of organohalogen compounds, the possiblity of biogenic breakdown or the occurrence of partly unknown breakdown products must be considered.

All these chemical transformations are strongly dependent on the other environmental conditions in the ecosystem. For example, the redox potential and pH in the bottom layers of lakes depend on periods of circulation and stagnation, and also on changing discharge levels and relative amounts of waste water in flowing waters and reservoirs. Changes may also be due to wave action in shallow water. Chemical transformations of pollutants can be stimulated or inhibited by all these changes in the environmental conditions; in particular, the possibility of mobilization of flocculated or sedimental pollutants must be considered.

A special problem exists in the hyporheic region (the interstitial water) that forms the transition between surface water and groundwater, because of local enrichment of toxic substances. This layer is the spawning area and nursery for many flowing-water organisms. Biological damage in flowing waters often starts in the hyporheic region. If organic pollution exists, anaerobic conditions occur first in this layer. Thus, in this layer, many heavy metals can be mobilized by reduction processes and can be transported to the nearby groundwater.

A.3.2.3. Short- and Long-Term Sinks for Sediment and Pollutants in Lake and Harbor Beds

Due to decreasing current velocity, sedimentation takes place where rivers enter into lakes. Harbors situated near the mouths of large rivers are areas of intensive sedimentation of both marine and river-carried suspended matter as a result of a number of different sediment transport processes that characterize most estuaries.

Sedimentation is selective with respect to grain size and density; smaller particles are less likely to be trapped in the sedimentation process. Organic matter is broken down in bottom sediment by chemical and microbiological processes; their rates and effectiveness, and thus the changes in E_h and pH induced, are influenced by the abundant availability of oxygen and/or sulfate ions in sea water.

Anaerobic conditions, even in the very top layer of bottom sediment, are characteristic of many areas in which intensive sedimentation of material rich in organic matter is taking place. These conditions can have an important influence on the behavior of pollutants that are associated with the sediment particles. Metals can be transformed from inactive sites, either adsorbed or included in structural units of inorganic sediment particles, into a reduced form from which they may be more readily available to the aquatic and biotic environment. Moreover, it has been observed that interstitial water may be enriched compared to the overlying water, particularly in polluted areas. As sedimentation continues, relatively thick layers of polluted, anaerobic material can be built up.

Metals can be kept in solution as complexes with inorganic or organic ligands, or they may form insoluble solid phases (e.g., sulfides). From bottom layers, metals in chemical forms characteristic of the anaerobic environment can be introduced into the overlying water system either by diffusion or by mechanical forces from the interstitial water. Alternatively, adsorbed metals can be released unintentionally by mechanical and by wind force action on the bottom layers, or by dredging activities.

A.3.2.4. Interactions in Estuaries

Metals associated with suspended matter can undergo several types of interaction in the estuarine environment. Adsorbed trace elements can be exchanged for the major elements found in sea water, causing a certain fraction to be dissolved. Colloidal particles of iron hydroxide may be formed, and may act as scavengers of trace elements. These particles may, in turn, adhere to larger particles and be sedimented in the marine environment. Usually, in an estuary, a sediment particle on its way to the sea will exhibit a complex dynamic behavior before it either escapes to the sea or is trapped somewhere in the estuary.

A.3.2.5. Entry and Distribution in the Marine Environment

Usually the mixing process between fresh water and sea water is relatively slow and ineffective. The fresh-water distribution is very often confined to an area relatively close to the coast, due to hydrographic conditions. Therefore, water and suspended matter in coastal areas of the industrialized parts of the world tend to show increased levels of pollutants.

The heavier particles are deposited on the continental shelf and only the smallest particles may escape to the sea. The deposited material can again undergo mobilization processes in bottom layers (Chapter 8); this may interfere with the biological events in these highly productive coastal areas. In cases where systematic studies of the distribution of trace metals in sea water and suspended matter have been performed, a rather complex pattern is observed in coastal regions.

Relatively little is known about the changes that man has caused in the trace element composition of open ocean water.

A.3.3. Summary and Recommendations

The following problems are suggested as subjects for further intensive research.

A.3.3.1. Mass Balance Studies

Studies of total entry, accumulation, and removal of heavy metals and organochlorine compounds need to be made on aquatic systems of different size ranges. These should include studies of estuaries, harbors, entire rivers, sections of rivers, coastal regions, and enclosed and open seas spanning concentrated sources. Knowledge of boundary conditions is critical for these regions, and requires general agreement between neighboring nations. The primary object of these studies should be to ensure that all important pathways have been identified, and, by implication, to estimate the importance of pathways which are themselves not well understood, such as water–atmosphere interchange and input of material from soil or from unidentified natural or artificial sources. Another result should be better information on rate of accumulation in bed sediments.

Understanding of mass balance and fluxes depends largely on analytic determination. In these studies attention needs to be paid to analytic protocols in at least two senses. First, mass balances depend on fluxes being known with comparable total accuracy, and the differing relative precision required in various pathways needs to be described in detail. Second, standard methods of sample gathering and preparation need to be adhered to in order to achieve comparability of results on a world-wide basis.

A.3.3.2. Distribution of Pollutant and Sediment Transport

Much remains to be learned about the distribution of pollutants between the dissolved state and that part bound to particles of various size fractions, and about how the different particles are transported in different flow regimes. More specifically, it is not understood how pollutant distribution changes with time, and with different physical and chemical conditions such as may be encountered when water together with its pollutant load flows into regions of different organic content or salinity. Research should be undertaken to describe the phenomena involved. In connection with sediment transport, specific questions that need further investigation are the ratio of sedimentation and flocculation in estuaries and coastal regions and interchange of sediment between rivers and adjoining regions of slow-moving or relatively still water.

A.3.3.3. Bottom Layers and Interstitial Waters

Nearly all the chemical transformations that have been discussed above need much more research, and their dependence on ecological conditions should be investigated. The properties of the region involving the bottom water layers and the upper sediment layers are different during periods of stagnation and circulation. In flowing water (rivers, estuaries, and seas), properties depend also on flow rates, circulation patterns, and changing amounts of discharge. In still waters, microstratification in the bottom water layer can occur with high concentration gradients. More research is needed in order to understand the solubility ratios of the different pollutants and their daughter products in different water types, the equilibria that govern adsorption and desorption processes with respect to the more important components of suspended matter and sediment, and the conditions under which the interstitial water can be enriched.

A.3.3.4. Dynamics at the Estuary–Sea Interface

The mobilization of metals, especially in estuarine parts of rivers, is one of the most striking phenomena found in some estuaries of the temperate climatic region. An important cause of these mobilization processes (transfer of material from the suspended matter to the aqueous phase) is the intensive decomposition of organic matter from the suspended material, especially as far as the mouth of the estuary. The mobilization processes can be so intensive that great quantities of a number of metals in the suspended matter of a very polluted river system (upper reaches of a river) are reduced to lower quantities in the lower courses of such an area (de Groot, 1973).

No evidence for such processes has been found in estuaries in tropical regions, probably as a result of lack of organic matter in the areas examined. On the other hand, it is questionable for rivers whether mobilization occurs under arctic conditions, when organic matter breakdown processes will be slow as in the Mackenzie River in Canada.

The kinetics of the mobilization processes are not very well known. In laboratory experiments, some evidence has been found that decomposition products of the organic matter (molecular weight mainly between 1000 and 10,000) form soluble organometallic complexes with the metals from the suspended matter.

It is doubtful, however, if the processes under consideration occur generally in estuaries in the temperate regions and to what extent they occur elsewhere. It is important to assemble more evidence on the existence of estuaries contrasting in this respect, and to carry out intensive investigations in these estuaries.

Detailed investigations on the processes of mobilization of metals may also throw more light on the constitution of organic and also inorganic metal compounds in the water of the various coastal regions. Also important in this respect is knowledge of the fate of trace materials after they have been solubilized; and this requires a better knowledge of interactions between coastal seas and oceanic regions. These undeveloped fields of research must be considered of prime importance for studies of bioaccumulation of heavy metals.

A.3.3.5. Realism of Predictive Models

When modeling studies are carried out involving many interacting compartments, validation is a long and expensive process, and assessment of reliability of predictions is difficult. As more complete quantitative information is accumulated, modeling studies which require a continuous multidisciplinary approach will become more attractive still; an essential part of such studies should be the continued development of validation techniques (Nihoul, 1975).

A.4. Studies of Pollutant Distribution and Fate in the Physical Environment—Summary of Research Recommendations

There was substantial agreement among the participants concerning the areas in need of further research within the general subject of physical distribution, notwithstanding the different toxic substances and pathways considered. Three problems emerge as having highest priority:

1. *Mass Balances of Pollutants.* This specifically refers to an examination of pathways and overall transport among the air, water, and soil compartments on a fully quantitative basis but not limited to specific transport mechanisms. The chemical speciation of the pollutants is to be considered in the formulation of mass balances.
2. *Distribution by Particle Size.* Specific studies are required on the amounts of pollutants bound to particles according to particle size and the amounts in the dissolved state (in water) or vapor phase (in air), including how these distributions change with time.
3. *Transformations while Resident in the System.* This includes the study of photochemical, chemical, and microbiological degradation processes, especially those which affect the future transport or distribution of the pollutant.

In addition, the following general problems arose in some contexts and may be regarded as supported by the group:

4. *Setting of Uniform Criteria.* This includes quality criteria for soils and acceptance criteria for new chemical products. This is at present being studied at the international level, but its importance still needs to be stressed.
5. *Alternatives to Use of Manufactured Chemicals.* General support needs to be expressed for continued research in solid waste recycling, biological control techniques, and other methods whereby introduction of contaminants to the environment can be avoided.
6. *Model Formulation.* In cases where large, multicompartment models are contemplated, data requirements are critical and improvements are required in validation techniques.

References

Aitkins, D. H. F., and Eggleton, A. E. J. (1971) "Studies of atmospheric washout and deposition of γ-BHC, dieldrin and *pp'*-DDT using radiolabelled pesticides," in *Nuclear Techniques in Environmental Pollution,* pp. 521–533 IAEA, Vienna.

Bidleman, T. E., and Olney, C. E. (1974) "Chlorinated hydrocarbons in the Sargasso Sea atmosphere and surface water," *Science*, 183, 516.

Cohen, J. M., and Pinkerton, C. (1966). In *Advances in Chemistry Series*, 60, 163, ACS, Washington, D.C.

de Groot, A. J. (1973). "Occurrence and behaviour of heavy metals in river deltas, with special reference to the Rhine and Ems rivers," In *North Sea Science*, pp. 308–325, MIT Press, Cambridge, Massachusetts.

Duce, R. A., Hoffman, G. L., Fasching, J. L., and Mayers, J. C. (1974). "The collection and analysis of trace elements in atmospheric particulate matter over the North Atlantic Ocean," in *Proceedings of the WMO/WHO Technical Conference on the Observation and Measurement of Atmospheric Pollution*, Helsinki, Finland.

Edwards, C. A. (1966). *Residue Reviews*, 13, 83.

Emmelin, L. (1973). "Sewage treatment in Sweden," in *Environmental Planning in Sweden (Current Sweden)*, No. 42.

Gibbs, R. J. (1973). "Mechanisms of trace metal transport in rivers," *Science*, 180, 71.

Halstead, R. L., Finn, B. J., and MacLean, A. J. (1969). "Extractability of Ni added to soils and its concentration in plants," *Can. J. Soil Sci.*, 49, 335.

Kloke, A. (1972a). "Immissionschäden an Pflanzen–Aufgabe der Immissionforschung," *Mededelingen Fakulteit Landbouw-Wetenschappen Gent.*, 37(2) 329.

Kloke, A. (1972b). "Die Belastung der gärtnerischen und landwirtschaftlichen Produktion und Erntegüter durch Immissionen," *Berichte über Landwirtschaft*, 50(1), 57.

Kloke, A. (1972c). "Zur Anreicherung von Cadmium in Böden und Pflanzen," *Stand und Leistung agrikulturchemischer und agrarbiologischer Forschung*, 22, 200.

Lagerwerff, J. V. (1967). "Heavy metal contamination of soils," in *Agriculture and the Quality of Our Environment* (ed. Brady, N. C.), (Amer. Assoc. Adv. Sci. Symposium Proc.), 85, 343.

Lagerwerff, J. V., and Specht, A. W. (1970). "Contamination of roadside soil and vegetation with cadmium, nickel, lead and zinc," *Environ. Sci. Technol.*, 4, 583.

Lisk, D. J. (1972). "Trace metals in soils, plants and animals," in *Advances in Agronomy*, Vol. 24, p. 267 (ed. Brady, N. C.), Academic Press, New York.

Liss, P. S., and Slater, P. G. (1974). *Nature (Lond.)*, 247, 181.

Lovelock, J. E., Maggs, R. J., and Mace, R. J. (1973). *Nature (Lond.)*, 241, 194.

MacLean, A. J. (1974a). "Effects of soil properties and amendments on the availability of zinc in soils," *Can. J. Soil Sci.*, 54, 369.

MacLean, A. J. (1974b). "Mercury in plants and retention of mercury by soils in relation to properties and added sulfur," *Can. J. Soil Sci.*, 54, 287.

MacLean, A. J., Halstead, R. L., and Finn, B. J. (1969). "Extractability of added lead in soils and its concentration in plants, *Can. J. Soil Sci.*, 49, 327.

Murozumi, M., Chou, T. J., and Patterson, C. C. (1969). "Chemical concentrations of pollutant lead aerosols, terrestrial dusts, and sea salts in Greenland and Antarctic snow strata, *Geochim. Cosmochim. Acta*, 33, 1247.

Nihoul, J. C. J. (ed.) (1975). *Modelling of Marine Systems*, Elsevier, New York, 272 pp.

Poet, S. E., Moore, H. E., and Martell, E. A. (1972). "Lead-210, bismuth-210 and polonium-210 in the atmosphere: accurate ratio measurement and application to aerosol residence time determination," *J. Geophys. Research*, 77, 6515.

Stanley, C. W., Barney, J. E., Helton, M. R. and Yobs, A. R. (1971). "Measurement of atmospheric levels of pesticides," *Environ. Science Technol.*, 5, 430.

Su, Chih-Wu, and Goldberg, E. D. (1973). *Nature (Lond.)*, 245, 27.

Webber, L. R. (1973). "Non-agricultural pollutants and their significance in agriculture," in *Environmental Quality Work Planning Meeting, Canada Dept. Agriculture, Ottawa*, p. 112.

Wilkniss, P. E., Lamontagne, R. A., Larson, R. E., Swinnerton, J. W., Dickson, C. R., and Thompson, T. (1973). *Nature, Physical Science,* **245,** 45-47.

Yule, W. N. (1973). *Proc. Pesticide Accountancy Workshop, NRC, Ottawa (Canada), AFA Tech. Report,* **13,** 123.

Zoller, W. H., Gladney, E. S., and Duce, R. A. (1974). "Atmospheric concentrations and sources of trace metals at the South Pole," *Science,* **183,** 198.

B/C
Uptake, Fate, and Action of Heavy Metals and Organohalogen Compounds in Living Organisms

HEAVY METALS

Chairman: D. V. Parke

Members: G. C. Butler, N. T. Davies, G. L. Eichhorn,
G. L. Gatti, J. Klaverkamp, I. Munro,
J. K. Miettinen, G. Nordberg, M. Webb

ORGANOHALOGENS

Chairman: E. M. Cohen

Members: J. Barstad, A. Disteche, D. J. Ecobichon,
J. R. Gillette, J. Greig, N. Nelson,
W. H. Stickel, P. Toft, A. Verloop,
R. T. Williams

Rapporteur: P. N. Magee

B/C.1. Introduction

The danger, ultimately for man himself, from production of large quantities of persistent toxic materials, such as organohalogen compounds and heavy metals, is twofold: (1) a perturbation might be caused to the total ecosystem that could escape man's control because of the sudden or gradual removal of populations essential to the stability of the system or parts of it; (2) large amounts of accumulated toxic material might be introduced into the human food supply. The study of uptake, fate, and action of organohalogens and heavy metals in the biosphere should be expedited in order to reach an evaluation of the risks involved as soon as possible.

The biosphere as a whole displays, on an enormous scale, all the properties and functions of the individual living species. The ecologist evaluates the sizes and the interactions of the different populations, both plants and animals. The physiologist and toxicologist have already gained a profound knowledge of life functions and their relationships from observations and experiments on single species, especially man. They should now turn their attention to similar functions in other parts of the ecosystem, to locate vulnerable spots at the level of communities, individuals, organs, and cells, and thus help to explain the problems encountered by the ecologist.

B/C.2. Uptake and Fate (Pharmacokinetics) of Metals

B/C. 2.1. Scope

In this section the discussion of the pharmacokinetics of metals will be limited to their behavior in target organisms, in most cases animals.

B/C.2.2. Chemical Forms

In general it can be stated there is a lack of information about the chemical forms of metal pollutants in the air, in fresh or marine waters, or in foods of either plant or animal origin.

1. *Air*—Metals in air may be present either as vapors (limited to elemental mercury and organometal compounds) or as particulate matter. In special cases the chemical form of a local pollutant has been determined but, in general, little is known about the chemical forms of metals bound in or on airborne particles.

2. *Water*—In natural waters metals may be present in four possible forms: (a)

as dissolved species, (b) as soluble complexes, (c) in inorganic or organic particles, and (d) adsorbed to particles—either as (a) or (b).

The relative proportions of each form will be different for individual metals and waters. It is essential in studies on metal toxicology to have adequate knowledge of the chemical nature of each of these forms and their relative proportions in a particular environment.

3. *Food*—It is impossible to generalize about the chemical form of metals in food material but, undoubtedly, the chemical nature of the metal compounds will influence their availability. In addition to the chemical form of the metal, dietary components such as phytic acid, alginates, and porphyrins may also modify the availability of ingested metals.

Especially relevant to grazing animals are the chemical forms of heavy metals in topsoil which may be ingested. This will be of special significance where domestic animals may graze soil contaminated with local industrial or urban fallout or agricultural and domestic sewage sludge.

B/C.2.3. Routes of Entry and Uptake

The possible routes of entry for the heavy metals are: (1) transdermal, (2) via respiratory membranes (gills of aquatic animals and lungs of terrestrial animals), (3) absorption following ingestion, and (4) passage through placenta and embryonic membranes.

B/C.2.3.1. Transdermal

This route is probably of minor environmental significance to terrestrial animals except for industrial or occupational exposures. The relative importance of this route for marine and aquatic species is not known.

B/C.2.3.2. Via Respiratory Membranes

a) Terrestrial Animals

Gaseous Metal Forms. The inhalation of metals in gaseous states is limited to mercury vapor and heavy metal organic compounds. Although representing only a small percentage of the total inhaled metals, these may be significant toxicologically because their fractional uptake from inhaled air is comparatively high.

Particle Forms. A quantitative model for the deposition of particles in the respiratory tract and subsequent uptake of deposited material is provided by the lung model of ICRP (1966). The major features of this model demonstrate the importance of particle size in determining the extent of deposition in various parts of the respiratory tract. The subsequent absorption of the particulate matter may be by three routes: the intestinal tract, the lymphatic system, and directly to the blood. The model describes the relative amounts absorbed by these different routes for particles of different solubility. The fate of material deposited in the alveoli as predicted by this model needs further study both in relation to transport by the "mucociliary escalator" and to other means of removal from the alveoli, e.g., solubility in pulmonary fluids and uptake in structures.

The precise figures derived from this model are valid for *"Reference Man"* (ICRP, 1975). With suitable modification this model could be used for human beings and other terrestrial animals. It is important that this model should be adapted to permit its application to domestic agricultural animals maintained in areas in close proximity to metal-emitting industrial complexes.

(b) Aquatic Animals

Fish may absorb metals directly from water through their gills, and mollusks may do so through their sieve tubes. When applicable, these routes of absorption apply mainly to dissolved chemical species. Since metal compounds often exist bound to particles in natural waters, the extent of uptake of such forms of metal via gills and sieve tubes merits further investigation. Moreover, binding of metal-containing particles to gills may be an important route of entry of potentially toxic materials into fish.

B/C.2.3.3. Absorption Following Ingestion

Metals may enter the gastrointestinal tract following ingestion or by transfer of deposited material from the lungs. Intestinal absorption varies with the element, its valence, its chemical form (organic or inorganic), and with the composition of the diet.

Values for the fractional absorption of metals from the gut have been given by ICRP (1975) for *Reference Man* and by Underwood (1971) for domestic and experimental animals. These values should be considered as only a first rough estimate and may be very different in any specific case because of the enormous variability in the behavior of ingested heavy metals.

In the case of marine animals there have been many estimates of the direct absorption from the water through the gills but fewer quantitative studies on absorption from the gastrointestinal tract.

In no instances are the molecular mechanisms involved in intestinal absorption of metal compounds sufficiently well known for even a single species of animal. Areas deserving of further study include examination of the possible role of "carrier" molecules in the mucosal membranes, consideration of interaction with intestinal transport systems for essential trace metals (Cu, Zn, Fe), and the possible role of naturally occurring or man-made chelating agents which may either increase or decrease the fractional absorption of ingested metals.

Further factors which may be of significance in determining the extent of absorption of heavy metals, particularly those which may be absorbed by processes common to the nutritionally essential metals, include generally: (a) nutritional state of the animal (protein and caloric intake), (b) specific mineral status (e.g., effect of Ca and vitamin status on Pb absorption), (c) effects of pregnancy and lactation (e.g., Zn uptake in pregnancy, Pb uptake in lactation), (d) age and sex differences (e.g., Pb uptake in children), and (e) species differences (e.g., fate of Mo in ruminants vs. nonruminants).

The variations due to these factors apply to all aspects of pharmacokinetics of metals and will subsequently be referred to as "biological modifications."

B/C.2.3.4. Passage through Placenta and Embryonic Membranes

Heavy metals and particularly organometallic compounds may vary widely in rate of transplacental transfer. Species differences in placental structure, gestational age, and availability of particular metals in maternal blood are some of the factors influencing the rate of placental transfer. For the transfer through the membranes of embryos of aquatic animals, temperature, salinity, hardness of water, pH, oxygen content, other metal ions present, other stresses, previous treatment, and, particularly, the age and the stage of development are variables that must be considered.

B/C.2.4. Biotransformation, Transport, and Deposition

There is a possibility that carbon–metal bonds (e.g., with mercury, lead, tin, and arsenic) may be cleaved or formed by intestinal microflora, especially in ruminants. After absorption the carbon–metal bond in organic metal compounds may be broken, resulting in other organic forms or inorganic metal species. The new metal compounds so formed may differ from the original ones with respect to transport, distribution, storage, and excretion. The transport of metals from the site of uptake to the tissue of deposition occurs in blood and interstitial fluid. Metals in blood will be distributed between corpuscles and plasma, but the latter is more important for transport. In plasma, metals are often largely bound to plasma protein, e.g., for Hg and Cd this fraction may account for more than 99% of plasma metal. Nevertheless the remaining, small, "diffusible" fraction may be of great importance for transport (cf. Task Group on Metal Accumulation, 1973).

The fate of many metals is often substantially influenced by the existence of relatively specific processes or carriers involved in transport and tissue distribution. Examples are (i) the transport of iron by transferrin and the possible involvement of metallothioneines in the transport of Cu, Zn, Cd, and Hg; (ii) the concentration of lead and methyl mercury in red blood cells; (*iii*) the transfer of insoluble materials from the lungs to the lymphatic system.

It is important to have as much information as possible about such mechanisms to understand the biological behavior of heavy metals. One important area of research would be the relative importance of the blood on the one hand, and other extracellular fluids on the other, in the transport of heavy metals.

B/C.2.5. Uptake and Release from Organs and Specific Localization in Tissues

The distribution of a metal compound among the various organs is dependent on transport across cell membranes from interstitial fluid as well as upon the varying affinities of ligands present in the cells. Variation in ligand affinity and transport processes may also account for uneven distribution within an organ, cell, or subcellular organelle, creating "hot spots" which may be of toxicological significance. The occurrence of such localized concentrations is insufficiently known for many metals. Moreover, the distribution of a metal compound among organs or within organs may be subject to biological modification. In many but not all instances, the harmful effect arises in the organ accumulating the greatest concentration of metal. Other organs, because of their relatively high sensitivity, may be affected at a lower concentration. For example, for inorganic Pb the greatest concentration will be in the skeleton, whereas the primary lesions are found elsewhere. The organ first suffering damage from a particular type of exposure is usually defined as the "critical organ" (Task Group on Metal Accumulation, 1973). The risks of harmful effects can be estimated by calculating, or directly measuring, the concentration in the critical organ.

B/C.2.6. Mathematical Description of Retention

For each species of interest it is useful for predictive purposes to have a formula describing the retention of the metal in the whole organism as a function of time (Task Group on Metal Accumulation, 1973). In practice it is found that these retention equations contain several exponential terms with coefficients adding up to unity. The integral of the retention equation multiplied by the rate of uptake is used to calculate the amount of metal present in the body at a given time (Butler, 1972) and from this the concentration in the tissue of interest. To do this with confidence it is necessary to know the retention equation for the critical organ itself. Failing this, it is possible in some cases to calculate the organ concentration by multiplying by some factor the concentration for the whole body or, in exceptional cases, only one term of the whole body retention equation which applies to the tissue in question. The use of a single set of parameters to describe the retention in a species is a representation of the average behavior, and it should be recognized that these parameters are subject to biological modification. A systematic knowledge of these interrelations would be most useful for predicting ecological behavior and effects of metals.

B/C.2.7. Excretion

The excretion of metals occurs by four principal routes in mammals and birds, viz., urine, feces, exhalation, and the shedding of integumentary structures.

Exhalation is significant only for volatile forms of metal such as dimethyl mercury. For some metal compounds, such as methyl mercury, the loss in integumentary structures such as hair and feathers constitutes a major route of excretion.

Urinary excretion results from three processes: glomerular filtration, transtubular transport, and the shedding of tubular cells containing metals. Fecal excretion may result from biliary excretion, pancreatic and glandular secretion, transmucosal transport, and the shedding of mucosal cells.

The information about the mechanisms and controlling factors of all these routes is fragmentary. However, in mammals most (ca. 90%) heavy metals are excreted in urine and feces, but the distribution between these two routes varies markedly with the metal and with the time after intake. Therefore, in metabolic studies it is important to measure the total excretion in urine and feces.

The routes of excretion in aquatic animals are probably analogous, but there is very little information on the subject and this would be a fruitful area for research.

In laboratory studies the total excretion is frequently measured for as long as possible after the cessation of intake, in order to determine the retention equation. The rationale for this approach is that the retention equation can be obtained by integrating the excretion equation. The application of the equations so obtained to animals in the natural state is subject to the same limitations as described previously for the derivation of retention equations.

B/C.2.8. Problems Fundamental to Pharmacokinetics

Passage through membranes and binding to ligands are two phenomena fundamental to the biological transfer and location of all metal compounds.

The mechanisms by which highly charged metal species are transported through cellular membranes at the level of uptake (alveolar, gut, and gill-cell membranes), embryonic uptake (placental and embryonic membranes), transfer to milk, and the cells responsible for some metal-excreting processes are poorly understood. Further investigation on the possible role that specific "carrier" proteins or low-molecular-weight natural chelating agents (e.g., amino acids) may play in these processes should illuminate many aspects of the pharmacokinetics of heavy metals.

Ligands bind metals through a number of chemical groupings such as hydroxy, amino, carboxyl, sulfhydryl, etc. The concentration of a metal in a tissue depends upon the occurrence and availability of such metal-binding chemical groupings. Their occurrence varies with type of tissue, type of cell within tissue, and even with the type of subcellular structure. The availability of ligands to bind metals depends on their organization in macromolecules and on other metal or nonmetal substances that can compete for the binding sites. The detailed pattern of binding and interaction of metals in tissues is not well described or understood at the present.

B/C.2.9. Recommendations for Research

1. Further studies on retention functions for metal compounds in the whole body and in critical organs in species of ecological significance, are needed because such information is fundamental to quantitative treatment of the fate of metals in food chains. The model for pulmonary absorption should be modified for application to domestic animals. Studies on the clearance of metal compounds from alveoli are needed for a correct quantification of pulmonary absorption.

The development of better model systems for individual species is required, taking into account the following biological factors affecting metal absorption, distribution, and excretion: (a) nutritional state (particularly protein and calorie intake), (b) mineral status, (c) effects of pregnancy and lactation, and (d) effects of age, sex, and stage of development.

A further area deserving more research concerns the role of naturally occurring and man-made chelating agents which may modify the uptake, distribution, and excretion of metal compounds.

2. Further information on the nature of the binding of metals to ligands is fundamental to our understanding of mechanisms of transfer across cellular and subcellular membranes, transport in body fluids, and disposition and storage within cells. Areas of specific interest warranting further research include (a) transfer through placental and embryonic membranes during the period of greatest susceptibility, (b) the role of specific metal-binding proteins, e.g., metallothionein in the pharmacokinetics of toxic metals, and (c) the uneven tissue distribution of heavy metals in critical organs.

3. Studies on the chemical forms of metal pollutants in air, fresh and marine

waters, food, and soil are needed because this information is fundamental both to our understanding of the biological behavior of metals and for the design of realistic experimental studies.

4. More information is required on the relative roles of direct absorption of metal compounds from water, absorption via gills, sieve tubes, or skin, and absorption from the gastrointestinal tract, in aquatic animals.

5. For evaluation of risks it is essential to determine the metal content in readily accessible biological materials (urine, blood, hair, etc.) that may serve as indices of critical organ or total body content of metal. Their suitability for this purpose must be further elucidated. Studies on the mechanisms of urinary excretion are important for understanding of variation of metal content in urine.

6. Little is known so far about the biotransformation of organic metal compounds. Further studies in various species are needed for understanding of pharmacokinetics and effects.

B/C.3. Toxic Action of Metals

The current status of the toxicology of certain metals has been reviewed in detail in several symposia and reports such as the EEC Symposium on lead, held in Amsterdam in 1972, and the Luxemburg EEC Conference on mercury and cadmium, in 1973, as well as in a WHO Report in 1973. In the present context, recommendations for further study will be made with only cursory reference to already accomplished investigations. It is recognized that the chemical form of the metal (e.g., organometals) may have profound effects on the nature of observed toxicological responses. Because of the dearth of information on this subject the present report will be confined mainly to general recommendations that apply to most chemical forms.

Toxicological effects of metals may be "acute" or "chronic." To describe the former the dose should be given in terms of the maximum amount of toxic agent to which the organism was briefly exposed. "Chronic" toxicity may result from accumulation of the agent in the organism (dose being the concentration in the "critical organ") or accumulation of biological damage from repeated sub-threshold exposure (dose being the accumulated exposure to the "critical organ").

B/C.3.1. Criteria for Selection of Species for Study of Adverse Effects

Present knowledge indicates that there are considerable variations in toxicological effects among species. We believe that it is impossible, with present knowledge of ecological interrelationships, to maintain rigid criteria for the selection of species to be studied. In addition to the FAO/WHO Joint Committee's recommendations for man, which include (1) high sensitivity to the metal under investigation and (2) similarity to metabolism in the human, we suggest that, when dealing with the total ecosystem, the selected species should handle the test metal in a manner *pharmacokinetically* similar to that observed or anticipated in the species of ultimate concern. For example, it has been demonstrated that pharmacokinetic behavior of methylmercury differs in rat and man, and thus the former is not a good model for the evaluation of safe levels of the metal for the latter species.

B/C.3.2. Toxicological Effects at Various Levels of Biological Organization

B/C.3.2.1. Whole Organisms

A variety of studies have revealed that heavy metals can produce numerous toxic effects upon living organisms, e.g., Parkinson-like symptoms from manganese; kidney damage and respiratory problems from cadmium and inorganic mercury; behavioral, CNS, teratogenic, and embryotoxic effects from methylmercury; dermatological effects from nickel and chromium; carcinogenic effects from nickel; antihemopoietic, neurotoxic, and nephrotoxic effects from lead. Recommendations for additional study are as follows:

(a) The accumulation of improved dose–response data, particularly in relation to the routes of administration of environmental significance. In addition, where there is more than one route of exposure (e.g., inhalation and ingestion) toxicological studies should encompass all routes.

(b) Studies of the effects of chronic low-level exposure.

(c) Effects of specific geographically localized factors such as apparent resistance or adaptation, e.g., from boron toxicity in inhabitants of Lardarello, Italy.

(d) The effect on response to heavy metals of (*i*) age and (*ii*) sex.

(e) Effects of genetic variations, e.g., race, strain, etc., on response to heavy metals.

(f) Studies on mutagenicity with particular reference to the establishment of valid tests.

(g) Metal-induced teratogenic and embryotoxic effects.

(h) The development of improved methodologies for epidemiological and toxicological studies on populations.

(i) Special attention should be given to the development of methods that serve as indicators of subclinical, or early toxicological, changes.

B/C.3.2.2. Organ Systems

Physiological, biochemical, and pathological changes have been demonstrated in many organs as the consequence of the administration of heavy metals. Some metals (e.g., Pb, Cd, and Hg) have received a great deal of attention, whereas others have been neglected. We recommend:

(a) Studies on the pathogenesis of metal intoxications that have not received enough attention to describe in detail the specific toxic response leading to the ultimate lesion.

(b) Studies of the effect of duration and level of exposure on critical target organs with regard to the development of altered structure and functions. Previous studies have generally been qualitative with inadequately controlled quantification.

B/C.3.2.3. Cellular Level

Studies on the content and distribution of metals in cells by microprobe analysis and autoradiography have been carried out to a limited extent. The effects of metals on subcellular particles (e.g., mitochondria, lysosomes, endoplasmic reticulum, ribosomes, the nucleus, etc.) have also been studied in isolated instances, using the electron microscope and biochemical subcellular fractionation methods. We recommend:

(a) A concentrated effort to evaluate metal content and distribution in cells by the above techniques and the development of newer techniques for more sensitive measurement.

(b) Further studies on the effects of metal ions on subcellular particles and cell membranes.

(c) Studies on the displacement of functional metals by the accumulation to abnormally high concentrations of other metals in subcellular components.

(d) Studies on the effects of metals on biochemical events within the cell, such as the identification of molecules with which metals react.

(e) *In vivo* studies (cell culture) in parallel with *in vitro* studies of the molecular events discussed in Section B/C.3.2.4.

B/C.3.2.4. Molecular Level

It is known that essential metals can be displaced from active sites by toxic metals, that enzyme-activating metals in excess can inhibit enzymes, and that metals can form cross-links in biomacromolecules and depolymerize them—they can produce mispairing of nucleotide bases and errors in protein synthesis. In isolated instances, studies at the molecular level have helped to explain specific toxic effects at higher levels of organization. Examples are the effect of metals in cross-linking of collagen and elastin and studies on the molecular basis of manganese-induced Parkinson-like disease. We recommend:

(a) Studies to describe, at the molecular level, the events leading to other important specific pathological changes in organs. Examples are: (*i*) the molecular basis for the decrease in δ-amino levulinic acid dehydratase induced by lead, and the determination of its significance in lead toxicity; (*ii*) the mechanism of the decreased level of ceruloplasmin arising from high dietary intake of zinc and of cadmium.

(b) Further studies on the effects of metal ions on small molecules such as vitamins and hormones, in addition to studies of macromolecular interactions designed as models for toxicological processes.

B/C.3.3. Categories of Metals to Be Studied

The metals can be subdivided into essential elements and those elements which are accumulated from the environment with no essential biochemical requirement. The differentiation between categories will change with time, as new elements are added to the "essential" list, and furthermore there are no differences in the toxicological methods for studying these two groups. A large number of examples of protection against the toxicity of one metal by another have been documented. We recommend:

(a) That "essential" and "nonessential" elements be treated similarly in toxicological studies.

(b) That the impact of interactions between metals in their toxic effects be further investigated, with the object of elucidating the mechanisms of such interactions. In this context it is important to bear in mind that pollution from several metals may occur simultaneously and that this may result in both adverse and beneficial effects in certain ecological systems. Also, exposure to metals and organohalogen compounds together is possible and has been reported already in several species of birds and mammals, e.g., seals.

B/C.3.4. Prevention and Treatment of Metal Toxicity

It is important that precautions be taken to prevent metal pollution by development of adequate environmental controls and legislative action. When pollution does occur, means of diminishing toxic states may be used for individuals and sections of the population. A variety of complexing agents have been employed in the treatment of metal toxicity. Examples are EDTA, EGTA, and derivatives of these, penicillamine, desferrioxamine, thiol resin for Hg and methyl Hg, and oligopeptides that have been synthesized for complexing copper. Limited studies have demonstrated that methylmercury may be removed in part from fish products by the use complexing agents such as cysteine. We recommend:

(a) A search for complexing agents, preferably natural, that are as specific as possible for toxic metals, and which are nontoxic in their original form and after complexation. This could include the utilization of micro-organisms for production of specific complexing agents, at least for certain metals, as in the development of desferroxamine.

(b) A search for nontoxic, preferably natural, metal complexing agents that might be used to reduce high levels of toxic metals in some parts of food chains.

(c) Studies on the combined toxic effects of metals and organohalogen compounds.

B/C.4. Action of Organohalogen Compounds

B/C.4.1. Introduction

The compounds considered in this section are the chlorinated cyclodienes, DDT, polychlorinated biphenyls, polychlorinated terphenyls, and the chlorinated benzenes, naphthalenes, cyclohexanes, dibenzofurans, and dibenzodioxins. These materials have the following properties: high oil/water partition coefficients, chemical stability, persistence in the environment, and prolonged storage in the body. Compounds such as carbon tetrachloride, *bis*-chloroalkyl ethers, and vinyl chloride, although recognized as hazards to health, do not possess the appropriate properties and were not considered.

It is recognized that in most species the nervous system is affected. In vertebrates, damage to the liver is found and other organs such as kidneys, adrenals, and skin are frequently involved. The acute and chronic toxic effects include teratogenicity, carcinogenicity, and mutagenicity.

B/C.4.2. The Present Position

To date, emphasis in research has been placed on studies using easily available laboratory animal species, unrepresentative of species in ecological systems. Some species, for example the mink, are extremely sensitive to changes in their prey population brought on by pollutants. Thus a toxic effect at one level of a food chain can be reflected in behavioral changes of a higher member of the chain. Field studies have often only considered a small part of the food chain and have usually been confined to the measurement of residue levels. The significance of such data is difficult to assess in the absence of reliable toxicological studies on the appropriate species. Acute toxicity, not infrequently found in environmental situations, is relatively easy to identify. Chronic toxicity, which is much more difficult to associate with a particular compound, may be even more important. It is known that a number of factors can influence the toxicity of these substances. Some of these are listed below:

1. *Species and group differences*—These can involve differences in the response to, or metabolism of, toxic agents or can be due to differences in exposure caused by varying food habits.
2. *Stresses*—Including change in environmental temperature, restricted (Ecobichon and Saschenbrecker, 1969) or unbalanced dietary intake, infection, migration, parturition, and lactation. These will all have a direct influence on fat mobilization and redistribution of stored residues.
3. *Age*—This can markedly influence both acute and chronic toxicity. As an example of the latter, the slow-maturing peregrine falcon can accumulate sufficiently high levels of organochlorine compounds to impair its reproductive capability (Ratcliffe, 1970).
4. *Sex differences*—These have been found in acute toxicity studies with laboratory animals. There are indications of differences in chronic dieldrin toxicity to quail. In addition, a higher incidence of hepatomas has been observed in male mice exposed to low dietary levels of DDT (IARC Monograph, 1974). Alterations in levels of the sex hormones can alter the hepatic metabolism of xenobiotics.
5. *Synergism*—The interactions in the organism of these compounds, among themselves or with other agents, can result in enhanced toxic effects. As an example, the synergism between the teratogenic effects of 2,3,7,8-tetrachlorodibenzo-*p*-dioxin and 2,4,5-T results in an increased incidence of cleft palate in mice (Neubert et al., 1973). A different example is the influence of one compound on the storage of another.
6. *Genetic differences*—Hypothetically, these might influence the distribution of an agent in a food chain if genetic variants of one or more species were unable, or more able, to degrade the compound, hence altering bioaccumulation.

B/C.4.3. Recommendations

For Ecological Studies
  (a) More toxicological studies should be undertaken on species representing components of the food chains, so as to better assess data on residue

levels. Where man is considered as a member of the ecosystem, efforts should be made to find species which respond pharmacokinetically and/or pathologically in a manner similar to man.

(b) There should be searches for sensitive indicator organisms which could be used to signal environmental contamination. Such an organism could accumulate the agent and/or show characteristic toxic signs.

(c) Although not considered in detail in this report, further information about the environmental fate of, and hazards due to, materials such as halogenated solvents, vinyl chloride, the *bis*-chloroalkyl ethers, and the perhalogenated aerosol propellants and refrigerants is required.

For Human Studies

(a) Extensive observations have been made on individuals chronically exposed to these chemicals in industrial and agricultural environments (Morgan and Roan, 1974); better epidemiological use should be made of these groups. Prospective epidemiological studies of newly developed chemicals should be undertaken in people at risk. Collaborative research in these areas between industrial and other scientists should be encouraged.

(b) Investigations should provide more information as to whether the induction of hepatomas in mice by DDT and dieldrin is a reliable criterion for the assessment of carcinogenicity of these compounds in other species, particularly man (IARC Monograph, 1974).

For Laboratory Studies

(a) Many of the organohalogen pollutants are complex mixtures for which a good toxicological assessment requires investigation of the individual congeners. Studies in this direction should be expanded. The modes of action of many of these compounds, as well as those of toxic trace contaminants, e.g., chlorinated dibenzofurans in PCBs, are unknown and should be clarified.

(b) In laboratory studies, variables which can influence toxicity should be recognized. Routes of administration should correspond to modes of exposure in the environment.

(c) Morphologic studies at the light and electron microscope level should be undertaken in parallel with chemical and biochemical studies. After exposure to these compounds, particular attention should be paid to the organs involved in excretion.

(d) Since there are indications (Kimbrough, 1974) that these chemicals or their metabolites can affect the immune system, more work sould be performed in this field.

(e) Techniques for testing for mutagenicity in higher animals are not well developed. Research in this field should be supported.

B/C.5. Uptake and Fate (Pharmacokinetics) of
Organohalogen Compounds

The uptake, distribution, and excretion (pharmacokinetics) of some of the more commonly used organochlorine compounds, such as DDT, dieldrin, and polychlorinated biphenyls have been widely studied in a variety of species of mammals, birds, and fishes (Kenaga, 1972) and also in natural and model ecosystems (Kapoor et al., 1972). A few organohalogen solvents, such as trichloroethylene, have been studied in mammals, particularly laboratory species. However, for many classes of organohalogens, e.g., the halogenated biphenyls and terphneyls, the existing knowledge of pharmacokinetics is minimal, and for many others, such as the chlorodibenzodioxins, halogenated oligophenyl and alkyl ethers, and perhaloalkanes (freons), practically nothing is known.

In both terrestrial and aquatic ecosystems, major pharmacokinetic determinants are the microflora and microfauna (plankton, bacteria, yeasts, fungi and protozoa) which facilitate transfer of organohalogen pollutants into higher organisms and initiate food chains. However, the pharmacokinetics of organohalogen compounds in microorganisms have been determined for only very few substances. Moreover, the pharmacokinetics of numerous, unidentified organohalogen by-products of industrial processes which find their way into the environment in chemical effluents, have not been studied in any species.

B/C.5.1. Entry into Living Organisms

The persistent, lipid-soluble, organohalogen compounds are readily absorbed by all species, are slowly metabolized, stored in fatty tissues and eggs, and excreted via the bile, intestinal mucosa, and urine. Exceptions are, for example, the highly polar chlorophenoxy acids, herbicides which are readily absorbed but also rapidly excreted unchanged in the urine with little or no storage in the body's tissues, and the rodenticides fluoroacetate and fluoracetamide, which, although polar, may become incorporated into tissues by "lethal synthesis" (Peters, 1963).

Organohalogen compounds may be taken up by means of food chains or by direct uptake from the surrounding media, particularly in aquatic systems. Most are unlikely to be free in water but are absorbed or adsorbed onto particulate, and often living, matter. Fish and mollusks process large amounts of water and may absorb these substances via the gills and the gastrointestinal tract; the skin of fish is covered in mucus which may prevent absorption. Absorption in birds may also occur to a small extent through the skin of the feet. The main entry of organohalogen compounds in plants is usually in the leaves, but they may also be taken up from the soil by the roots, particularly in the case of the

halogenated phenylureas. Special cases of high oral intake that merit consideration are fish-eating birds and aquatic mammals, and nursing mammalian young.

B/C.5.2. Distribution in Tissues

The pesticide DDT is metabolized to DDD, DDE, and DDA; only DDA is
readily excreted, while DDE and DDD, like the parent pesticide, are highly
lipid-soluble and remain stored in the adipose tissues. High intakes of DDT into
the body of mammals occur immediately after birth and are associated with
lactation (Tomatis et al., 1971); high levels of DDT and metabolites have been
found in the milk of many species, including human beings. Apart from o,p'-DDT,
a minor component of technical DDT, there is a direct relationship between the
concentration of each metabolite in each organ and the dose to which the animal was exposed; highest concentrations are found in the fat and then the
kidneys, liver, and reproductive organs at approximately the same level, with
lower concentrations in the males than in females (Tomatis et al., 1971).

Aldrin and its epoxide metabolite, HEOD (dieldrin), are similarly stored in
adipose tissue and to a lesser extent in liver and brain (Robinson et al., 1969);
a sex difference in storage occurs in rat, with dieldrin having a biological half-
life ($t_{1/2}$) of 10 days in male and 30 days in female, probably due to sex differences in the metabolism (Matthews et al., 1971). The metabolism of hexachlorocyclohexane, and hence the tissue storage and turnover rates, vary with
the isomer studied. As this compound is metabolized into chlorophenols and
chlorophenylmercapturic acids it is excreted, by rats, more in urine (80%) than
in bile (Koransky et al., 1964).

The chlorinated hydrocarbon pesticides are highly bound to plasma proteins
and probably also to hepatic proteins; plasma dieldrin is >99.9% bound to
protein (Eliason and Posner, 1971).

These highly lipid-soluble, halogenated pesticides cross the placenta into the
fetus (Eliason and Posner, 1971), and this would similarly be expected for other
lipophilic organohalogen compounds.

B/C.5.3. Excretion

The chlorinated pesticides and their metabolites, as compounds of high
molecular weight and highly bound to plasma proteins, are excreted to only a
small extent in the urine but are extensively excreted in bile. More than 65%
of orally administered DDT and its metabolites are excreted in the bile of rats
and are exposed to enterohepatic circulation and enterobacterial metabolism.
Similarly, the major fractions of aldrin, dieldrin, perthane, and endosulfan are

excreted in the bile of rats (Smith, 1973). Heptachlor and endrin, although more readily excreted and less persistent than DDT or dieldrin, are also excreted primarily via the bile. The metabolites of chlordane, however, are excreted mainly in the urine.

Chlorobiphenyls, similar to DDT and aldrin, are slowly metabolized and excreted and are stored in adipose and other tissue (Yoshimura et al., 1971). In contrast, the less-halogenated benzenes and lower alkanes are readily metabolized with excretion of polar metabolites in urine and of unchanged hydrocarbon and nonpolar metabolites in the expired air.

B/C.5.4. Factors Affecting Distribution and Excretion

Factors which affect the metabolism of organohalogen compounds will consequently affect their excretion rates and tissue turnover and storage. Mobilization of lipid reserves has only a modest effect on excretion rates, though competitive displacement of these compounds from protein-binding sites, probably hepatic, has been shown to have some effect. Metabolism thus seems to be the most significant factor in determining rates of tissue turnover and excretion.

Inhibitors and inducers of metabolism may therefore affect tissue storage and excretion of these persistent chemicals. Since many chlorinated pesticides are inducers of the hepatic drug-metabolizing enzymes the simultaneous administration of a mixture of these compounds may lead to more rapid metabolism and excretion with correspondingly lower body burdens (Chadwick et al., 1971), and human patients on drug regimens have significantly lowered tissue levels of DDT and its metabolites (Watson et al., 1972). However, examples are known where the converse occurs, and dieldrin, for instance, may increase the body storage of DDE in some species (Ludke, 1974).

B/C.5.5 Recommendations for Future Study

B/C.5.5.1. Species

The marked species differences in toxicity to the lipophilic, persistent organohalogen compounds may reflect differences in pharmacokinetics metabolism, or receptor sites, and are of the greatest importance. Representative examples of sensitive species, e.g., crustacea, should be compared with examples of insensitive species, e.g., ciliates, mollusks, annelids, some fish (e.g., carp), and mammals. Highly sensitive species, albeit to only selected compounds, such as the mink, should be especially studied in the hope that knowledge of the pharmacokinetics, particularly when compared with closely related but resistant animals, will reveal abnormalities of turnover or location in a particular organ or subcellular fraction that would give a clue to the heightened toxicity.

Pharmacokinetics in microorganisms, including bacteria, yeasts, fungi, zooplankton, and phytoplankton, have too long been neglected and urgently need study, both as individual species and in ecosystems. Studies in these species may reveal particular organisms with high rates of uptake, metabolism, and turnover which, by training or selection of mutants, might prove valuable in the future treatment of sewage and chemical effluents.

Studies of a variety of species in natural and artificial ecosystems, both aquatic and terrestrial, would focus attention on the more sensitive species, indexed by the diversity of species in relationship to the concentration of total biomass. A study of such ecosystems might also reveal compartments with high storage levels of organohalogens. A greater knowledge of the population turnover in these ecosystems and their rates of uptake, metabolism, and release of organohalogen compounds would also be helpful, especially in the case of the high rates exhibited in aquatic systems.

B/C.5.5.2. Chemicals

The chlorinated dibenzodioxins and dibenzofurans have received some attention but merit further study of pharmacokinetics. Halogenated aliphatic ethers, naphthalenes, and alkanes, and other lipophilic persistent organohalogen compounds, particularly those numerous contaminants already detected in the ecosphere but as yet unidentified, merit urgent investigation. The freons, although generally gaseous and largely confined to the atmosphere in low concentrations, are nevertheless manufactured and dispersed in very large quantities and are chemically inert. Little is known of their pharmacokinetics, particularly in ecosystems, and they merit study.

Because many previous pharmacokinetic studies have been conducted at relatively high dosages, future investigations should be made with concentrations of chemicals comparable to those found in the ecosphere, and the effects of dosage on the pharmacokinetics of these persistent substances should be further investigated.

B/C.5.5.3. Distribution

Although the tissue distribution for common halogenohydrocarbons, such as DDT, dieldrin, and the PCBs, is known in a few species of birds, fishes, and mammals, more information is needed in crustaceans and other vulnerable species. This is important with species consumed for food, where identification of organs of high storage, say, for example, fish livers, could lead to their exclusion from human diet and other usage.

Distribution studies, in particularly vulnerable and resistant species, should be extended to subcellular studies in the hopes of revealing the causes of toxicity.

B/C.5.5.4. Excretion

Particular routes of excretion such as the bile, and secretion into the gastro-intestinal lumen, should be studied with all important organohalogen compounds. DDT and other chlorinated hydrocarbons may have sufficient vapor pressures to be codistilled in the breath and consequently may be excreted in small amounts in the expired air. Plants also may lose these compounds by transpiration from the leaves. This route of excretion should be investigated particularly in mammals.

B/C.5.5.5. Factors Affecting Distribution and Excretion

The effects of highly active inducing agents of the drug-metabolizing enzymes, and potent inhibitors, are deserving of study. Pesticide synergists, such as piperonyl butoxide and other methylenedioxyaryl compounds, although not themselves highly persistent in the ecosphere, are relatively stable in the animal body and may markedly inhibit metabolism. Their effects on pharmacokinetics of organohalogens compounds should be further investigated.

Sex differences in certain mammalian species have been observed for the rates of turnover of certain chlorinated hydrocarbon pesticides. Similar studies to examine possible sex differences should be undertaken when the kinetics of other oganohalogen compounds are investigated.

The effects of temperature on the pharmacokinetics of organohalogen compounds in poikilothermic animals should also be studied.

B/C.5.5.6. Reproduction

DDT is known to affect population growth in phytoplankton, particularly at high concentrations, and may be a problem even at low concentrations with other organohalogen compounds.

The concentration of organohalogen compounds in the gonads of crustacea and fish merits study. Embryonic mortality in fish, just prior to the free-swimming stage, may be associated with high uptake of these compounds in the yolk sac of ova. Embryonic mortality in birds is similarly associated with high concentration of organohalogen compounds in the egg, and the concentrations or organohalogen contaminants in the yolk sac should be determined in several species of birds to reveal individual susceptibility to this toxicity.

Aquatic mammals, such as the seal, are experiencing toxicity associated with absorption of organohalogens and require pharmacokinetic investigation. Placental transfer of all classes of organohalogen compounds is likely to occur if they are sufficiently lipophilic, and will be important if these substances are embryotoxic.

The secretion of organohalogen compounds in milk reflects the concentration in maternal tissues. Differences observed between tissue and milk levels of DDT and PCBs in cow and human beings are also likely to be found with other persistent organohalogen compounds and must be considered in relationship to possible hazard to the nursing human infant.

B/C.5.5.7. Measure of Persistence

A major need is a standardized measure and description of biological persistence of chemicals. Persistence and toxicity are the cardinal traits by which we appraise environmental pollutants. Toxicity data are obtained early in the study of a chemical, persistence data, however, are not regularly obtained, are seldom comparable, and are often hard to find. We suggest that it would be desirable and practicable to measure persistence in the rat, at the time of the early toxicity tests, by determining the whole-body turnover rate on an agreed standardized basis. The intervals between samplings would, of course, have to be decided upon with some knowledge of the chemical.

This type of study would not be expensive, and as regulatory agencies now require analytical methods for all new chemicals and their major metabolites, there should be no chemical obstacles to this proposal.

This immediate proposal for persistence studies in the rat is minimal by design. Eventually, persistence of a chemical must be determined for various forms of life, as persistence varies widely in different species. Model ecosystems offer a sophisticated means of testing persistence and it should be possible to operate them to provide comparable data on half-lives. As different ecosystem models will yield different results, it would be desirable to test important persistent chemicals in fresh water, salt water, and terrestrial models, where these have been validated against natural ecosystems for known persistent compounds.

Desirable as such ecosystem studies may be, they should not be allowed to obscure the basic need for a quick, early evaluation of biological half-life obtained from rats at the time of the first toxicity listing.

B/C.6. The Metabolism of Organohalogen Compounds

B/C.6.1. Introduction

The environment contains not only the persistent organohalogen compounds discussed in Section B/C.4 but also large amounts of chlorinated phenoxyacetic acids and chlorinated alkanes and alkenes, including halogenated solvents. The reactions undergone by both the persistent and the nonpersistent compounds in mammals include hydroxylations, epoxidation, hydration of epoxides, dehydrochlorination, glucuronic acid conjugations, and mercapturic acid synthesis (Williams, 1959; Brodie and Gillette, 1971; Hathway, 1972).

With chlorinated benzenes, naphthalenes, and biphenyls, the initial reaction is probably epoxidation catalyzed by enzymes in the hepatic endoplasmic reticulum, and the resulting epoxides are converted to phenols, dihydrodiols, catechols, and mercapturic acids. Monochlorobenzene is rapidly metabolized in mammals by these reactions. However, the dichloro- and polychlorobenzenes, -naphthalenes, and -biphenyls are metabolized at considerably slower rates. Indeed the rate of conversion tends to be inversely proportional to the number of chlorine atoms added. Moreover, the position of the chlorine atoms is important. For example, polychlorinated benzenes and biphenyls that have two vicinal unsubstituted carbon atoms are metabolized more rapidly than those which do not.

In many species of insects, DDT is metabolized mainly by dehydrochlorination to DDE. In mammals, DDT is also converted to DDE, but to a relatively minor extent. The major route of metabolism of DDT in mammals is by reductive dechlorination to DDD, presumably by microorganisms in the gut and by tissue enzymes followed by oxidative dechlorination to DDA. The rate of these reactions is slow compared with that of monochlorobenzene epoxidation.

Chlorinated cyclodienes include aldrin and heptachlor. The initial metabolites of these insecticides in mammals are epoxides; for example aldrin is converted into dieldrin. Dieldrin then undergoes a series of reactions including the formation of dihydrodiols to form several different metabolites. The formation and further metabolism of the epoxides, however, are slow, and thus the epoxides as well as the parent compounds persist in the tissues of most mammalian species.

Benzene hexachloride is metabolized to 2,4-dichlorophenylglutathione by an enzyme in houseflies and grass grubs. The primary product is thought to be pentachlorocyclohexylglutathione, which subsequently undergoes dehydrochlorination. In mammals, the compound is converted to chlorinated phenols and glutathione conjugates.

Chlorinated phenoxyacetic acid derivatives are rapidly excreted into the urine of mammals and thus undergo little biological transformation. Soil microorganisms readily convert these substances to relatively simple nontoxic materials.

Chlorinated alkanes and alkenes are metabolized in mammals by a variety of different reactions. Carbon tetrachloride is converted first to a trichloromethyl free radical that promotes lipid peroxidation and then to chloroform. Chloroform may be metabolized to unknown intermediates which lead to carbon dioxide. Dichloromethane is converted to carbon monoxide. In mammals

1,1,2-trichloroethylene is converted to trichloracetaldehyde and then to trichloro-ethanol. The reaction is unusual in that a chlorine atom migrates from one carbon to another. Monochloro and terminal dichloro moieties normally undergo dechlorination reactions by either oxidation or reduction reactions.

Although the general pathways by which organohalogens are converted to their metabolites are similar in most mammalian species, the relative rates of metabolism and the relative proportions of the metabolites vary markedly among different species. Moreover, the rates of metabolism and the relative proportions of metabolites may also differ with the strain, age, sex, diet, and physiological state of the animal. It is especially important to realize that the activity of the enzyme systems that catalyze these reactions may be markedly increased or decreased by many different substances, a great number of which occur in the environment, and that the effects of these substances differ with the animal species. Many of the organohalogens are known to be inducers of xenobiotic metabolism; in fact 2,3,7,8-tetrachlorodibenz-p-dioxin is the most potent inducer known. Thus, these compounds, in large doses, can alter their own metabolism when animals are continuously exposed to them. In addition, many of the enzymes that catalyze the metabolism of these compounds are hemoproteins, and thus, in large doses, various heavy metals, including lead and cobalt, can alter the activity of these enzymes by inhibiting their synthesis.

Although many substances, including organohalogen compounds, may evoke toxicities by combining reversibly with vitally important physiological control mechanisms and biochemical processes, other substances may evoke toxicities indirectly. Some substances may induce the synthesis of enzymes that metabolize endogenous steroids and vitally important steroid derivatives in food such as vitamin D. Some compounds such as fluoroacetate may be toxicologically inert by themselves, but may be transformed to chemically inert metabolites that evoke toxicological responses. Other substances may be converted to transient chemically reactive metabolites that combine irreversibly with tissue components and thereby result in various kinds of toxicities. It is important to determine whether the toxic responses of organohalogen compounds are caused by the compounds themselves or by their metabolites, because such knowledge may suggest ways of treating threatened species, particularly when the toxicity is mainly impaired reproduction.

B/C.6.2. Recommendations

1. Metabolic studies should be carried out, where possible, on pure compounds or mixtures of known composition, using acute and chronic dosing.
2. More information is required on metabolic pathways in the less com-

monly studied mammalian species such as ruminants and in nonmammalian species including birds, reptiles, fish, invertebrates, microorganisms, and terrestrial and aquatic plants and algae.

3. Comparative metabolic studies should be carried out in resistant and susceptible organisms.
4. The effect of environmental temperatures on the metabolism of xenobiotics in poikilotherms should be examined.
5. Metabolic studies should be carried out in combined biological systems such as the soil–plant systems and the liver enzymes–gut flora system associated with enterohepatic circulation in mammals.
6. The metabolism of various analogs and derivatives of known persistent compounds should be investigated so that more biodegradable but still effective compounds can be designed for the future.

B/C.7. Uptake, Fate, and Action of Heavy Metals and Organohalogen Compounds in Living Organisms— Summary of Recommendations for Future Study

B/C.6.1. Metals

1. Determination of the chemical forms of metal pollutants in animals, air, waters, food, and soil, and study of the mechanisms of absorption and the factors which may affect this.
2. Study of the nature of metal binding to proteins and nucleic acids, how this may affect metal transport across biological membranes, absorption, tissue distribution, storage, and excretion; the role of natural and synthetic chelating agents should also be investigated to ascertain how they may affect the biological properties of metals, particularly with regard to the reduction or increase of toxicity.
3. Determination of metal content in critical organs and the correlation of toxic hazard with metal content in biological tissues and fluids, particularly in species of ecological importance.
4. The development of methods to serve as indicators of subclinical or early toxicological changes, and improvement of methods for epidemiological surveys of metal toxicity. Studies on mutagenesis, carcinogenesis, embryotoxicity, and teratogenicity of metals and metal complexes.
5. Accumulation of dose–response data, by experimental methods, and epidemiological studies of populations with various levels of exposure to metals, including chronic low-level exposure. Special reference should be made to apparent resistance to toxicity, geographical factors, and the

effects of species, strain, race, age, and sex in individuals and also in natural and artificial ecosystems.

6. Studies on the pathogenesis of metal toxicity, particularly in target organs; correlation of tissue, cellular, and subcellular concentration of the metal with toxicity. Studies on the biochemistry and molecular pathology of metals and the displacement of physiologically functional metals by toxic metals.

7. Influence on toxicity of the interaction between different metals and between metals and organohalogen compounds in living organisms.

8. In relation to prevention and treatment of metal poisoning, further search for specific complexing agents which are nontoxic *per se* and after complex formation is recommended.

B/C.7.2. Organohalogen Compounds

1. Routine evaluation of new chemicals for biological persistence in the environment should be made during the early toxicological studies.

2. Studies of pharmacokinetics and toxicity should be conducted in a wide variety of species, particularly microorganisms, and those species which are specially sensitive or resistant. Sensitive organisms should be selected as indicators of environmental contamination and studied in both natural and artificial ecosystems.

3. Much further work is required on metabolic pathways, particularly in compounds not yet adequately studied and particularly in a greater variety of species including microorganisms. Further study of mechanisms of excretion is required, especially via the bile and expired air, and the significance of enterohepatic circulation.

4. Pharmacokinetic and metabolic studies should also be undertaken in artificial and natural ecosystems. They should also be performed in vulnerable and resistant species and strains, to correlate differences with toxicity. If the toxicant affects the metabolism of endogenous hormones or food factors such as vitamins, the toxicity of other substances which cause similar changes should be compared with that of the organohalogen compounds.

5. Studies should be made of the fate and toxicity of the less-studied organohalogen compounds such as the halogenated solvents, halogenated alkanes used as propellants and refrigerants. Study should also be made of the unidentified organohalogen contaminants and by-products present in industrial effluents. Studies comparing the effects of known mixtures of the major components in the effluents with those of the naturally occuring effluents should be performed in order to determine

the necessity of identifying minor components in industrial products and effluents.

6. New organohalogen chemicals should be introduced only after suitable animal toxicity studies have been performed. Any new organohalogen that is introduced should be monitored for toxicity, particularly in human populations at risk. Collaborative research in this area between industrial and other scientists should be encouraged.

7. Further studies are required concerning the effects of these compounds on reproduction, mutagenicity, and carcinogenicity, and their effects on immunological responses, with emphasis on techniques and interpretations.

8. More studies are required in molecular toxicology of organohalogen compounds, including the correlation of morphological with biochemical changes.

9. Factors affecting toxicity should be studied, particularly with respect to uptake, metabolism, and excretion, e.g., species and strain, pesticide synergists, age, environmental temperature, nutrition.

10. The possibility should be examined of utilizing microorganisms exhibiting high rates of metabolism of organohalogen compounds for the treatment of sewage and industrial effluents. Nontoxic biodegradable substitutes for persistent organohalogen compounds should be sought.

Bibliography

National Research Council of Canada (1973). Report of an Associate Committee on Scientific Criteria for Environmental Quality, *Lead in the Canadian Environment*, No. 13682.

The Environmental Mercury Problem (1972). (ed. D'Itic, F. M.). Chemical Rubber Co., Cleveland.

Friberg, L., Piscator, M., and Nordberg, G. F. (1971). *Cadmium in the Environment: An Epidemiological and Toxicologic Appraisal*, Chemical Rubber Co., Cleveland.

References

Brodie, B. B., and Gillette, J. R. (1971). *Concepts in Biochemical Pharmacology*, Vol. 28/1, Heffter-Heuber Handbuch der experimentellen Pharmakologie (ed. Eichler, O. O., Farah, A., Herken, H., and Welch, A. D.), Springer-Verlag, Berlin.

Butler, G. C. (1972). In *Assessment of Radioactive Contamination in Man*, Int. Atomic Energy Agency, Vienna.

Chadwick, R. W., Crammer, M. F., and Peoples, A. J. (1971). *Toxic. Appl. Pharmacol.*, **20**, 308.

Ecobichon, D. J., and Saschenbrecker, P. W. (1969). *Toxicol. Appl. Pharmacol.*, **15**, 420.

Eliason, B. C., and Posner, H. S. (1971). *Amer. J. Obstet. Gynecol.*, **111**, 925.

Hathway, D. E. (1972). In *Foreign Compound Metabolism in Mammals*, Vol. 2, p. 285, The Chemical Society, London.

IARC (1974). *The Evaluation of the Carcinogenic Risks of Chemicals to Man*, IARC Monograph, H.M.S.O., London.

ICRP (1966). *Task Group on Lung Dynamics, ICRP, Health Physics*, **12**, 173.

ICRP (1975). *Reference Man: Anatomical, Physiological and Metabolic Characteristics* (Publication No. 23), Pergamon, Oxford.

Kapoor, I. P., Metcalf, R. L., Hirwe, A. S., Lu, P-Y., Coats, J. R., and Nystrom, R. F. (1972). *Agric. Fd. Chem.*, **20**, 1.

Kenaga, E. E. (1972). *Residue Reviews.*, **44**, 73.

Kimbrough, R. D. (1974). *Critical Rev. Toxicol.*, **2**, 445.

Koransky, W., Portig, J., Vohland, H. W., and Klempau, I. (1964). *Naunyn-Schmiedebergs Arch. Exp. Pharmak.*, **247**, 49.

Ludke, J. L. (1974). *Bull. Environ. Contam. Toxicol.*, **11**, 297-302.

Matthews, H. B., McKinney, J. D., and Lucier, G. W. (1971). *J. Agric. Fd. Chem.*, **19**, 1244.

Morgan, D. P., and Roan, C. C. (1974). *Essays in Toxicol.*, **5**, 39-99.

Neubert, D., Zens, P., Rothemwaller, A., and Merker, H. J. (1973). *Environ. Hlth, Perspectives*, **5**, 67-79.

Peters, R. A. (1963). *Biochemical Lesions and Lethal Synthesis*, pp. 88-130, Pergamon Press, Oxford.

Ratcliffe, D. A. (1970). *J. Appl. Ecol.*, **7**, 67-107.

Robinson, J., Roberts, M., Baldwin, M. and Walker, A. I. T. (1969). *Food Cosmet. Toxicol.*, **7**, 317-332.

Smith, R. L. (1973). *The Excretory Function of Bile*, pp. 182-186, Wiley, New York.

Task Group on Metal Accumulation (1973). *Environ. Physiol. Biochem.*, **3**, 65.

Tomatis, L., Turusov, V., Terracini, B., Day, N., Barthel, W. F., Charles, R. T., Collins, G. B., and Boiocchi, M. (1971). *Tumori*, **57**, 337-396.

Underwood, E. J. (1971). *Trace Elements in Human and Animal Nutrition*, 3rd ed., Academic Press, New York.

Watson, M., Gabica, J., and Benson, W. W. (1972). *Clin. Pharmacol. Therap.*, **13**, 186-192.

Williams, R. T. (1959). *Detoxication Mechanisms*, 2nd ed., Chapman and Hall, London.

Yoshimura, H., Yamamoto, H., Nagai, J., Yae, Y., Uzawa, H., Ito, Y., Notomi, A., Minakami, S., and Ito, A. (1971). *Fukuoka-Igaku Zasshi*, **62**, 12.

D

Movements of Heavy Metals and Organohalogens through Food Chains and Their Effects on Populations and Communities

Chairman: B. H. Ketchum

Members: R. G. V. Boelens, N. Fimreite, E. E. Kenaga,
Q. Laham, H. Metzner. F. Moriarty, I. C. Munro,
H. Remmer, D. Saward

Rapporteurs: R. J. Pentreath and H. Windom

D.1. Introduction

This report deals with the effects of chemical pollutants on populations and communities as affected by physical, chemical, and biological processes in the environment. Evaluation of these effects eventually requires an assessment of the toxicity of residues to species existing in the total environment including plants, animals, air, water, and sediments.

The direct effects of chemicals in the environment are those occurring immediately subsequent to their first introduction into a specific ecosystem, resulting in the exposure of living individuals to lethal or sublethal concentrations. We have some knowledge of the lethal toxic effects which can be measured in a short-term laboratory bioassay. However, there is a need to know more about sublethal effects such as those on genetics, breeding habits, orientation and migration, energy transfer, feeding behavior, competition for habitat, and ability to escape predation. These effects, which in the short term are sublethal, may be reflected ultimately in population dynamics and in the ability of a species to survive as a population in contrast to the survival of an individual within that population.

The appearance of a chemical in the environment may subject individual organisms or populations to acute, chronic, or intermittent exposure. The study of potentially toxic materials should adequately reflect these situations, and the overall evaluation of effects should be based on the impact upon the most sensitive life stage of the most sensitive organism which is an essential component of the ecosystem under consideration. This has rarely been done.

The ecological consequences of pollution by heavy metals and organohalogen compounds are ultimately determined by four characteristics of the pollutant:

1. The amount reaching the environment.
2. The persistence and ultimate fate of the substance in the environment.
3. The toxicity of the pollutant to the organisms which constitute the populations and the communities.
4. The extent to which the pollutant is subject to bioaccumulation or degradation and transfer through the ecosystem.

Although population and community changes are ultimately mediated by the direct effect on the individual organism, a minor change may have no measurable ecological effects, since it merely increases the "death and predation" component of the population dynamics equations. This component normally shows large natural variations, and a small incremental change in response to a pollutant may be compensated for by an enhanced reproduction or survival component. A large change may, of course, eliminate a population and modify the structure of the community or ecosystem.

The first effect of a major pollution stress may thus be the elimination of the most sensitive population(s) with a consequent reduction in the diversity of the system. If the eliminated population is an essential link in the food web, the indirect effect will be the elimination or decrease of the food supply of higher trophic levels. This effect may cascade to produce an ecosystem totally different from the one originally present. In estuaries and other confined bodies of water such drastic modifications have already occurred in many parts of the world.

Even chronic, sublethal concentrations of pollutants may have long-term effects which are difficult to evaluate or predict from laboratory toxicity tests. Breeding and feeding behavior may be modified so as to endanger the survival of the species in a given locality. Migratory species may be excluded from their customary routes. The pollutant may modify the genetics of the species with unpredictable results; the offspring may be more adaptable to the pollutant, but less adapted to survive natural stresses, for example. Resistance of species to toxicants may, however, result from natural selection for resistant strains within the population, rather than from genetic changes. This is probably the explanation for the emergence of insect populations resistant to DDT.

Once a pollutant reaches the environment it may be bioaccumulated so that the concentration within the tissues of an organism is greater than that in the environment. The consumer may further concentrate the pollutant with resultant increases in "body burden" at successive trophic levels, a process known as biomagnification. In contrast, exclusion from the tissues may also occur with a progressive reduction in concentrations within the organisms. These effects are clearly dependent upon the relative rates of uptake and elimination. Some pollutants are metabolized and rendered harmless; others are bound within a specific tissue, such as some heavy metals in bones.

Laboratory tests can give important information on the relative toxicity of various pollutants, but are generally inadequate to evaluate or predict the long-term changes in behavior, genetics, or food chain dynamics. These more subtle effects are also more difficult to evaluate in the field. Studies are needed of controlled or confined systems which include multiple generations of the critical species which constitute the community.

This report elaborates on these concepts, gives examples of the variation in effects of different pollutants in different environments, and enumerates six major categories of problems for which more precise information is felt to be needed.

D.2. Accumulation, Transfer and Fate

The concepts of bioaccumulation (or exclusion) and transfers through food webs are important to the understanding of pollutant movement and impact on ecosystems. The accumulation and possible transformation of a pollutant in one biological compartment of the web may have a significant effect on its subsequent transfer to higher trophic levels. The flux of pollutants through an ecosystem is mediated by food web transfers and its evaluation requires a knowledge of the biomass at each trophic level, the effects of changes in pollutant concentrations on the productivity, turnover rate, and food conversion efficiencies at each trophic level, the concentration of the pollutant at each level, and "leaks" of pollutants from each level such as excretion followed, in aquatic environments, by sedimentation of particulate matter and thereby removal from the water. It is possible, with this information, to assess the flow of a pollutant through a food chain when uptake at any level affects productivity as well as pollutant accumulation. There is, however, no example for which all of these characteristics and processes are adequately known.

D.2.1. Microbial Activities

Most of the fluxes of matter in biogeochemical cycles depend to a large extent upon microbial activities in sediments or water. Bacteria are an important biological component of detritus-based terrestrial and coastal marine food chains. They are the dominant decomposers and are responsible for nutrient regeneration and cycling in all ecosystems by such processes as remineralization, nitrogen fixation, or denitrification. Although the accumulation in bacteria does not account for a major portion of a pollutant in an ecosystem, microorganisms may be responsible for the transfer of pollutants in food webs, and may exert a significant influence on the accumulation and transfer in other food chain members, by conversion of a pollutant to a more or less available or toxic form, for example, in the conversion of inorganic mercury to methylmercury (Jensen and Jernelöv, 1969).

Clearcut evidence exists for inhibitory effects of heavy metals and chlorinated hydrocarbons on microbial activities under laboratory conditions. Chloroform and carbon tetrachloride, for example, exert a 50% inhibition of methane-producing bacteria in concentrations between 1 and 100 mg/liter (Thiel, 1969). Toxic effects on algae have been noted for concentrations ranging from 1 to 1000 ppb, depending on the species examined, indicating a great diversity of susceptibility (Cairns and Lansa, 1972). It is recommended that special efforts be devoted to the effects of these pollutants on microbial activities under natural conditions, with special emphasis on possible alterations in fluxes of matter and on the effects of changes of population composition and concomitant modifications of food webs.

D.2.2. Primary Producers

Uptake of heavy metals by vascular plants is probably dominated by the root system. The metals are subsequently translocated to other parts of the plant, where they associate with connective tissue and protein. Environmental factors affect pollutant uptake and translocation. For example, air humidity influences both transpiration and metal uptake. Direct adsorption of both metals and halogenated hydrocarbons from the atmosphere, soil, or water may occur in vascular and lower terrestrial plants. Subsequent to adsorption, however, DDT and the cyclodiene group of organochlorine insecticides are not translocated to other parts of the plant in amounts toxic to animals (Finlayson and MacCarthy, 1973).

In aquatic ecosystems unicellular plants, the phytoplankton, rapidly accumulate pollutants such as heavy metals and halogenated hydrocarbons from water. Uptake is primarily by adsorption and is therefore a function of surface area rather than biomass, with smaller cells accumulating more than larger ones of equal biomass. Plants having acid polysaccharide cell walls, such as brown algae, adsorb metals much faster than those whose cell walls are composed of other membrane materials (Fogg, 1952). The highest accumulations of some heavy metals and halogenated hydrocarbons in aquatic food chains are commonly found in unicellular plants; others may be more concentrated in herbivores (Lowman et al., 1971). Some heavy metals and halogenated hydrocarbons accumulated by phytoplankton can be reversibly removed by ion exchange or by physical desorption.

D.2.3. Higher Trophic Levels

In the aquatic environment the concentration of heavy metals is generally less in the pelagic herbivores than in phytoplankton on which they feed. Some small crustacea, however, due to their large surface area, act like the primary producer by adsorbing metals on the surface. The classification of herbivore/carnivore is sometimes arbitrary in aquatic environments, especially for benthic invertebrates which filter large volumes of water. Under these circumstances both food and water contribute to the accumulation of heavy metals, although concentrations in the filter-feeders are generally lower than in the food organisms. Exceptions are often found where selective metal absorption occurs; for example, Zn in oysters is related to a high intake of Ca (Wolfe, 1970a,b; Coombs, 1972).

The higher aquatic herbivores and carnivores, fish, can potentially accumulate metals from both food and water. Many elements, such as Ce, Z₁, and Nb, are not absorbed through the gill or gut, while some, like Ru, are slightly retained. For transition metals such as Zn, Mn, Co, and Fe, water input plays only a minor role, with the major contribution being from food in marine species (Pentreath, 1973a,b,c). As a consequence, when feeding rates are low, retention less than 100% and with reasonably short biological half-life, the food commonly has a higher concentration than the fish. Thus the metal concentration at this end of the food chain decreases.

For other elements, such as Cs, the uptake from food and water is approximately equal, resulting in some enrichment (Pentreath and Jefferies, 1971). Current information on Hg indicates that both inorganic and organic forms are taken in through the gill, and that the latter form is readily absorbed from food (Hannerz, 1968; Keckes and Miettinen, 1972; Olsen et al., 1973). Also, mercury may accumulate with time within the organism so that the concentration is directly related to the size of the fish (Bache et al., 1971; Barber et al., 1972), but Westöö (1973) was unable to demonstrate age-dependence for the methylmercury fraction. Practically all the mercury in fish of the size normally eaten exists in the methyl form (Westöö and Rydälv 1969; Fimreite and Reynolds, 1973), but there is conflicting evidence on the methylation processes. Since there is little evidence for the presence of methylmercury in sea water itself, it is assumed that this form could be accumulated via the food chain. For freshwater fish, both food and water pathways may be important. The application of a total budget approach would be of value here. Studies with metals on fish eggs suggest that, with the possible exception of methylmercury, accumulation is largely by adsorption.

Terrestrial species accumulate metals from food, although for some, such as Pb, other routes may play a part. Higher vertebrates can regulate their body burdens of many of the essential trace elements, by balancing absorption and excretion with differing levels of intake. For some metals, however, including those which are more toxic (e.g., Pb, Cd), an increased intake with the same proportional absorption is not compensated for by an increase in excretion. Such metals therefore progressively accumulate in particular tissues. In addition, the effect of one metal on the absorption of others is poorly understood. As a consequence of such mechanisms the levels of many metals in the predator differ from those of the food species.

The organohalogens differ in many important respects from metals, in that they accumulate selectively in tissues high in lipids, and body burdens are frequently expressed in relation to lipids. In the aquatic environment the accumulation of such substances directly from water by all organisms is rapid (Reinbold et al., 1971; Sanders and Chandler, 1972). The ultimate ratio of an organo-halogen and its residues, in either herbivores or carnivores, will depend on the ratio taken in with the food, as well as its metabolism by the consumer. Present information on these aspects is limited to some organohalogens.

It is frequently found that the ultimate level of organohalogens in any member of a food chain is related to the lipid content of that species. Such lipid reserves may be mobilized under differing conditions so that concepts of steady state and food chain accumulation may be difficult to apply (Moriarty, 1972).

D.3. Biological Effects on Individuals and Populations

The effects of pollutants on populations are mediated either directly or indirectly by the effects on individuals. It is usually assumed that all effects of pollutants are deleterious, but for relatively low exposures this is not always demonstrably true. For example, one study reports that small doses of methyl-mercury have a beneficial effect upon pheasants (Fimreite, 1971). It is convenient to consider toxic effects as lethal or sublethal. To some extent the distinction is arbitrary; the longer the period of exposure, the greater the risk of adverse effects, since the impact of a pollutant depends upon both the concentration and the duration of exposure. The distinction between acute and chronic exposure is also arbitrary in many cases. The characteristics of the physical environment and the selection of the test organism (i.e., species, sex, strain, developmental stage) may also greatly modify the observed effect.

A sublethal effect can be critical for the survival of a population, even though not fatal to the specimen tested. For example, an embryo toxin may not harm an individual, but may kill its offspring or produce malformations and poor survival. Pollutants can be lethal at relatively low exposures, and we know that lesser doses can have deleterious effects, but we need to know much more about sublethal effects if we are to assess the potential impact of pollution. Many types of sublethal effects have been recorded (Stickel, 1968; Moriarty, 1969; McKim et al., 1973; Water Quality Criteria Data Book, 1971), but their significance in the field situation is often very difficult to assess. Among the effects which can have adverse consequences upon population survival are teratogenic (Miyoshi, 1959; Ferm and Carpenter, 1967), mutagenic (Ramel and Magnusson, 1969; Fishbein et al., 1970), reproductive (Cooke, 1973; Burdick et al., 1964; Mount et al., 1969), and behavioral effects (Sprague et al., 1965; McEwen and Brown, 1966; Jeffries and Prestt, 1966), and modification to normal physiological processes, e.g., the inhibition of photosynthesis in fresh-water algae by heavy metals (Harris, 1971; Menzel et al., 1970; Wurster, 1968).

Short-term toxicity tests, or bioassays, are useful in determining the concentrations which will be lethal to a fixed fraction of a population in a known period of time—LC_{50}, for example. (LC_{50} is the concentration lethal to 50% of the tested population in a fixed period of time, commonly 96 hours.) These are obviously not "safe" concentrations in the environment. Consequently, "application factors" of 0.1 to 0.01 (or even less) are used to extrapolate from the toxic concentration to a concentration that is presumed to offer minimal hazard of deleterious effect to the populations of concern. Long-term bioassays, generally in flowing systems extending over the complete life cycle of the organism, are needed to confirm the validity of the application factors used (Sprague, 1971). Also, it is important to know whether or not a bioassay on one organism can be applied to other species in the environment.

The key factors that control population size need not be direct effects on mortality. Although a pollutant may reduce a population directly by its effects on individuals within that population, it may also have indirect sublethal effects on that species, or may directly modify other species essential for the maintenance of a food chain or other environmental essentials for population survival. Normally it is very difficult to demonstrate that a pollutant is responsible for a change in population size. Even if a proportion of individuals is killed, the population size in subsequent generations may be unaffected (Dempster, 1974) because, as previously mentioned, a small increase in mortality may be compensated for by increases in fecundity or survival of larvae. However, pollutants that kill some individuals in successive generations may alter the population's genetic constitution by selection rather than mutation. Resistance of insects to organochlorine insecticides is probably the result of selection for resistant strains rather than mutation and genetic changes. Except for their resistance to the pesticide, these strains may be less well adapted to the environment than the original susceptible strain.

At present there are many controlled laboratory studies of toxicity of heavy metals and organohalogens, and many field observations. The great difficulty is to make valid extrapolations from the controlled laboratory experiment to the field, or to interpret the field work independently. Studies of the effects of heavy metals and organochlorines on individual species range from the determination of lethal concentrations for short periods of exposure to the effects of the pollutant on various physiological and behavioral processes.

Short-term toxicity studies, such as the LC_{50}, have been criticized for many years, but it cannot be denied that these bioassays provide an evaluation of toxicity which can be useful when discussing quality criteria or considering longer-term experiments. The chemical, physical, and biological variables should be realistically represented and carefully controlled in such studies. Toxicity tests should be extended, and there is perhaps scope for choosing other test organisms such as bacteria and protozoa or even tissue cultures as more sensitive indicators of toxicity. Criteria less drastic than mortality, such as changes in photosynthesis or respiration, might also be valuable.

Little attention has been paid to toxic effects on embryos. Although there have been some studies on the effects of a variety of pesticides and heavy metals on birds, fish, and the rabbit (Allison et al., 1964; Swensson, 1969; Villeneuve et al., 1971), we lack knowledge for most animal groups. In recent years, placental transfer of mercury, lead, and cadmium has been studied (Suzuki, 1967; Ferm and Carpenter, 1967; Barltrop, 1969) because this gives an initial body burden which will be augmented by later environmental exposures. In general, ease of passage is related to the intimacy of the placental relationship between mother and offspring.

In dealing with embryonic forms the effects of any element or substance on development depends upon the nature of the compound, the dose, route of administration, duration of exposure, and the stage of development. There are recognized critical stages when the embryo is more sensitive which are the same for most species, and include the period within 24 hours of fertilization, during gastrulation, at the onset of liver function, and at hatching or birth.

In general, inorganic salts of heavy metals exert toxic effects only in nonplacental forms after hatching and then probably due to the loss of the physical barrier formed by the capsule. In contrast, methylmercury is accumulated from the onset by the embryo and is teratogenic or lethal to fish exposed during development. Examples of these effects have been noted from both the marine and fresh-water environments.

D.4. Models and Monitoring

Models for the effects of pollution of an environment should include, as discussed by Ketchum for the aquatic environment (Chapter 3), assessment of the inputs to and exports from the system, and all the changes and effects of the pollutant within the system. No such complete model has ever been developed for any pollutant in any environment.

Partial models have been constructed for the transfer of pollutants in all environments, and atmospheric models are at an advanced stage of development. However, models for atmospheric transport of organohalogens and readily volatilized compounds are, in general, poorly developed, in part because the atmospheric content of the pollutant is poorly known. Terrestrial models are also well developed and researchers are at an advantage in the ease with which the data can be obtained. In aquatic systems, models of physical circulation and mixing are often of overriding importance since the distribution of the pollutant and the distribution of organisms (e.g., primary producers) bearing a pollutant load are influenced by these physical processes. Submodel kinetic data are required for all models and, particularly for metals, many already exist in all environments as a result of studies in radioecology. The behavior of some metals is poorly understood and information on organochlorines in the marine environment is considerably less than in fresh-water systems. However, Harvey et al. (1972) reported substantial amounts of organohalogens in organisms collected from the open sea, supporting the postulated atmospheric transport. Also, radioisotopes from fallout have been measured in waters of all oceans many miles from shore (NAS, 1971). These partial models help to identify gaps in our knowledge and areas of research which should be vigorously pursued.

Computer analysis of large models is ultimately limited by operational time and expense. More precise submodels would greatly narrow the necessary range of limits due to unknown correlations. Ultimately, for predictive calculations, food chain transfers should incorporate data on lethal and sublethal effects; limits could thus be set on maximum transfer coefficients to provide for total budget calculations. One should also capitalize on the presence of existing contaminants to study various ecosystem processes, as has been done using radioisotopes to follow large-scale water movements, sediment transport, and energy transfer in ecosystems (Reichle, 1967; Preston et al., 1972).

Finally, since we cannot yet predict the effects of pollutants on populations, we must monitor the environment. Monitoring programs must be designed for more than the mere accumulation of data. With proper planning they can provide information on local regions of relatively high levels, general environmental contamination, patterns of distribution of pollutants, and changes in populations. Monitoring could also provide data for the submodel kinetics, especially if it is closely linked with controlled studies of cause–effect relationships.

D.5. Research Needs

Various research needs have been identified throughout the text; these are summarized here under five main groupings. The ultimate objective of the recommendations is to develop the capability to achieve adequate prediction of the impact of an added pollutant in an ecosystem. We do not include research needs which are covered in other sections of this volume, such as the inputs to the environment, the persistence and ultimate fate in the environment, and the toxicity to individuals, except insofar as this information is needed for ecosystem analysis or the development of precise and accurate analytical methods.

D.5.1. Biological Effects

Short-term bioassay tests are useful to determine the toxicity of a pollutant to a selected test organism. Extrapolation of these results to derive the long-range impact on populations and communities (the ecosystem) requires use of an "application factor," which is frequently little more than an educated guess. Most particularly, the short-term test cannot evaluate chronic sublethal effects, which may take one or more generations to become evident but which can influence the survival of the population as much as, or even more than, the death of some individuals in the population. These long-term effects, as identified in the text, include teratogenic, mutagenic, reproductive, and behavioral effects, each of which could be critical for population survival.

More long-term studies should be initiated, preferably including one or more generations of the test organism. Long-term tests on a simplified food chain would provide information on the dose–accumulation–effect relationships. They would also enable us to study the dynamics of the action of pollutants, whether, assimilated from the water or the food. These studies would also emphasize the interactions that exist between species. The chemical speciation of the pollutant in the natural environment and possible synergistic and antagonistic effects may be very important, so that it is critical to conduct these tests with isolated but realistically representative portions of the natural environment. Studies of effects in reproduction and development behavior (e.g., feeding, avoidance, and migrations) and key physiological and metabolic processes such as respiration and photosynthesis should be expanded. They are of obvious importance in terms of populations and communities.

A greater understanding of food chain interactions is needed in both terrestrial and marine environments. In studies of pollutant transfer through food chains, a greater understanding of the life history of member organisms must be integrated with data on pollutant levels. Information on such things as food conversion efficiencies between trophic levels and feeding habits are extremely important in understanding pollutant transfer. Along with productivity and turnover rate data, this information can lead to a more fundamental understanding of biomagnification within food chains.

D.5.2. Environmental Modification of Pollutant Character

The character of the pollutant may change with time in the environment in ways which are not detectable in short-term (days or weeks) studies and are difficult to reproduce in short-term bioassays. These changes may be mediated, for different pollutants, by microbial action, by photo- or chemical oxidation or degradation, by hydrolysis, by adsorption onto living or nonliving particulates, or by metabolic processes of the organisms assimilating the material. These processes can increase the toxic effect, as in the methylation of mercury or the production of more toxic by-products; they can decrease the toxicity, by the oxidation of an organic material to CO_2 and water; or, without influencing toxicity, they may modify the distribution (e.g., by sedimentation in aquatic systems). All these processes are being studied in connection with ecosystem analysis programs, but not necessarily with respect to heavy metal and organohalogen pollutants. Specific studies for these purposes should be initiated.

D.5.3. Mechanisms of Accumulation and Transfer

Accumulation of pollutants in individuals and transfer along food chains are among the more important processes which must be evaluated in order to help predict pollution effects. Partition coefficients of pollutants and their degradation products which describe their distribution within lipid–water, soil–water, air–water, air–soil, air–plant, soil–plant, water–plant, and plant–animal systems are useful in assessing the potential accumulation of a substance within various organisms in the environment (Kenaga, 1972, 1974). The uptake and excretion of many substances are controlled by physiological processes which, for essential substances, can result in homeostatic control. Other substances can be combined and immobilized so that the body content can gradually increase with age or size. Thus, organisms may accumulate some substances to a concentration greatly exceeding that in the environment, or, conversely, may exclude the substance. For some substances, the fact of accumulation or exclusion is known, but generally the mechanisms are not well understood.

The extent to which compounds become adsorbed to environmental surfaces or absorbed by organisms should be determined for predictive purposes, since these properties, in addition to persistence and stability, account for the likelihood of accumulation in the food chain organisms and determine whether they will continue to accumulate stepwise in the food chain.

D.5.4. Background Pollutant Levels, Baselines, and Monitoring

Data on the concentration of pollutants in complete food chains exist for only a few ecosystems. There is probably more known about levels in terrestrial than in marine aquatic ecosystems. It is clear that more information on the levels of pollutants in members of food chains from many areas is required. In areas such as the North Sea, the English Channel, and the coastal environment of the United States much information exists. Even here, however, more baseline data could be beneficial in designing meaningful laboratory experiments. With the exception of the Antarctic Ocean, data on background levels of pollutants in the southern oceans are almost completely lacking. The collection of more background data on the levels of pollutants in unique marine and terrestrial environments of the Northern Hemisphere is also recommended.

Monitoring programs should be maintained in environments where man's impact is increasing or diminishing. Information from these studies should include changes in pollutant levels within the food chain, changes in population dynamics and community structure, and changes in productivity and turnover rates. Data from such monitoring programs would be beneficial not only to the understanding of the ecosystem under study, but would also provide useful information for developing predictive models in other environments.

D.6. Ecosystem Models and Prediction

A model which faithfully reflects nature is an indication that the critical processes are adequately understood, and will permit prediction of the effects of changes imposed upon the system. All the previously discussed research needs would provide the essential input data for an ecosystem model.

Terrestrial accumulation of pollutants is largely via food, although some are inhaled. For aquatic systems, assessment of the relative contributions of food and water to each compartment is required and it must be recognized that these differ in fresh-water and marine environments. In order to improve the existing expertise, more precise kinetic values, for specific biotic groups, are required from specialists in these fields. The data obtained should be in a form that is readily utilized in computer models. More attention to the development of total budget models will highlight these areas where more precise kinetic data are most urgently required. This is of special importance for the organohalogens, where their metabolic products are particularly persistent in the ecosystem. The transport of these metabolites must be more closely studied.

The total budget model would also emphasize the relevant importance of studying the fate of pollutants, particularly in the biota in either a local or a global context. Those pollutants which are not conservative in the vectors of air and water are best studied locally at the source. It might be expected that organohalogen budgets, particularly within the biota and the products of its decay, are related to the total lipid content of the compartment.

References

Allison, D. R., Kallman, B. J., Cope, O. B., and van Valin, C. (1964). "Some chronic effects of DDT on cutthroat trout," *U.S. Fish Wildl. Serv. Res. Rept.*, No. 64, 1–30.

298   Working Group Reports

Bache, C. A., Gutermann, W. H., and Lisk, D. J. (1971). "Residues of total mercury and methylmercuric salts in lake trout as a function of age," *Science*, 172, 951-952.

Barber, R. T., Vijayakumar, A., and Cross, F. A. (1972). "Mercury concentrations in recent and ninety-year-old benthopelagic fish, *Science*, 178, 636-639.

Barltrop, D. (1969). "Environmental lead and its paediatric significance," *Postgrad. Med. J.*, 45, 129.

Burdick, G. E., Harris, E. J., Dean, H. J., Walker, T. M., Skea, J., and Colby, D. (1964). "The accumulation of DDT in lake trout and the effect on reproduction," *Trans. Am. Fish. Soc.*, 93(2), 127-136.

Cairns, J., and Lansa, G. R. (1972). "Pollution controlled changes in algal and protozoan communities," in *Water Pollution Microbiology*, p. 245 (ed. Mitchell, R.), Wiley-Interscience, New York.

Cooke, A. S. (1973). "Shell thinning in avian eggs by environmental pollutants," *Environ. Pollut.*, 4, 85-152.

Coombs, T. L. (1972). "The distribution of zinc in the oyster *Ostrea edulis* and its relation to enzymatic activity and other metals," *Mar. Biol.*, 12, 170-178.

Dempster, J. P. (1974). "Effects of organochlorine insecticides on animal populations," in *Organochlorine Insecticides: Persistent Organic Pollutants* (ed. Moriarty, F.), Academic Press, London.

Ferm, V. H., and Carpenter, S. J. (1967). "Teratogenic effect of cadmium and its inhibition by zinc," *Nature (Lond.)*, 216, 1123.

Fimreite, N. (1971) "Effects of dietary methylmercury on ringnecked pheasants," *Can. Wildl. Service Occ. Paper*, 9.

Fimreite, N., and Reynolds, L. M. (1973). "Mercury contamination of fish in north-west Ontario," *J. Wildl. Manage.*, 37, 62-68.

Finlayson, O. G., and MacCarthy, M. R. (1973), "Pesticide residues in plants," in *Environmental Pollution by Pesticides* (ed. Edwards, C. A.), Plenum Press, New York.

Fishbein, L., Flamm, W. G., and Falk, H. L. (1970). *Chemical Mutagens*, Academic Press, New York.

Fogg, G. E. (1952). "The production of extracellular nitrogenous substances by a blue-green algae," *Proc. Roy. Soc. London, Series B* 139, 372-397.

Hannerz, L. (1968). "Experimental investigations on the accumulation of mercury in water organisms," *Fishery Bd. of Sweden Inst. Freshwater Res. Rep.*, No. 48, 120-176.

Harris, R. C. (1971). "Ecological implications of mercury pollution in aquatic systems," *Biol. Conserv.*, 3, 279-283.

Harvey, G. R., Bowen, V. T., Backus, R. H., and Grice, D. G. (1972). "Chlorinated hydrocarbons in open-ocean Atlantic organisms," in *The Changing Chemistry of the Oceans*, p. 177 (ed. Dryssen, D., and Jagner, D.), Nobel Symposium 20, Almquist and Wiksell, Stockholm and Wiley, New York.

Jeffries, D. J., and Prestt, I. (1966). "Post mortems of peregrines and lanners with particular reference to organochlorine residues," *Br. Birds*, 59, 49-64.

Jensen, S., and Jernelöv, A. (1969). "Biological methylation of mercury in aquatic organisms," *Nature (Lond.)*, 223, 753-754.

Keckes, S., and Miettinen, J. K. (1972). "Mercury as a marine pollutant," in *Marine Pollution and Sea Life*, p. 276 (ed. Ruivo, M.), Fishing News (Books) Ltd.

Kenaga, E. E. (1972). "Guide lines for environmental study of pesticides: determination of bioconcentration potential," *Residue Reviews*, 44, 73-111.

Kenaga, E. E. (1974). "Partitioning and uptake of pesticides in biological systems," 167th

American Chemical Society National Meeting, Los Angeles, California, April 1–5 (to be published in *Advances in Chemistry Series*, ACS).

Lowman, F. G., Rice, T. R., and Richards, F. A. (1971). "Accumulation and redistribution of radionuclides by marine organisms," in *Radioactivity in the Marine Environment*, p. 161, National Academy of Sciences, Washington, D.C.

McEwen, L. C., and Brown, R. L. (1966). "Acute toxicity of dieldrin and malathion to wild sharp-tailed grouse," *J. Wildl. Manage.*, **30**, 604–611.

McKim, J. M., Christsen, G. M., Tucker, J. H., and Lewis, M. J. (1973). "Effects of pollution on freshwater fish," *J. Wat. Pollut. Cont. Fed.*, **45**, 1370–1467.

Menzel, D. W., Anderson, J., and Randke, A. (1970). "Marine phytoplankton vary in their response to chlorinated hydrocarbons," *Science*, **167**, 1724.

Miyoshi, Y. (1959). "Experimental studies on the effect of toxic substances on pregnancy," *Med. J. Osaka Univ.*, **8**, 309–318.

Moriarty, F. (1969). "The sublethal effects of synthetic insecticides on insects," *Biol. Rev.*, **44**, 321–357.

Moriarty, F. (1972). "The effects of pesticides on wildlife: exposure and residues," *Sci. Total Environ.*, **1**, 267–288.

Mount, D. I., and Stephan, C. E. (1969). "Chronic toxicity of copper to the fathead minnow (*Pimephales promelas*) in soft water," *J. Fish. Res. Bd. Can.*, **26**, 2449–2457.

NAS (1971). *Radioactivity in the Marine Environment*, National Academy of Sciences–National Research Council, Washington, D.C.

Olsen, K. R., Bergman, H. L., and Fromm, P. O. (1973). "Uptake of methylmercuric chloride and mercuric chloride by trout: a study of uptake pathways into the whole animal and uptake by erythrocytes *in vitro*," *J. Fish. Res. Bd. Can.*, **30**, 1293–1299.

Pentreath, R. J. (1973a). "The roles of food and water in the accumulation of radionuclides by marine teleost and elasmobranch fish," in *Radioactive Contamination of the Marine Environment*, p. 421, IAEA, Vienna.

Pentreath, R. J. (1973b). "The accumulation and retention of ^{65}Zn and ^{54}Mn by the plaice (*Pleuronectes platessa* L.)," *J. Exp. Mar. Biol. Ecol.*, **12**, 1–18.

Pentreath, R. J. (1973c). "The accumulation and retention of ^{59}Fe and ^{58}Co by the plaice (*Pleuronectes platessa* L.)," *J. Exp. Mar. Biol. Ecol.*, **12**, 315–326.

Pentreath, R. J., and Jefferies, D. F. (1971). "The uptake of radionuclides by 1-group plaice (*Pleuronectes platessa* L.) off the Cumberland coast, Irish Sea," *J. Mar. Biol. Ass.*, **51**, 963–976.

Preston, A., Jefferies, D. F., and Pentreath, R. J. (1972). "The possible contributions of radioecology to marine productivity studies," in *Conservation and Productivity of Natural Waters* (ed. Edwards, R. W., and Garrod, D. J.), *Symp. Zool. Soc. Lond.*, No. 29, 271–284.

Ramel, C., and Magnusson, J. (1969). "Genetic effects of organic mercury compounds," *Hereditus*, **61**, 208–254.

Reichle, D. E. (1967). "Radioisotope turnover and energy flow in terrestrial isopod populations," *Ecology*, **48**, 351–366.

Reinbold, K. A., Kapoor, I. P., Childers, W. F., Bruce, W. F., and Metcalf, R. L. (1971). "Comparative uptake and biodegradability of DDT and methoxychlor by aquatic organisms," *Ill. Natur. Hist. Surv. Bull.*, **30**, 405–417.

Sanders, H. O., and Chandler, J. H. (1972). "Biological magnification of a polychlorinated biphenyl (Arochlor 1254) from water by aquatic invertebrates," *Bull. Environ. Cont. Toxicol.*, **7**, 257–263.

Sprague, J. B., Elson, P. F., and Saunders, R. L. (1965). "Sublethal copper-zinc pollution in a salmon river—a field and laboratory study, *Proc. Int. Conf. Wat. Pollut. Res.*, Tokyo, pp. 61-82.

Sprague, J. B. (1971). "Measurement of pollutant toxicity to fish. III Sublethal effects and safe concentrations," *Water Research*, **5**, 245-266.

Stickel, L. F. (1968). "Organochlorine pesticides in the environment," *Spec. Scient. Rep. U.S. Fish. Wildl. Serv. Wildlife*, No. 119.

Suzuki, T. (1967). "Placental transfer of mercuric chloride, phenylmercury acetate and methyl acetate in mice," *Ind. Hlth.*, **5**, 149-155.

Swensson, A., (1969). "Comparative toxicity of various organic mercury compounds," *J. Japan Med. Soc.*, **61**, 1056-1059.

Thiel, P. G. (1969). "The effect of CH₄ analogues on methanogenesis in anaerobic digestion," *Water Research* **3**, 215-223.

Villeneuve, D. C., Grant, D. L., Phillips, W. E. J., Clark, M. L., and Clegg, D. J. (1971). "Effects of PCB administration on microsomal enzyme activity in pregnant rabbits," *Bull. Environ. Contam. Toxicol.*, **6**, 120.

Water Quality Criteria Data Book (1971). "III. Effects of chemicals on aquatic life," *Water Pollut. Cont. Res. Ser. 18050 GWV E.P.A.*, Washington, D.C.

Westöö, G. (1973). "Methylmercury as percentage of total mercury in flesh and viscera of salmon and sea trout of various stages," *Science*, **181**, 567-568.

Westöö, G., and Rydälv, M. (1969). "Kvicksilver och methylkvicksilver i fisk och kraftor," *Vär Föda*, **21**(3), 18-111.

Wolfe, D. A. (1970a). "Levels of stable Zn and ⁶⁵Zn in *Crassostrea virginica* from North Carolina, *J. Fish. Res. Bd. Can.*, **27**, 47-57.

Wolfe, D. A. (1970b). Zinc enzymes in *Crassostrea virginica*, *J. Fish Res. Bd. Can.*, **27**, 59-69.

Wurster, C. F. Jr. (1968). "DDT reduces photosynthesis by marine phytoplankton," *Science*, **159**, 1474.

E

Analytical Methodology

Chairmen: H. V. Morley and J. L. Monkman

Members: H. J. M. Bowen, T. L. Coombs, C. S. Giam, F. Korte, K. H. Palmork, C. C. Patterson, P. W. West, V. Zitko

Rapporteur: H. V. Morley

E.1. General Introduction

It must be recognized that many problems still exist in the tasks of characterizing and obtaining quantitative assessment of those heavy metals and organohalogen compounds which, directly or indirectly, may be harmful to man and other members of the ecosystem. The points emphasized by this working group on analytical methodology as meriting further research broadly fall into such categories as basic studies of the chemical properties of the pollutants, procedures for their isolation, identification, and quantitative determination, and, particularly, the need for adequate consideration of pollutant metabolites and degradation products in the above contexts. The priorities accorded to these studies will be determined by such aspects as the gross quantities of potential pollutants produced, usage and commercial distribution patterns, persistence, bioaccumulation potentials, and the toxicity of these materials and their metabolites or transformation products.

The reports of other working groups emphasize how ignorance of the forms in which many of the heavy metals enter the environment and undergo modification before and during passage through individual organisms and food chains hinders assessment of their significance. In many instances the design of realistic experimental studies of toxicity is entirely dependent upon the adequacy with which existing analytical methodology is capable of describing these transformations in quantitative terms. While, for example, it is known that the total trace metal content of a soil, plant, or animal tissue may often bear little relationship to the content of "biologically available" metal, the development of suitable techniques for the determination of the "available" component is contingent upon the chemical identification of such components. Description of the biological transformation undergone by mercury promoted rapid progress toward an understanding of the potential toxicity of this element. Regrettably, similar progress has not been made with the other heavy metals even though the need for such study is apparent, if only by virtue of the fact that biochemical studies clearly suggest that the free ionic species of many of the potentially toxic metals are likely to be of trivial importance compared with the products of their interaction with organic ligands in biological systems.

A large amount of information on compounds such as DDT, dieldrin, heptachlor epoxide and PCB has been accumulated and, in spite of the fact that many of the early data are questionable due to lack of positive identification and nonspecific methodology (Morley and McCully, 1973), the general patterns of these compounds in the environment are reasonably well established. The use of some of these persistent organochlorine compounds has been either banned or severely restricted, and analyses indicate that the concentration of these compounds in food and biological samples remains more or less constant or is slowly decreasing. Little is known about the environmental properties of the majority of organohalogen compounds. Knowledge is mostly limited to the recognition that many of these compounds are, or may be, discharged into the environment as economic poisons, industrial chemicals, or by-products of industrial processes (involving the production of or utilization of other halogenated compounds or chlorine). Some of these compounds may also be generated during the chlorination of waste water and sewage plant effluents. Many of them have not been identified or isolated. The complexity of the problem is well illustrated in a recent publication which identifies some of the by-products produced in the manufacture of vinyl chloride (Palmork and Wilhelmsen, 1972).

E.1.1. Monitoring

Since monitoring analyses are designed to determine temporal trends, the analytical technique should be as simple as possible, should be precise, and should not be changed during the program unless absolutely essential. Experience with the OECD wildlife monitoring program for PCBs, DDT (and metabolites), mercury, and cadmium has shown that the variability in content between individual biological specimens is very high, in spite of the fact that samples were collected under conditions as uniform as possible. Biological samples may be more suitable and meaningful for the monitoring of persistent materials than samples of the physical environment, especially air and water. For the less persistent compounds, measurement of biological parameters, such as enzyme inhibition, rather than the search for residues may be more useful, since an unknown toxic transformation product may be indicated even though the parent compound is no longer detectable.

E.1.2. By-products

The possible significance of the great quantities of by-products entering the environment has not been fully assessed. The production of organic chemicals is based on chemical syntheses the yields of which vary a great deal, in some cases being as low as about 25%. In such an example the production of 100,000 tons of a product will result in approximately 300,000 tons of by-products.

By-products contain a mixture of the starting materials and results of side reactions. Such mixtures are, inevitably, very complex. To illustrate this, the production of vinyl chloride (the basis for PVC) may be cited (Palmork and Wilhelmsen, 1972; Jensen et al., 1970). This production results in approximately 2-4% of by-products, and in Europe alone this amounts to between 70 and 100 kilotons per year. The by-product (ethylenedichloride-tar, also called EDC-tar) consists of a black tarry material and differs in composition depending on the manufacturing process used. Twenty-five organohalogens have been identified in the steam-volatile portion of the EDC-tar resulting from one manufacturing process and 27 in that resulting from another. Many of these compounds are widely distributed in the sea, and results of a recent survey of the North Atlantic suggest that they originate from industries on both sides of the ocean. Some of the components of EDC-tar are known to be accumulating in marine organisms (Jensen and Renberg, 1974). The preceding discussion indicates only some organohalogen compounds which should be studied according to the priority criteria mentioned earlier.

E.2. Purpose of Analysis

The design of any analytical method will be governed to some degree by the purpose of the investigation proposed. This purpose must be clearly defined before a selection of possible analytical techniques can be made. Thus, for example, identification of a particular pollutant in a selected environment may require more complex analysis at exceptionally low concentrations, than is later demanded for continuous assessment, i.e., monitoring at an established level. It is therefore recommended that prior discussion between the analyst and the primary investigator (ecologist, toxicologist, etc.) be arranged so that the limitations of the analytical system to be employed can be clearly outlined and understood by both parties.

While all types of analysis require good precision and accuracy, it should be recognized that analytical results are not absolutely precise and accurate, and in all cases there is an acceptable minimal error imposed by the chosen procedure, for example, approximately ±20% for organohalogen compounds present in concentrations in the range of 0.5–1.0 mg/kg in biological samples when determined by gas chromatography.

E.3. Sampling

It is most important that any sample be accurately representative of the larger bulk which it is intended to assess. If the sample is not representative no meaningful analysis can be made subsequently, in spite of all possible care in the sample preparation and analysis. In particular, the introduction of contamination during the sampling process must be avoided, and procedures to ensure this must be clearly set out. In addition, the sampling process should not introduce segregation of any sample constituent, nor should it alter the physical or chemical character of the constituents. On the other hand, it is legitimate and may be expedient to concentrate the sample at the sampling site.

If separation and concentration of the material of interest is complete, the larger bulk of depleted sample matrix may then be left behind.

Factors affecting biological variation are not always appreciated. More attention should be paid to recording information such as time of sampling, temperature, season, and so on.

In any assessment situation, it is necessary to prepare sound guidelines as to the frequency of sampling with time or in space, which is required to maintain true representation of the bulk sample.

A recent publication has discussed the difficulties inherent in the sampling of biological materials, together with recommendations for the preparation, transport, and preservation of samples (Morley and McCully, 1973).

E.4. Preparation of Sample

Problems involved in the preparation of samples are those of contamination and loss. Contamination is a serious problem, especially for liquid samples which may dissolve metals from sampler and container surfaces. Thus mammalian blood can dissolve substantial amounts of manganese, molybdenum, and tungsten from metal hypodermic needles. Metallic soaps used as lubricants during the extrusion of plastics frequently give rise to contamination of samples stored in new plastic containers. Many of the pigmenting agents used in colored plastics have a high metal content. PCB may occur in appreciable quantities in plastic wrappings, in some batches of organic solvents, and in inorganic reagents such as sodium sulfate. Contamination during processing may involve a ten- or hundredfold increase of trace constituents.

Losses are often overlooked. Drying of sediments at 100°C can result in losses of some chlorobiphenyls and is therefore best avoided. Mercury can be lost when samples are heated, as during drying or ashing. The analysis of tissues for mercury presents many opportunities for losses of the element under reducing conditions below 100°C, opportunities for contamination of the agent used for trapping volatile mercury species, and risks arising from incomplete breakdown of organic mercury compounds during wet ashing. Cadmium and zinc may be lost if ashing temperatures exceed 425°C, while biologically active complexes of chromium and selenium may be lost during oven drying of samples.

All analytes tend to be lost from very dilute solutions by sorption onto particles or container walls during storage. Losses of metals can be minimized either by adding dilute nitric acid or potassium cyanide. It has been found that mercury can penetrate the walls of polyethylene containers. Analysts should be aware of these and other problems when preparing, storing, or transporting both samples and standards.

To determine submicrogram amounts of those constituents which are widely disseminated contaminants (e.g., lead, mercury, PCB), clean laboratory techniques must be developed. These should aim at consistent and accurately measured blanks that do not significantly interfere with the determination required. The use of radioisotopes as internal standards for yield determination is recommended.

In environmental studies, it is important to determine whether a toxic substance originates from natural or industrial sources. Thus for lead, more refined techniques indicate that more than 99% of the lead ingested by the population of the United States originates from industrial sources; the amount ingested amounts to 20 tons per year. There is a requirement to measure lead in dietary items in the range 0.1–0.001 mg Pb/kg. Atomic absorption spectrometry using a graphite furnace and spark source mass spectrometry with isotope dilution have adequate sensitivity to achieve this. However, to achieve accuracy in the determination of lead and other metals at these concentrations it is necessary to pay careful attention to blanks and to laboratory cleanliness.

E.5. Identification

As a part of the determinative process, unequivocal identification of the material should be sought. Whenever possible, several approaches should be used to increase the certainty of identification. If, at the same time, the identification process can be made to yield more information as to the chemical speciation than a total elemental analysis, this should be done.

In the case of organochlorine compounds, heavy reliance is placed upon gas-chromatographic techniques. It is often forgotten, however, especially by the nonanalyst, that gas chromatography is primarily a separation technique. Reliance upon gas chromatography to identify a substance positively is thus fraught with danger and results in many misidentifications. Ancillary methods of identification, such as the chemical preparation of derivatives and the use of mass spectrometry, should be routinely applied. (For the same reason, alternative methods of quantitation should also be used wherever possible.)

E.6. Standards, Reference Materials, and Interlaboratory Comparisons

1. The purity of standards and the stability of standard solutions are very important, and the attention required by these cannot be overemphasized.

Standard solutions of metals are readily prepared and offer few problems, apart from storage. On the other hand, standards of many organohalogen and/or organometallic compounds are not readily available. Some technical products and effluents are exceedingly complex mixtures of compounds. All individual components of these mixtures may not be available, and the mixtures may have to be analyzed in terms of the technical product which they more or less resemble. In such cases the results may be precise, but not accurate. However, the precision may be adequate for monitoring purposes, and there may be no need to determine the individual components.

Analytical chemists and toxicologists should keep in mind that technical-grade compounds may contain impurities, not normally present in purified materials used as standards. These impurities should be identified, tested for biological activity, and, if biologically active, included in the analytical procedures.

2. The importance of interlaboratory comparisons is well recognized, and most established laboratories participate in some type of comparison program using reference materials. Reference materials are relatively few in number, and it would be useful to have more of these, especially materials with very low concentrations of lead (dried milk might be suitable). Among reference materials available for metal analysis, bovine liver (National Bureau of Standards), flour, bone, and dried blood (IAEA), and kale (Bowen, 1966) may be mentioned.

3. It would be useful to prepare reference materials, with and without added organohalogen compounds, and to make these available to all interested analytical laboratories. Suitable matrices might be animal or vegetable lipids and dried soil or sediment. Little is known about the long-term stability of organohalogen compounds in any type of matrix. Such materials are important in testing the accuracy of new methods, in interlaboratory comparisons, and in quality control work where large numbers of analyses are required continuously. Their production is no easy undertaking as 50–100 kg of homogeneous powder is usually required.

4. Guidance is needed on the frequency of quality control checks. The National Bureau of Standards recommends that one sample in five and the International Atomic Energy Agency that one sample in ten should be a reference material inserted at random in any series of samples to check quality control. These are probably reasonable figures where the cost of analysis is low, e.g., in atomic absorption spectrometry, or when using an autoanalyzer.

E.7. Presentation of Data

The present procedure of data presentation commonly used in reporting environmental pollution leaves much to be desired in terms of presenting meaningful results for comparative purposes. Suitable procedures have been compiled previously by the International Union of Pure and Applied Chemistry (IUPAC), and we recommend that such procedures be used routinely. The following items merit particular emphasis:

1. Accuracy of data should be checked by two or more techniques, preferably employing different analytical principles.
2. The number of significant figures given should agree in a realistic manner with the known precision, accuracy, and sensitivity of the method employed.
3. Standard deviation and the number of determinations on which this is based should always be given.
4. The preferred units are mg/kg dry weight, with a conversion factor to fresh weight where this is applicable, and in the case of organochlorine compounds, mg/kg extracted lipid, together with the relevant conversion factor.

E.8. Determination

The determination step should not be confused with the term "analysis." The finish is only a part of the analysis, consisting, as it does, of some chemical or physical process that is assumed to give a measure of the substance being measured. Classical analytical methods are based upon chemical reactions. These are typified by precipitation, neutralization, oxidation–reduction, and color formation. Reliability of the chemical methods is usually dependent on the use of the proper conditioning of reactions to eliminate or minimize interferences. In some instances, the material to be determined is isolated before measurement. In other cases, the interfering agents are separated or, better, are masked as unreactive complexes.

There is a trend toward the use of sophisticated, expensive, analytical procedures, such as neutron activation analysis and mass spectrometry, which utilize physical rather than chemical principles. Optical methods, such as emission spectroscopy, atomic absorption spectroscopy, x-ray fluorescence, and infrared spectrometry, are especially popular. Electrochemical techniques and the use of chemiluminescence reactions fall generally between the chemical and the physical methods. It should not be overlooked that the physical methods and instruments used often depend upon preliminary steps that are chemical operations and are subject to matrix interference. Calibration of the methods and reference procedures is usually based upon established chemical techniques, and quite often chemical reactions are an adjunct to the final physical measurement.

In conclusion, a word of caution should be applied to the concept of accuracy. For example, it is common practice to claim accuracy for an instrument based upon electronic sensitivity. This sensitivity, in turn, is established on the basis of an arbitrary signal to noise ratio, such as a ratio of two to one. Overlooked, usually, is the lack of specificity of the quantitating sensor, the high proportion of spurious signals, the recurring need for calibration, and the fact that sampling and sample treatment have far more effect on the overall accuracy than the measuring device itself.

E.9. Future Studies

The discussions above have been concerned only with weaknesses and gaps in present analytical techniques. We shall end this report with recommendations for developmental studies in areas at present unexplored.

Heavy Metal Studies
1. *Determination of the Chemical Form of Metals in the Environment.* Techniques are rudimentary and information scanty on this important topic, which may influence profoundly the biological importance of any metabolism. Basic research is required on separation and identification techniques for metal complexes using possibly gas or high-pressure liquid chromatography, electrophoresis, or solvent extraction. This information is essential for the realistic appraisal of survey data and to facilitate the development of experimental studies of toxicity intended to reproduce situations pertaining in the natural environment.

2. *In Situ Techniques.* By sampling *in situ*, problems of contamination, loss, or storage can be minimized. Examples where this is already under study include CO determination in air by reaction with hot HgO, determination of Hg in water by reaction with ^{110}Ag dibutyldithiocarbamate in chloroform, and determination of Cd in human kidney by γ-emission counting after neutron irradiation.

3. *Simultaneous Determination of More than One Element.* A metal may exert its metabolic or toxic effect indirectly by affecting other essential metals present. Simultaneous determination of a limited number of these metals may uncover hitherto unsuspected relationships. Present techniques require further development in terms of resolution, sensitivity, and suppresssion of interference effects.

4. *Range of Metals Determined.* Elements have been listed according to their toxicity to small mammals. These data suggest that more attention be given to the following in addition to Cd, Pb, and Hg: As, Be, Cr (VI), Pd, Pt, Sb, Se, Te, Tl.

5. *Cycling of Volatile Elements.* From a biogeochemical point of view, there is a need to know more about the cycling through the atmosphere of organic derivatives of As, Se, Hg, S, and F. While the trace element composition of coal is well known, knowledge of the fate of volatile elements released after burning is fragmentary.

6. *Destruction of Organic Matter Previous to Inorganic Analyses*. There is an urgent need for the development of standardized, efficient methods for mineralization techniques and for the wider recognition of the particular limitations of existing procedures.

7. *Automation*. In order to handle the large numbers of environmental samples the ability to process by automated techniques is becoming increasingly important.

Organic Compounds

1. *Improvement of Existing Methods*. The development of new and the improvement of existing analytical methods will undoubtedly continue and lead to increased sensitivity and specificity of the methods. However, there is an urgent need for more sensitive analytical methods for the determination of chlorinated dibenzodioxins and dibenzofurans, because of the extreme toxicity of some of these compounds.

2. *Extending the Range of Compounds Which May Be Determined*. Methods should be developed for industrial chemicals such as chlorinated paraffins, alkylchlorobiphenyls, chlorofluorobiphenyls, chlorobiphenylols, other halogenated compounds, and industrial wastes containing halogenated compounds which, according to the criteria mentioned earlier, are or may become environmentally important.

Chemical methods are generally suitable for persistent compounds, but not applicable to nonpersistent ones, for which biochemical or biological methods need to be developed. These methods would also be useful in the case of persistent compounds and would facilitate the evaluation of the biological significance of the concentrations found.

In the case of persistent compounds, more attention should be given to establishment of level–effect relationships, so that biological significance of analytical results can be better evaluated.

References

Bowen, H. J. M. (1966). *Trace Elements in Biochemistry*, Academic Press, London.

Jensen, S., and Renberg, L. (1974). *Scientific Report to the Oslo Commission Working Group on Degradability*.

Jensen, S., Jernelφv, A., Lange, R., and Palmork, K. H. (1970). *F.A.O. Technical Conference on Marine Pollution and Its Effects on Living Resources and Fishing, Rome*, FIR: MP/70/E-88.

Morley, H. V., and McCully, K. A. (1973). *Methodicum Chimicum* (Vol. 1, Part 1), Chapter 11.1, pp. 850–904. Georg Thieme Verlag and Academic Press, New York.

Palmork, K. H., and Wilhelmsen, S. (1972). *Fisken og Havet, Series B*, No. 5, 1–13.

Participants

Cochairmen: Dr. A. D. McIntyre
Department of Agriculture and
Fisheries for Scotland
Marine Laboratory
PO Box 101
Aberdeen AB9 8DB, Scotland

Dr. C. F. Mills
Nutritional Biochemistry Department
The Rowett Research Institute
Greenburn Road
Bucksburn, Aberdeen AB2 9SB, Scotland

Dr. J. Barstad
Statens Inst. for Folkhelse
Geitmyrsveien 75
Oslo 1, Norway

Dr. K. I. Beynon
Tunstall Laboratory
Shell Research Ltd.
Sittingbourne, Kent, England

Dr. R. G. V. Boelens
Biologist in Charge, Toxicity Unit
Ontario Ministry of Environment
PO Box 213
Rexdale, Ontario, Canada

Dr. H. J. M. Bowen
Department of Chemistry
Reading University
Whiteknights
Reading, Berks., England

Dr. G. C. Butler
Director, Division of Biological
Sciences
National Research Council of Canada
100 Sussex Drive
Ottawa K1A OR6, Canada

Prof. E. M. Cohen
President, Organization for Health
Research TNO
148 Juliana van Stolberglaan
PO Box 297
The Hague, The Netherlands

311

Dr. T. L. Coombs
Institute of Marine Biochemistry
St. Fitticks Road
Aberdeen, Scotland

Prof. S. Dalgaard-Mikkelsen
Royal Veterinary and Agricultural
  College
Department of Pharmacology and
  Toxicology
13 Bulowsvej
Copenhagen V, Denmark

Dr. N. T. Davies
The Rowett Research Institute
Greenburn Road
Bucksburn, Aberdeen AB2 9SB,
  Scotland

Dr. A. J. de Groot
Instituut voor Bodemvruchtbaarheid
Oosterweg 92
Haren (Groningen), The Netherlands

Prof. A. Disteche
Institut E. van Beneden
Section: Océanologie
Université de Liège
22 Quai van Beneden
4000 Liége, Belgium

Dr. R. Duce
Graduate School of Oceanography
University of Rhode Island
Kingston, Rhode Island 02881, USA

Dr. J. Duinker
Netherlands Institute for Sea Research
Horntje, Texel, The Netherlands

Dr. D. J. Ecobichon
Department of Pharmacology
Dalhousie University
Dartmouth, Nova Scotia, Canada

Dr. G. L. Eichhorn
National Institutes of Health
Gerontology Research Center
Baltimore City Hospital
Baltimore, Maryland 21224, USA

Prof. Dr. H.-J. Elster
Limnologisches Institut
Mainaustrasse 212
775 Konstanz-Egg, Germany

Dr. N. Fimreite
Biology Department
University of Tromso
9000 Tromso, Norway

Prof. G. L. Gatti
Istituto Superiore di Sanita
Viale Regina Elena 299
00161 Rome, Italy

Dr. C. S. Giam
Chemistry Department
Texas A & M University
College Station, Texas 77843, USA

Dr. J. R. Gillette
Laboratory of Chemical Pharmacology
National Heart and Lung Institute
National Institutes of Health
Bethesda, Maryland 20014, USA

Dr. E. D. Goldberg
Scripps Institution of Oceanography
University of California
La Jolla, California 92037, USA

Dr. J. Greig
MRC Toxicology Unit
MRC Laboratories
Woodmanstern Road
Carshalton, Surrey, England

Dr. R. L. Halstead
Research Coordinator (Soils)
Research Branch
Canada Agriculture
K. W. Neatby Bldg.
C. E. F. Ottawa, Ontario K1A OC6,
  Canada

Dr. P. Heurteaux
Centre d'Ecologie de Camargue
Le Sambul
13200 Arles, France

Dr. E. E. Kenaga
Ag-Organics Department
Dow Chemical Co.
Midland, Michigan 48640, USA

Dr. B. H. Ketchum
Associate Director
Woods Hole Oceanographic Institution
Woods Hole, Massachusetts 02543,
  USA

Dr. J. Klaverkamp
Research Scientist
Freshwater Institute
Fisheries and Marine Service
501 University Crescent
Winnipeg, Manitoba, Canada

Prof. Dr. A. Kloke
Biologische Bundesanstalt für Land-
  und Forstwirtschaft
Königin Luise-Strasse 19
1 Berlin 33 (Dahlem), Germany

Prof. Dr. F. Korte
Institut für Oekolgische Chemie der
  Technischen Universität
München–Weihemstephan, Germany

Prof. J. W. M. La Riviere
c/o International Courses
Oude Delft 95
Delft, The Netherlands

Dr. Q. Laham
Biology Department
University of Ottawa
Ottawa, Ontario, Canada

Prof. P. N. Magee
Courtauld Institute of Biochemistry
The Middelsex Hospital
Medical School
London W1P 5PR, England

Prof. H. Metzner
Institut für Chemische
  Pflanzenphysiologie der
  Universität Tübingen
Auf der Morgenstelle
Tübingen, Germany

Prof. J. K. Miettinen
Department of Radiochemistry
University of Helsinki
Unioninkatu 35
00170 Helsinki 17, Finland

Dr. D. R. Miller
Division of Biological Sciences
National Research Council
Ottawa, Ontario K1A OR6, Canada

Dr. J. L. Monkman
Department of National Health and
  Welfare
Occupational Health Centre
Tunney's Pasture
Ottawa, Ontario K1A OH3, Canada

Dr. F. Moriarty
Monks Wood Experimental Station
Abbots Ripton
Huntington PE17 2LS, England

Dr. H. V. Morley
Research Branch
Agriculture Canada
Ottowa, Ontario K1Z OC6, Canada

Dr. I. Munro
Head, Toxicology Division
Health Protection Branch
Health and Welfare Canada
Tunney's Pasture Bld.
Ottawa, Ontario K1A OA2, Canada

Dr. N. Nelson
Director, Institute of Environmental
*   Medicine*
New York University Medical Center
550 First Avenue
New York, New York 10016, USA

Dr. G. Nordberg
Department of Environmental Hygiene
The Karolinska Institute
104 01 Stockholm 60, Sweden

Dr. H. K. Palmork
Institute of Marine Research
PO Box 2906
5011 Bergen, Norway

Prof. D. V. Parke
Department of Biochemistry
University of Surrey
Guildford, Surrey, GU2 5XH, England

Dr. Clair C. Patterson
Division of Geological and Planetary
*   Sciences*
California Institute of Technology
Pasadena, California 91109, USA

Dr. R. J. Pentreath
Fisheries Radiobiological Laboratory
Hamilton Dock
Lowestoft, Suffolk, England

Ms. I. Price
Canadian Wildlife Service
Environment Canada
Ottawa, Ontario K1A OH3, Canada

Prof. H. Remmer
Institut für Toxikologie der
*   Universität Tübingen*
Lothar-Meyer-Bau
Wilhelmstrasse 56
74 Tübingen, Germany

Dr. L. Renberg
National Swedish Environment
*   Protection Board*
Special Analytical Laboratory
Wallenberglab
University of Stockholm
104 05 Stockholm 50, Sweden

Dr. D. Saward
Marine Laboratory
PO Box 101
Victoria Road
Aberbeen, Scotland

Dr. W. Stickel
Patuxent Research Center
U.S. Fish and Wildlife Service
Laurel, Maryland 20810, USA

Dr. P. Toft
Environmental Health Directorate
Health and Welfare Protection Branch
Department of Health and Welfare
Ottawa, Ontario K1A OL2, Canada

Prof. R. Truhaut
Université René Descartes
Laboratoire de Toxicologie et
* d'Hygiène Industrielle*
4 Avenue de l'Observatoire
Paris, France

Dr. A. Verloop
Biochemical Department
Philips-Duphar B. V.
Postbox 4
's Graveland, The Netherlands

Dr. M. Webb
MRC Toxicology Unit
MRC Laboratories
Woodmansterne Road
Carshalton, Surrey, England

Prof. P. W. West
College of Chemistry and Physics
Louisiana State University
Baton Rouge, La. 70803, USA

Prof. R. T. Williams
Department of Biochemistry
St. Mary's Hospital Medical School
London W2 1PG, England

Dr. H. L. Windom
Skidaway Institute of Oceanography
PO Box 13687
Savannah, Georgia 31406, USA

Dr. R. Wollast
Laboratory of Industrial Chemistry
Université Libre de Bruxelles
Av. F. D. Roosevelt, 50
1050 Bruxelles, Belgium

Dr. W. N. Yule
Chemical Control Research Institute
Canadian Forestry Service
25 Pickering Place
Ottawa, Ontario K1A OW3, Canada

Dr. V. Zitko
Biological Station
St. Andrews
New Brunswick E0G 2XO, Canada

Conference Organization and Support

Dr. E. G. Kovach
Deputy Assistant Secretary General
for Scientific Affairs
NATO
1110 Bruxelles, Belgium

Miss E. I. Austin
Scientific Affairs Division
NATO
1110 Bruxelles, Belgium

Dr. R. W. Durie
Director
Advanced Concepts Centre
Environment Canada
Ottawa, Ontario K1A OH3, Canada

Mrs. D. Smith
Environment Canada

Mrs. V. Bourdon
Environment Canada

Miss M. Fraser
Environment Canada

Mr. W. Parks
Environment Canada

Mrs. J. Burns

Miss S. Rusenstrom

316

Index

317